Whole Language Intervention for School-Age Children

School-Age Children Series

Series Editor
Nickola Wolf Nelson, Ph.D.

Children of Prenatal Substance Abuse
Shirley N. Sparks, M.S.

What We Call Smart: A New Narrative for Intelligence
and Learning
Lynda Miller, Ph.D.

Whole Language Intervention for School-Age Children
Janet Norris, Ph.D., and Paul Hoffman, Ph.D.

Whole Language Intervention for School-Age Children

Janet Norris, Ph.D.
and
Paul Hoffman, Ph.D.
Louisiana State University
Baton Rouge, Louisiana

S SINGULAR PUBLISHING GROUP, INC.
SAN DIEGO, CALIFORNIA

Singular Publishing Group, Inc.
4284 41st Street
San Diego, California 92105-1197

© **1993 by Singular Publishing Group, Inc.**

Typeset in 10/12 Palatino by CFW Graphics
Printed in the United States of America by BookCrafters

Library of Congress Cataloging-in-Publication Data

Norris, Janet.
    Whole language intervention for school-age children / by Janet
Norris, Paul Hoffman.
      p.   cm. — (School-age children series)
    Includes bibliographical references and index.
    ISBN 1-56593-070-3
    1. Learning disabled children — Education — Language arts.
2. Language experience approach in education.   3. Language disorders
in children — Treatment.   4. Speech therapy for children.   5. Oral
communication — Study and teaching (Elementary)   I. Hoffman, Paul.
II. Title. III. Series.
LC4704.85.N67   1993
371.9′0446 — dc20   92-40679
                                                     CIP

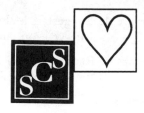

Contents

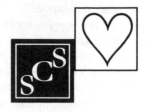

Foreword

In school, children and adolescents face language demands and opportunities that are unequaled elsewhere. Children who arrive at school prepared with a competent set of oral language abilities closely matched to the language expectations of classrooms have a considerable advantage over those who do not. For children with weaker oral language abilities, school must seem a maze of confusing expectations and unreachable goals. The goal of learning to read and write may be particularly frustrating; yet, it is often viewed as the central goal of formal education.

In *Whole Language Intervention for School-Age Children*, Norris and Hoffman offer a way to address this discouraging scenario. The authors provide both a philosophical framework and a set of practical strategies for serving children.

The text fits beautifully within the series on school-age children. The series is designed to guide speech-language pathologists and other professionals, teachers, and parents, working with school-age children with communicative disorders to build on the students' successes. The series encourages a view of language intervention as a process of fostering normal development. The approach described by Norris and Hoffman for keeping language intervention whole is a prime example of intervention based on this philosophy.

The authors base their writing on expertise gained with real children in real intervention contexts. Thus, they are able to ground their intervention approach in theory while making it applied in focus. Their clear explanations of complex material also incorporate the four major theories of this series — collaboration, contextually based intervention, change, and relevance.

Whole Language Intervention for School-Age Children educates readers about Whole Language, one of the hottest topics in the field of general education today. Norris and Hoffman's special application of Whole Language philosophy is designed to make school more accessible for youngsters who otherwise would be at high risk for school failure. The authors start by explaining language acquisition as a whole-to-part process. This insight provides a key to unlocking some of the mysteries about why earlier language intervention methods often yielded such poor results in real-life contexts. In the second chapter, Norris and Hoffman present a model for integrating aspects of language using the three dimensions — situational, discourse, and semantic. In the third chapter, they offer an integrated view of assessment, intervention, and accountability that maintains their whole-to-part philosophy and provides examples of how to make it work. The last two chapters are filled with suggestions for implementing the model with children who are operating at lower and higher academic levels. In these final two chapters, Norris and Hoffman develop their argument that school-age children at different academic levels need different degrees of focus on the explicit and implicit understandings of language.

With this book, Norris and Hoffman fill a void in resources for professionals who are serious about making Whole Language principles work for children and adolescents with language-related learning difficulties. The authors show respect for their readers and for the skills demanded of Whole Language interventionists by making their arguments careful and thorough. I am deeply pleased that they agreed to present their work in this format. I am honored to introduce their book as part of the series on school-age children.

Nickola Wolf Nelson, Ph.D.
Series Editor

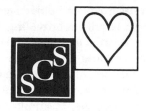

Preface

The purpose of this book is to provide a practical guide to the design and implementation of whole language-based assessment and intervention for school-age children with less integrated and flexible language systems. These children experience difficulty in the development of oral and written language and fail to process the subtleties and complexities of language used in context, even when the form and content have been acquired. These children are often identified in preschool or kindergarten because their oral language is not developing as rapidly as that of their peers. They are provided intervention by a speech-language specialist who seeks to improve their oral language abilities, typically by targeting specific aspects of language form, content, and use within goal-directed activities and conversational interchanges. After a while, the oral language abilities improve to meet normative expectations, and most children are released from intervention by first or second grade.

Unfortunately, at school-age many of these same children begin to fail in the development of written language abilities and are identified as learning disabled or as exhibiting poor readiness abilities for reading and writing. They are either referred back to the speech-language specialist, or more often, to a reading specialist. The speech-language specialist then turns her attention to subtle metalinguistic abilities such as phonemic awareness, metaphoric language, or the appreciation of the language ambiguities that form the basis of humor. The reading specialist provides practice in discrete reading abilities, such as letter-sound correspondences and rhyming, that are thought to prepare the child for true reading. The classroom teacher, reading specialist, and speech-language specialist each approaches the problem from a different perspective, and each has goals and objectives that may be unrelated to the others. This strategy results in providing more curriculum goals and approaches and less integrated learning time to the children who are having the most difficulty keeping up with the demands of the classroom curriculum and generalizing information that is acquired.

This book advocates the intergration of curriculum goals and intervention strategies to simultaneously facilitate the development of oral and written aspects of language. Within this approach, the speech-language specialist, reading specialist, and classroom teacher seek to change the dynamics within learning contexts, such as the classroom, to maximize the children's ability to learn using their existing language system. At the same time, written language is used as the forum for increasing the complexity of the child's language system so that the child can function as a more independent learner in both the short and the long term. Component abilities of oral and written language such as letter-sound correspondences are addressed as parts of the whole acts of reading and writing rather than as prerequisites to real reading and writing. The child with a less flexible language system is given assistance in dealing with the language demands of school, rather than learning a second set of skills that must be generalized before they are of use in school.

Chapter 1 introduces the basic principles of Whole Language philosophy and corresponding strategies for intervention. The primary underlying premise of this approach is that language is learned from whole to part. The whole referred to is the process of meaning making within whole events, such as a story recounted in a book. The parts include all aspects of the meaning-making process, from establishing letter-sound correspondences through the interpretation of metaphor. This premise presents a polar opposite to more traditional programs for these children that seek to gradually build toward the whole out of a collection of discrete skill parts.

Chapter 2 presents a contextual model of language that integrates three interrelated contexts: Situational, Discourse, and Semantic. These contexts each represent demands placed on children's language systems that require them to use language to impose interpretation of experience, to understand and respond to the language presented to them, and to communicate in order to affect the beliefs, behaviors, or attitudes of others. The model demonstrates how professionals seeking to facilitate oral and written language development can manipulate these interacting contexts to increase or reduce the demands on the child's language system. Understanding the dynamic interactions between the Situational, Discourse, and Semantic dimensions of a context of language use enables the facilitator to manipulate these contexts during assessment to gain insights into the child's language abilities, and during treatment to enhance the child's acquisition and flexible use of language.

Chapter 3 applies the contextual model to the analysis of the language abilities of two elementary school children — one whose academic performance is average and one whose reading and writing performance is significantly below grade level. Excerpts from oral reading and writing samples are used to demonstrate how the child's language system can be evaluated as a whole and integrated process.

Chapter 4 discusses the application of the contextual model in intervention for the low-achieving child. General principles of intervention are described and exemplified with respect to children who are at the beginning stages of reading. Specific strategies for facilitating language development and use through reading, writing, and oral discussion are presented.

Chapter 5 profiles children who have apparently mastered the mechanics of reading and elementary writing, but only at explicit levels of comprehension and expression. This chapter demonstrates how to facilitate interpretations of meaning at the more implicit critical levels of semantics and provides strategies for intervention through writing and reading.

Since assessment and intervention evolve from the same model of contextualized language in this book, from earliest stages of language development throughout the school years (and potentially beyond) continuity in development and, therefore, continuity in goals and objectives, is present within and across grade levels. The model allows for both short-term and long-term planning and monitoring of meaningful changes within the whole language system.

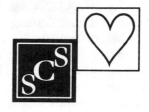

Acknowledgments

Our special thanks is extended to The Wright Company for allowing us the use of their books for purposes of this project.

The following books from **The Sunshine Series** are used by permission of The Wright Group Publishers, 19201 120th Avenue NE, Bothell, WA 98011-9512.

Biddulph, F. & Biddulph, J. (1992) *What Will Float?*
Boon, K. (1990) *The Big Fish*
Burleigh, L. (1990) *The Stranger from the Sea*
Ciantar, G. (1988) *The Goats and the Troll*
Cowley, J. (1988) *Cousin Kira*
Cowley, J. (1988) *Dragon with a Cold*
Cowley, J. (1988) *Huggle's Breakfast*
Cowley, J. (1988) *I Love My Family*
Cowley, J. (1988) *Just This Once*
Cowley, J. (1988) *Road Robber*
Cowley, J. (1988) *Soup*
Cowley, J. (1989) *Bogle's Feet*
Cowley, J. (1989) *Busy Baby*
Cowley, J. (1990) *The Secret of Spooky House*
Cowley, J. (1990) *Water Is My Friend*
Cutting, J. (1988) *Come On!*
Cutting, J. (1990) *To School*

Cutting, B. and Cutting, J. (1988) *Captain B's Boat*
Cutting, B. and Cutting, J. (1988) *The Dandelion*
Cutting, B. and Cutting, J. (1988) *Dreams*
Cutting, B. and Cutting, J. (1988) *It Takes Time To Grow*
Cutting, B. and Cutting, J. (1988) *The New Building*
Cutting, B. and Cutting, J. (1988) *Space*
Cutting, B. and Cutting, J. (1988) *Together*
Cutting, B. and Cutting, J. (1988) *The Tree*
Cutting, B. and Cutting, J. (1988) *Underwater Journey*
Cutting, B. and Cutting, J. (1988) *What Am I?*
Jackson, T. (1990) *The Wonderhair Hair Restorer*
Mahy, M. (1986) *The Man Who Enjoyed Grumbling*
Mahy, M. (1987) *The King's Jokes*
Mahy, M. (1987) *Tai Taylor and the Sweet Annie*
Mahy, M. (1990) *Crocodile! Crocodile!*
Vickers, K. (1987) *A Wizard Came to Visit*
Young, C. (1988) *The Gingerbread Man*
Young, C. (1988) *The Little Red Hen*
Young, C. (1988) *Shopping*

The following books from the **Storybox Series** are used by permission of The Wright Group Publishers, 19201 120th Avenue NE, Bothell, WA 98011-9512.

Cowley, J. (1983) *To Town*
Cowley, J. (1983) *Who Will Be My Mother?*
Cowley, J. (1990) *The Big Hill*
Cowley, J. (1990) *Grumpy Elephant*
Cowley, J. (1990) *Hairy Bear*
Cowley, J. (1990) *Houses*
Cowley, J. (1990) *The Hungry Giant*
Cowley, J. (1990) *I Want Ice Cream*
Cowley, J. (1990) *If You Meet a Dragon*
Cowley, J. (1990) *In the Mirror*
Cowley, J. (1990) *The Jigaree*
Cowley, J. (1990) *Just This Once*
Cowley, J. (1990) *Little Brother*
Cowley, J. (1990) *On a Chair*
Cowley, J. (1990) *The Red Rose*
Cowley, J. (1990) *Stop!*
Cowley, J. (1990) *Water is My Friend*
Melser, J. (1981) *Little Pig*
Melser, J. (1985) *One, One, is the Sun*

Melser, J. and Cowley, J. (1980) *The Big Toe*
Melser, J. and Cowley, J. (1990) *Boo Hoo*
Melser, J. and Cowley, J. (1990) *Obadiah*

The following books from the **TWIG Books Series** are used by permission of The Wright Group Publishers, 19201 120th Avenue NE, Bothell, WA 98011-9512.

Williams, R. (1990) *Underground*
Williams, R. (1990) *Who Lives in This Hole?*

The following books from the **Once Upon a Time Series** are used by permission of The Wright Group Publishers, 19201 120th Avenue NE, Bothell, WA 98011-9512.

Moon, C. (1988) *Goldilocks and the Three Bears*
Moon, C. (1988) *Jack and the Beanstalk*
Moon, C. (1988) *Little Red Riding Hood*
Moon, C. (1988) *The Three Pigs*

The following books from the **Tales from Long Ago Series** are used by permission of The Wright Group Publishers, 19201 120th Avenue NE, Bothell, WA 98011-9512.

Butterworth, B. (1986) *The Discontented Pig*
Butterworth, B. (1986) *The Giraffe Who Could Not Walk*
Butterworth, B. (1988) *The North Wind*
Butterworth, B. (1988) *The Two Windmills*

The following books from the **Fables from Aesop Series** are used by permission of The Wright Group Publishers, 19201 120th Avenue NE, Bothell, WA 98011-9512.

Biro, V. (1986) *The Donkey in the Lion's Skin*
Biro, V. (1990) *The Farmer and His Sons*
Biro, V. (1991) *The Fox and the Crow*

The following book from the **Readings in Science Series** is used by permission of The Wright Group Publishers, 19201 120th Avenue NE, Bothell, WA 98011-9512.

Moon, C. and Moon, B. (1986) *Look At An Ice Lolly*

The following books from the **Science Understandings: The Environment Series** are used by permission of the Wright Group Publishers, 19201 120th Avenue NE, Bothell, WA 98011-9512.

Lovett, S. (1992) *Extremely Weird Frogs*
Walker, C. (1992) *Ecology — Plants and Animals*
Walker, C. (1992) *Forests Forever*
Walker, C. (1992) *Oceans of Fish*
Walker, C. (1992) *Our Changing Atmosphere*

The following books from the **Traditional Tales from Around the World Series** are used by permission of The Wright Group Publishers, 19201 120th Avenue NE, Bothell, WA 98011-9512.

Berry, J. (1986). Hurricane. In E. Jones (Ed.), *Tales of the Caribbean: The Beginnings of Things* (pp. 32–33).
Candappa, B. (1986). The Three Dragon Eggs. In *Tales of South Asia: How Things Began* (pp. 24–32).
Candappa, B. (1988). Something Strange for Sale. In *Tales of the Far East: Daring Deeds* (pp. 4–10).
Candappa, B. (1988). How the Weather Gods Help. In *Tales of the Far East: Listen to Grandmother* (pp. 22–27).
Jones, E. (1986). Old Nelson Godon. In *Tales of the Caribbean: The Beginnings of Things* (pp. 16–26).
McLeish, K. (1986). Merpeople. In *Tales of the British Isles* (pp. 50–58).
McLeish, K. (1986). Guher and Suher. In *Tales of the Mediterranean: Turkey* (pp. 11–17).

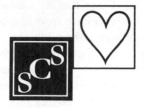

Prologue

Tommy was the only child of working professionals with eight flexible work schedules that allowed them to supply his care. He was 9 months to 1 year older than the other children in the neighborhood, and yet by the time he was 3, he was noticeably more timid than the others. He was also not as verbal as his younger friends. His parents enrolled him in a two morning a week preschool program to give him an opportunity to interact with children his own age. The first day, with all the parents and confusion, went okay. The second day was a disaster. As soon as his mother started to leave, Tommy started screaming. The teacher told her to go on home. She said that the first day jitters did not last long. She was wrong. Tommy, the usually quiet child, threw a tantrum all morning. Tommy's mother rearranged her schedule so that she could go to preschool too. She sat in the room for 4 weeks, leaving the room for longer and longer periods each day, until finally she was able to leave him there for the whole morning.

The next year, Tommy attended a half day, prekindergarten class with eight other children. The program was geared toward "seat work" that taught fundamental skills for reading and classroom performance. Near the end of the year, the class took the California Achievement Test. While Tommy scored above the 90th percentile on letter forms and letter names, skills that had been specifically taught in class, his overall pre-reading score was below the 10th percentile. On most of the subtests, he scored at the 1st or 2nd percentile. His teacher suggested that Tommy be evaluated by the school psychologist.

The school psychologist conducted a battery of educational and psychological tests and observed Tommy's behavior in the classroom. He found that Tommy actively avoided contact with other children. He did not seek help from the teacher, even when it was apparent that he did not understand what he was supposed to be doing. He did not follow instructions that involved two or more steps. When he finished an assignment, he would hug himself and rock in his chair. These observations and results from projective psychological tests led the psychologist to label Tommy as "socially isolated." He suggested a form of play therapy to increase his confidence and ability to socialize with others. Based on an average performance IQ score compared to a below normal verbal IQ, the psychologist suggested evaluation by a speech-language pathologist.

The speech-language pathologist evaluated Tommy's verbal interaction in play with his parents. Tommy focused more on the objects than on his parents. His symbolic use of the objects appeared to be at age level. However, his discourse skills were not well developed. Over 30% of his verbal interactions were problematic. Tommy's parents often had to use multiple prompts to get him to verbally respond. His speech attempts most often included linguistic nonfluencies and were semantically inappropriate to the context. Tommy's syntactic development was delayed by 12 to 18 months, with deficits in the expression of aspect and time. Over 75% of his language difficulties occurred when he was trying to use language for higher level semantic functions such as reordering perception or reasoning about aspects of the situation.

During the following summer and the fall of his kindergarten year, a speech-language pathologist worked with Tommy individually and in his classroom. Individually, she worked with Tommy on using language to reason about changes in objects and actions within common routines like cooking, shopping, eating, and storybook reading. At school, she sat with Tommy in the classroom and made suggestions to him about when it would be appropriate to respond to the teacher's requests and when he might make requests of the teacher or other children. She modeled these uses of language and the language forms that he could use in these situations. This approach appeared to have good effect on Tommy's development of oral language. His nonfluencies decreased, and his language became more semantically and syntactically appropriate. At the end of Tommy's kindergarten year, his California Achievement Test scores were all above the 50th percentile. Tests of his oral language performance all showed that he was within normal limits. Tommy's treatment was considered a success by the speech-language pathologist, who phased out her contacts with him.

Tommy was still noticeably shy. His parents actively kept him engaged in interactions with the neighborhood children. They enrolled him in sports programs to keep him in contact with other children as well. They helped him organize his oral language in social interactions in the manner that the speech-language pathologist had taught them.

Tommy started the first grade smoothly. It was his third year at the same school with mostly the same children. The first semester repeated many of the alphabet and single word recognition skills that he had learned in the previous 2 years.

Then, at the start of the second semester, the rules of the reading game were changed. He was no longer supposed to just read the words in a list, or circle the words that rhymed. He was a "shark," a member of the class' best reading group, because he had learned these skills well over the past 3 years. Instead, reading became something different. He was supposed to say what the words, sentences, and stories meant. Tommy could not do that. Instead, he started to look nervous again, making distracting noises and repetitively knotting and unknotting his fingers. Like so many others, Tommy's preschool oral language problem had apparently disappeared, only to reappear in a new guise. It had become a problem of poor reading comprehension and classroom distractibility.

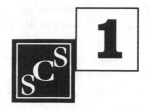

Language Learning as an Integrated Whole-to-Part Process

Whole Language is a philosophy of learning that guides decisions that are made while constructing curriculum, conducting assessments of language and learning, and providing intervention. This philosophy can be described in a small number of principles that are embodied in the assessment and intervention strategies applied to individual children. This chapter provides an overview of Whole Language principles, the nature of less integrated and flexible language learning, intervention strategies based on Whole Language principles, and a comparison of Whole Language learning to more traditional teaching strategies. The specific objectives include understanding

- That language is whole
- That learning occurs whole to part
- That oral and written language develop reciprocally
- That language increases in decontextualization

1

■ The early acquisition of written language
■ The nature of less flexible language learning
■ How to maintain whole learning environments
■ Oral and written language connections

Language intervention has often been viewed in the past as a "part-to-whole" process. Beginning with the smallest, and therefore presumably the "easiest" elements of language, discrete phonological, syntactic, morphological, semantic, or pragmatic skills have been identified, targeted, and taught, first in isolation and then gradually in longer or more complex contexts. Intervention is viewed as completed when the child exhibits all of the age-appropriate skills, or parts of language, according to some developmental continuum. While this view at first glance appears to be logical and based on sound principles of development, in fact, it violates principles derived from research that examines the actual *process* of development. Researchers such as Piaget (1952), Vygotsky (1962), Brown (1973), Nelson (1985, 1991), Snow (1972), Bruner (1978), Wells (1986), and many others have shown us that language learning is actually a "whole-to-part" process. From infancy children participate in whole, complex events that are goal oriented and meaningful. Over time, the child discovers the specific parts of the event and how they function within the whole. The purpose of this book is to demonstrate how language intervention can be viewed as a whole-to-part learning process for the school-age child.

The major theme throughout this book is that language is a process that involves complex whole-part relationships. The smaller parts of language are always embedded within, and related to, larger wholes. In normal development of both oral and written language, children learn about language parts by using them within larger wholes. They progressively learn more about language by refining their knowledge of the parts that exist within the wholes, the relationships that exist among the parts within a whole, and the relationships between a part and many different wholes. This expanding knowledge results in a *flexible language system*, because each language part has been extensively networked to a broad conceptual base. This network of connections among language parts allows normally developing children to creatively combine, contrast, and compare language parts in many different contexts. Their development of written language abilities is a seamless extension of their oral language abilities. From their earliest experiences, sitting in a parent's lap with a picture book, children learn that books contain pictures and print that also are parts of the language network.

In contrast, children who fail to develop flexible language systems become context bound. They creatively combine language elements only when the situation provides enough structure so that language can be used to refer to concrete and directly experienced information. When the situation demands that they devote more of their own cognitive resources to organizing information through language, their lack of flexibility results in language use that is static and constrained. These children often find the transition from oral to written language a daunting passage. They struggle with the decoding process that takes them from print to sound; then they fail to develop insights into the communicative function of print and the meaning reconstruction process by which they come to understand an author's intended message.

Traditional language intervention strategies play into the hand of the core problem. Rather than helping the child learn to flexibly use language to change focus from whole to part and back within meaningful contexts, practice is provided in isolated language skills. These skills, learned as discrete entities, lack the networked characteristics of the parts embedded within an integrated whole to part system. The interventionist then must try to build the individual skills into a system by progressively adding skills together. The meaning-making process is saved for last, or it is assumed to occur automatically once the appropriate component skills are mastered. The child comes to view these skills as isolated behaviors that are to be performed under specific task conditions, rather than internalizing them as part of an integrated system of thought and language. This leaves the interventionist with the problem of then "teaching generalization."

This chapter presents a description of some major principles that guide Whole Language learning and intervention. Included is a discussion of the less flexible language learner's problems and how the symptoms are manifested differently across time. Additionally, intervention strategies consistent with Whole Language principles are contrasted with traditional strategies to demonstrate the different mode of thinking that must be adopted regarding the purposes, goals, and methods of intervention within a Whole Language perspective.

◼◻ WHOLE LANGUAGE PRINCIPLES

Whole Language is not a teaching method or approach to intervention, but rather a philosophy of learning, or a set of beliefs regarding how people learn. This philosophy is based on a number of principles that are used to guide the development of curricula, teaching, or intervention strategies (Goodman, 1986). The following discussion examines three of these principles. First, language is whole. Second, language is learned from whole to part. Third, written language is developed in parallel with oral language, each serving to develop and refine an integrated language system.

Language is Whole

Function, Content, and Form

The central theme in Whole Language theory is that language is whole, and therefore cannot be meaningfully subdivided into components (Goodman, 1986). All real language simultaneously expresses function, content, and form. *Functionally,* we use language to inform, persuade, learn, command, and accomplish other goals within purposeful interactions with others. The *content* of language refers to the relationship between language and the language user's conceptual understanding of the physical nature of objects and actions, as well as the social intentions, plans, and emotions that motivate people's actions. Variable language *forms* are used to express content and function when people interact through spoken and written symbols. In everyday interactions, language forms are used to refer to things that are noticed, or needs that can be met by others within meaningful, whole events. The complexity of the whole events increases for contexts such as drama and literature, in which language forms are manipulated for the purpose of creating an emotional reaction to the language itself.

School-age children must possess sufficient language ability to coordinate the function, content, and form of language within highly complex contexts. Inasmuch as the meaning expressed by language forms depends on the context in which they are used, learning about language forms requires their use in realistic, or Whole Language, contexts. Isolated drills involving discrete language forms cannot approximate the richness of real language. Consider the referential usage of pronouns in the following passage from a fourth-grade-level book, *The Three Dragon Eggs* (Candappa, 1986).

> One of the merchants had seen the crow flying down with something in *his* beak. *He* was curious so *he* watched as the crow dived under the bush, left *his* bundle, and flew away. "I wonder what's in that bundle?" *he* asked *himself.* So curious was *he* that *he* crawled under the bush and opened it.

Two characters are presented in the first sentence, a merchant and a crow. The first use of "his" in "his beak" refers to the crow. A number of cues help a reader make this interpretation, including the occurrence of the pronoun "his" after "the crow," without mention of another character in between, and the reference to a beak, which is more likely a part of a crow than a human. The next two occurrences of "he" refer to the merchant, even though the merchant was not explicitly referred to since the introduction of the crow. Thus, the child must know that pronouns do not necessarily refer to the last character named. Instead, this determination must be made by understanding that the pronouns refer to a character who is watching the crow, and therefore logically cannot be the crow. The crow is named and then referred to by the pronoun "his" (i.e., "his bundle"), thus serving as the subject twice within the beginning of the same sentence. Next, the merchant, who has been explicitly mentioned only at the start of the passage, is referred to as "I," "he," and "himself." To understand these pronoun uses, the reader must learn from the pronouns used by the narrator that the merchant is talking to himself, thus referring to himself as "I," a language use requiring the child to simultaneously adopt two perspectives, neither of which is his own or the crow's.

As this passage makes clear, no word in a real context of language use has a meaningful interpretation that can be separated from the whole context. Thus, the wholeness of language is violated by teaching practices in which function, content, and form are separated from one another. Attempts to teach characteristics of pronoun use in decontextualized sentence exercises, such as using sentences to describe single pictures of boys and girls performing isolated activities as in "He is walking" or "She is walking," will fail to capture the more global aspects of pronoun use. Such practice may enable the young school-age child to use personal pronouns in conversational contexts in which the referents are observable to the participants; however, it will likely not be enough to enable the child to understand the passage above. In contrast to such exercises, the Whole Language intervention strategies seek first of all to maintain the wholeness of language acts by asking children to read, write, and talk about meaningful and, therefore, complex whole events.

Whole-to-Part Learning

Parsing

The second principle within Whole Language theory is that aspects of language content, form, and use are learned from whole to part (Goodman, 1986). That is, the smaller conceptual parts of language are constructed by gradually discovering how they function and refer to specific elements within larger wholes. Nelson (1985, 1991) describes this learning process using the term *parsing*. From the earliest months of infancy, the child engages in interactions with the objects and people encountered within the environment. The child's knowledge of objects and actions is limited to what can be immediately seen, touched, or heard and, therefore, bound to the individual contexts in which they occur. The earliest object concepts are undifferentiated parts of whole contexts. That is, the infant does not realize that a ball seen in the context of play in the playroom may be the same ball that later appears in the toy box in the child's bedtime routine.

However, by acting on the ball and discovering that it rolls, bounces, and flies through the air in both contexts, the child develops a mental concept of "ball," and this mental concept can be used independently of any particular context. The concept has been parsed, existing as an identifiable part of a number of whole contexts. This parsed concept for "ball" allows for new flexibility, enabling the child to classify newly encountered objects as balls, to label the concept with the word "ball," and to put that word into a variety of sentences that express different relationships of meaning. Simultaneously, the concept of this object is still networked to the situations in which the original experiences occurred, and to the many other actions and objects that were present in those situations. This network of knowledge enables generalizations and discriminations to be made so that the child learns that baseballs maintain both similarities and differences to basketballs.

While parsing occurs as an unconscious and automatic process of learning, it also can be brought under conscious control. In school, children are expected to perform parsing in contexts such as language arts exercises where grammatical structures are to be identified and named. Within the context of a sentence, a word is described as serving one or another syntactic function. This level of parsing also requires a whole-to-part consideration, since the syntactic function of a word cannot be determined without considering its relationships to the other words within the sentence. For example, in the sentence, "The boy is running," the word "running" functions as a verb. However, in the sentence, "The running boy fell down," the word "running" is a gerund. To determine the syntactic class of the word "running," its whole-to-part relationship with the sentence must be determined.

Refinement

The process of parsing enables *refinement* to occur within the child's interrelated system of concept formation and language. Each time a new object, or characteristic of an object, or action related to the object, or consequence of the action, or the agent performing the action, or the recipient of the action and so forth is parsed from the whole event, the event exists with greater specificity, detail, and complexity. The understanding or knowledge of the event is thus refined. The network of information related to the event is expanded to conceptually include these newly parsed actions, objects, states, attributes, and people and their roles. Language is inextricably part of this refinement process, both developing as a result of the parsing and serving as a catalyst for its occurrence. Pointing to a newly noticed object indicates that the concept of that object has been parsed from the whole event and exists without language. The existence of the unnamed concept creates the need for a word to refer to this new piece of information. Conversely, a word can create the need for conceptual information, as the child hears a new word and seeks to determine what is being referred to. The more specific the refinement becomes, the greater this process depends on language. For example, a concept such as "deciding" has no physical referent that can be pointed to, but rather is created through the use of language in a relevant context (Blank, Berlin, & Rose, 1978; Nelson, 1985).

Flexibility

Within the whole-part relationships that function in language, an important characteristic is substitutability. The question is whether one concept, word, or object can be substituted for another within a context. For example, the words "apple," "coffee," "cereal," "juice," and "bread" are all substitutable within the context "The grocery store had _____," but not "She ate the _____." Stated another way, *flexibility* of organization allows for different aspects of meaning to be focused on within different contexts. Flexibility allows the child to develop the ability to reorganize and recombine concepts in thought and language. It allows the child to use the same language in a variety of different contexts. Flexibility develops as the same language is used within a variety of different contexts for both similar and different purposes and as different language is used to refer to the same events within the same or different contexts.

To help children develop flexibility in language learning and use, the principle of parsing wholes into parts is critical to language intervention. This principle requires the interventionist to always maintain a meaningful and whole context in which language learning can occur. When language interventionists isolate parts of language from meaningful contexts, they essentially destroy the whole-part relationships that make language such a flexible system. To become a flexible language user, the child must experience the parts of language in a variety of whole contexts. They must use the parts of language in a variety of relationships to other parts within the unified and coherent contexts.

Contexts of intervention that are structured to give the child opportunities to learn about language must be meaningful to the child. Language is a process of giving and receiving linguistic information that is used by other participants to recreate and thus share meaning. Each person's system of concepts and language is unique, reflecting individual knowledge, interests, and abilities. But at the same time, each person's system must be sufficiently similar to that which is conventional within the cultural and social environment for meaning to be exchanged (Halliday, 1985). For children with less flexible language systems to successfully communicate with other children and adults, their organization of conceptual and linguistic knowledge must be sufficiently conventional. Intervention must support the meaning-making process.

Meaning Making

Meaning making involves understanding how specific objects, actions, or persons fit within a whole event. When this understanding exists, then information that is shared serves to develop the topic for some specific purpose. For example, when asked to tell a story about a ball, networks of whole-part relationships must be used to choose an appropriate event that unifies the ball within a larger whole, such as a baseball game. A coherent story would include not only a ball, but also a place, relevant people, and other objects found within the event. The resulting story can be interpreted by listeners who also activate their knowledge of the potential relationships within baseball games as they recreate the event by interpreting the language (Halliday, 1985). This process of creating and exchanging meaning through language must be the focus of intervention. When the context provided to children is not a coherent whole, but rather incoherent parts (i.e., a series of picture cards showing a dog barking, a cat sleeping, a child jumping, and a man eating for purposes of eliciting 10 trials of present progressive verb tense), children with less flexible systems are not helped to activate those higher order contexts that unite actions into whole events.

When asked to tell a story, these children often reply by describing a ball and giving one or two actions related to a ball. Without the organization provided by an understanding of the various interrelationships within a whole context, the "story" shifts from topic to topic. Listeners are lost because the story does not match their expectations of possible whole contexts. By making the language intervention process similar to the characteristics of normal language use, the child's conceptual networks will become structured more conventionally, consistent with listener expectations, and result in greater sharing and interpreting of meaning.

Scaffolded Assistance

Children are aided in the process of creating appropriate conceptual networks, including concepts related to language use, content, and form, when they engage in meaningful communication with a facilitative speaker of the language. Bruner (1978) described the adult's role as providing *scaffolded assistance* to the child. The adult first seeks to keep the child engaged in a social conversational format of providing relevant information and interpreting information given by the child as meaningful and relevant to the context. In early development, the adult provides all of the structure for these exchanges, but as the child takes a more active role in the interaction, the adult relinquishes control until the child is an equal partner. As the child demonstrates that she can do more, the adult increases demands on the child for participation. The end result is that the child progresses toward the adult model of performance in the situation. The whole conversational interaction serves as a framework that supports the child's learning about the components of the interaction, including aspects of language form that express a variety of conceptual relationships. Vygotsky (1962) suggested that this type of adult-child interaction allows the child to understand and produce language at a higher level than the child could accomplish on his own. Within assisted interactions, the child practices higher level abilities and subsequently develops the ability to perform at these higher levels without assistance. This type of scaffolded interaction is the primary method of providing intervention within Whole Language contexts.

Active Participation

The child's role is to be an *active participant* who is willing to use language for new purposes, to express new semantic-syntactic relationships, and to experiment with new words and new sounds. This adventuresome spirit is motivated by the child's desire to accomplish goals and is facilitated by the adults' willingness to regard child language as "work in progress." The people with whom the child interacts must be tolerant of language forms that are not yet adultlike so that the child will feel comfortable in taking such inventive risks. Rather than reacting negatively to the child's language form, the adult must seek to understand the child's goal. The adult reacts to the child's goal and expands on the topic, putting into words the attempts to achieve the goal and the results of those attempts. The language spoken by the adult supplies the child with models of appropriate language forms for the context. Children learn from these models by adjusting their language forms to more closely match those modeled by the adult.

Relevance

Learning occurs best when the information to be learned has *relevance* and is motivating to the learner. Thus, intervention should focus on the accomplishment of some meaningful and relevant goal, such as reading a book containing information that is interesting and important to the child, writing a poem for a specific occasion or to express personal feelings, or discussing the physical changes that occur in objects about which the child is curious. These basic goals are similar to those that are sought in the classroom. These goal-oriented activities provide the context and motivation for communication through oral and written language to occur. The children's desire to participate in these activities, to understand the information, and to make themselves understood serves as the underlying motivation to take risks in the formulation of language. The language facilitator fosters a risk-taking attitude by always acting to help the child communicate through scaffolding, rather than punishing the child's attempts with negative comments.

Oral and Written Language Develop in Parallel

A third Whole Language principle is that children's knowledge of written language is developed in parallel with, and in much the same manner as, oral language (Goodman, 1986). Written language shares a number of important characteristics with oral language. One obvious parallel is that it is used to accomplish goals. Street signs are constructed by the city government to provide information to drivers. Authors of novels seek to provide enjoyment to readers on topics that are familiar, unusual, humorous, adventuresome, frightening, or informative. The authors of children's expository texts seek to broaden the child's knowledge to include places the child has never seen, experiences from other cultures or time periods, and concepts that are too abstract to be learned through direct experience alone. To accomplish these goals, written language must represent a portion of the author's cognitive organization of the world in a manner that can be reconstructed by the reader. To be comprehensible, written language must utilize conventional relationships among language forms, content, and purposes consistent with oral language.

Decontextualization

While parallels exist between oral and written language use, there are a number of characteristics of written language that make its use more difficult than the oral language learned by the preschool child. Written language often represents a more *decontextualized* relationship between language form and the meaning expressed than does oral language (Westby, 1984, 1985). Oral language often refers to objects and actions present in the environment and visible to both the speaker and listener. The ability of two people to adequately refer to this content is enhanced by their ability to gesture toward objects and see that the listener has noticed them. Thus, the speaker can use relatively nonspecific language such as "that over there" while pointing to make reference to objects. In contrast, the author of written language must create the context using language, and the reader must reconstruct that context from the printed words. The author's references within the context must utilize specific language forms such as "that manila envelope on the top of the blue filing cabinet," rather than a gesture accompanying the general words "that over there."

A speaker can use intonation, stress patterns, and facial expressions to convey information about feelings toward a topic. A writer must convey this information through the words that are chosen to be read from the page. The writer's choice of syntax and words must be more highly organized than those of a speaker. A speaker can watch for a quizzical look on the face of a listener. When a speaker is not understood, the listener can ask for clarifications. Writers must try to anticipate the ability of their audience to reconstruct their meaning without the benefit of feedback. There is no opportunity for clarification, since readers cannot ask the author what was meant by a particular passage.

Early Acquisition of Written Language

Children from literate societies show early acquisition of written language. They acquire this knowledge of print through their daily exposure to print on labels, boxes, street signs, magazines, newspapers, and storybooks. Adults often scaffold the child's interactions with print by helping the child to understand the meaning intended by the print and the characteristics of the letters and words that are present in the environment. Storybook reading experiences start with the 1-year-old child sitting on a parent's lap playing the "naming game" (Ninio & Bruner, 1978). The adult scaffolds this interaction by presenting a repeated context of pointing to a picture, asking for a label for the picture, and providing feedback about the child's attempt to name the picture. The child learns to respond with labels and eventually takes on the role of the adult. The parent continues to scaffold reading by making use of oral conversational interaction patterns that aid the child's attempts to interpret the meaning expressed in the pictures and words in books.

Sulzby (1985) describes a sequence of stages through which children advance from the naming game to becoming proficient readers. In the first stage, the child's attention is directed toward the pictures, where first the objects and then the actions are labeled. The child and adult engage in a conversation about the pictures that are discussed as though the actions are occurring in the present. In the next stage, children tell disjointed stories related to the pictures that utilize oral language techniques such as changing voices to indicate dialogue and use of verb tense markers to indicate changes in the time of the actions. In the third stage, complete stories are told that use storytelling intonation. However, these stories are not complete enough to be interpreted without access to the pictures that are being discussed. The next stage involves telling stories that contain more characteristics of written language and that are actually based on the events that occur in the storybook as written (Teale, 1984). Later stages involve a shift in focus from the pictures in the book to the print. At first, children may refuse to try to read because they do not know the words on the page. Later, they may attend to particular aspects of print by reading certain words or particular letters. From these prereading experiences, children learn conventions of the reading process, such as the left to right orientation of print, the relationships between print and picture, spoken word to print correspondences, story structure, and letter to sound relationships. These are prerequisites to independent reading that are established by engaging in whole and meaningful language experiences with print.

Summary

Whole Language is a philosophy of learning that is based on principles of natural language learning as it occurs within both oral and written language experiences. To establish a Whole Language environment, interventionists must present children with complex, meaningful experiences that are unified or whole, must provide a scaffold or assistance to enable children to parse increasingly more specific and abstract parts from within the whole, and must provide coordinated experiences with oral and written language that work together to assist children with the language refinement process. The goal of whole language intervention is to assist the child in creating an interrelated network of concepts and language that will maximize the flexibility of language learning and use.

■□ NATURE OF LESS FLEXIBLE LANGUAGE ABILITY

Increasing Subtlety

Whole Language is not a curriculum, method, or set of strategies. Rather, it is a belief about how people learn. As indicated previously, this belief can be described according to a set of guiding principles. These principles hold that language is best represented as a whole-part system, that learning occurs from whole to part, and that written language is learned in parallel with oral language. Our choice to apply these beliefs to the facilitation of language development among children with less flexible language systems is supported by observations that have been made about the changing nature of children's language problems. As the child with less flexible language learning ability grows older, the manifestations of the problem become more *subtle*. Preschool oral language problems manifested in the acquisition of semantic-syntactic relationships become elementary school problems in classroom discourse, reading, and writing.

The preschool child with a language development delay produces language that is restricted to the concrete aspects of the situation, is bound to the here-and-now, lacks morphemic markers for temporal and spatial changes, and is restricted in length of utterance. As a result of intervention, or perhaps with the passage of time, these aspects of language apparently improve enough to be acceptable, or at least within the measurement error of available test instruments. But a disturbing trend has been noted in which these children evidence differing forms of oral and written language problems as time passes and as differing demands are placed on language processing (Westby, 1985; Wiig & Semel, 1984).

The language difficulties experienced by school-age children with language delays affect a wide range of language domains. These children evidence more communicative breakdowns, including pauses, repetitions, and abandoned utterances in their conversations (MacLachlan & Chapman, 1988). Their narratives contain less information (Merritt & Liles, 1989; Roth & Spekman, 1986) and are less cohesive (Norris & Bruning, 1988). They show problems in processing abstract vocabulary, figurative language, discourse structure, complex syntactic structures, and metalinguistic concepts (Crais & Chapman, 1987; Ripich & Griffith, 1988; Roth & Spekman, 1989).

The picture that emerges from these studies is that preschool oral language problems change form, becoming more subtle as the child progresses through the early grades. Their problems become less obvious because the children learn enough about elementary aspects of semantic-syntactic relationships to perform well in oral conversations with familiar partners and about familiar topics. The child's expectations about what will be discussed, the perception of objects and actions in the environment to support the formulation of language, and the partner's ability to help clarify the child's inaccurate language all make it possible for adequate communication to occur.

Increasing School Demands

School presents children with *increasing demands* to use language that is displaced from the situation, that incorporates more elements of discourse structure, and that represents more implicit understanding of a topic. Children with less flexible language systems may perform well enough in classroom situations as long as the tasks presented place minimal demands on learning primarily through language. Books depicting much of the information in pictures and concrete explorations of topics through experimentation and manipulation of objects and materials provide for language experiences that are sufficiently contextualized for learning to successfully occur. The concrete context and ability to interact with the teacher supports the child's language performance. However, subtle linguistic breakdowns are apparent in the form of nonfluencies that occur as the children try to express their observations using language. Their discussions or explanations are marked by a lack of cohesion, reflecting a limited whole-to-part understanding of the experiences. Poor narrative structure belies a disorganized whole or unifying structure for interpreting events, including the goals that people set, the plans they make to attain those goals, and the problems they encounter as they attempt to execute their plans. Lacking sufficient narrative structure to meet the demands imposed by much of the elementary school child's early reading experiences, the child with a less flexible language system struggles when asked to read and interpret the stories read in the classroom. Lacking sufficient knowledge of expository discourse structure, the child with a less flexible language system does not rapidly comprehend the relationships stated in their science and social studies texts.

Studies that have followed the progress of preschool children who were treated for language problems show that they are at risk for academic failure. Hall and Tomblin (1978) found that a high percentage of these children showed a history of below average performance on tests of reading and academic achievement during the elementary grades. Aram, Ekelman, and Nation (1984) found that 69% of the preschool language-impaired children with normal intelligence experienced grade retention, special tutoring, or placement in classes for the learning disabled. Over 75% of the preschool children who were treated for delayed speech in a university clinic required remedial educational services during the elementary grades (Shriberg & Kwiatkowski, 1988). Approaching the question from the other direction, Gibbs and Cooper (1989) administered speech and language tests to elementary school children who had been categorized as learning disabled. They found that over 90% presented current problems in oral language structure and function.

These observations support the principle that written language develops in parallel with oral language. Written language aspects of the child's problem become more apparent as the classroom situation becomes more oriented toward using print rather than oral language to set the context for learning. To effectively deal with these problems, educators must acknowledge these interactions and provide educational experiences that facilitate the development of language simultaneously through both oral and written modes of language.

■⊐ WHOLE LANGUAGE INTERVENTION STRATEGIES

The strategies for structuring Whole Language learning experiences are based on the following three principles: (1) maintaining whole learning environments, (2) whole-to-part learning, and (3) using oral and written language simultaneously. The first Whole Language principle is that all aspects of language form an indivisible and integrated system. Thus, the first intervention strategy is to structure and maintain learning environments where integrated language learning can occur. The second principle is that language is learned from whole to part. The corresponding strategy is to provide children with experiences that enable them to parse increasingly more specific and abstract information and language from the same context or event. The third principle, that written language develops in parallel with oral language, leads to the strategy of using oral and written language simultaneously to refine language. Each of these strategies is contrasted with more traditional strategies in the following section to demonstrate how Whole Language intervention differs from part-to-whole learning.

Maintaining Whole Learning Environments

Meaningful and purposeful language simultaneously integrates content, form, and use. The learning situation that is presented in intervention should be conducive to maintaining this integration. The interventionist must establish and maintain a central topic that can be explored through a variety of activities across an extended time period. This extended exploration of the same topic allows for the language refinement process to occur, as the same information is discussed with greater specificity and abstraction with repeated exposures.

The topics and language that are explored in intervention should be relevant to the demands presented by the school environment (Nelson, 1992). The language learning experiences provided should be consistent with the classroom and curricular uses of language, so that they reinforce rather than take time and effort away from the child's language learning in school. Since the school environment places demands for understanding a variety of narrative and expository discourse structures, and for learning many aspects of cultural and world knowledge, these should be used to structure intervention. A variety of topics that occur in the classroom are appropriate for use in language intervention, including topics from history, political science, geography, psychology, sociology, anthropology, physical science, and biological science. Each of these topics is encountered with varying degrees of complexity across the child's school years.

For example, a discussion of plants in the early grades may involve a visual examination of the primary parts of a flower and the creation of a chart to show the metamorphosis from a seed to a seedling and finally a flowering plant. The same topic at higher grade levels may involve a discussion of the interactions that occur between climate, geography, wind currents, and plant growth. The interventionist can control the level of complexity presented by manipulating aspects of the situation in which the information is presented, the complexity of the discourse that is used within the situation, and the level of semantic abstraction at which concepts are developed within the discussion.

Situational Context

The information and materials used to explore and discuss a topic constitute the *situational context* in which the child attempts to learn. These must be organized at an appropriate level of contextualization for learning to occur. The exploration of more difficult topics will require greater use of sensorimotor experiences that enable the children to manipulate concrete objects and observe the effects of their actions on them. More familiar topics may be explored through oral discussions or reading, with less dependence on direct experience or visual examples. Younger children, or those with less flexible language systems, will require greater use of concrete objects and action to learn, while those demonstrating greater flexibility will be able to engage in learning about a topic through oral discussion or reading. At the highest levels of organization, topics may be created through the logical use of language. Thus, the topic of "cooperation" may be explored by working together on a joint project at kindergarten, may be understood in relationship to a description of the first Thanksgiving Day dinner in fourth grade, or may be discussed as a theoretical construct in seventh grade.

Discourse Context

The topics discussed within a learning situation will be structured within a *discourse context*. The simplest form of discourse involves an unstructured expression of an individual's reactions to the topic. Many oral interactions that occur while exploring materials or negotiating turns and responsibilities would fall in this category. More complex discourse structures are used to organize actions or events into sequences that involve connections of time, causality, goal, transformation, or integration. These may involve narrative structures that reflect on a topic or experience, or expository structures that organize scientific or cultural knowledge about a topic. Each of these discourse structures specifies an overall organization for the information that will be included, the specific types of information that are important, and the language forms that should be used.

The distinction between narrative and expository discourse is more than a distinction among traditional forms of text organization, it represents a fundamental distinction in manners of cognitively organizing information (Bruner, 1986). Literary narratives represent a sequence of events, mental states, and physical changes that occur over time. The typical flow of events within a setting is interrupted by some novel occurrence that causes the characters to react mentally through emotional changes and planning to reach goals that have been motivated by the unusual event. The characters attempt to put their plans into action with a variety of possible outcomes. For example, in *Goldilocks and the Three Bears* (Moon, 1988a), the three bears each react to the arrival of Goldilocks into their home with surprise and even anger at the sequence of missing and broken items. They plan to search the house and then execute their plan by systematically moving from room to room, looking for a stranger. Bruner concludes that normally developing preschool children organize their memories for events in narrative format inasmuch as they tend to recall and talk about unusual events, the reactions that people had to those events, and their attempts to carry out plans in relation to the unusual events. Bruner maintains that narrative thought is used to code our knowledge of social norms and interpersonal interactions.

Development of narrative thought is obviously important to success in school experiences with literature. But it also undergirds understanding of social sciences in which the actions of groups of historical figures, as well as whole societies, can be understood with reference to critical events that motivated plans and attempts to fulfill those plans. For example, the heads of governments in Spain, England, and Portugal all desired to open trade routes to India and China in the 16th century because the growing class of craftsman and merchants in each country required expanding economic markets as well as raw materials that were rare in Europe. They formulated plans that resulted in sending Columbus, Cabot, and da Gama on different routes toward the Orient. The narrative form of thought can be applied whether the events are parts of cultural history, personal history, or imagined, as in fiction.

Children with less flexible language systems often demonstrate difficulties in organizing information in narrative form. Their play lacks organization and appears to be hyperactive. They fail to plan for the short and long terms, missing school assignments and making last minute attempts to complete homework. They have trouble comprehending and acquiescing to school rules and become labeled as behavioral problems. They fail to consider the perspectives of the people around them, causing failures in communication with adults, as well as arguments and even altercations with peers.

Bruner (1986) contrasts narrative thought with logico-mathematical thought in which physical characteristics of objects are explored, categorized, contrasted, and compared. Experiments are planned and executed to study the cause-effect relationships among objects and actions that can be applied to them. The development of this type of knowledge was the focus of Piaget's work. Bruner argues that this type of knowledge may result from the development of narrative thought, because children appear to demonstrate use of logical operations first when they are embedded within an ongoing story or typical event. Nelson's (1985) studies of preschool children suggest that the first abstract object categories developed by children are functional in nature with respect to fulfilling a role within common events. For example, one of the first object categories may be "things that are eaten at lunch time." Only later are objects such as bananas, hot dogs, applesauce, salami, and juice recategorized in classes such as "things that grew on trees," that is, fruits, versus things that were parts of animals.

Consequently, children who demonstrate difficulty with narrative thought and narrative language will exhibit more generalized difficulties with expository forms of thought and language. Thus, by focusing intervention on narrative forms of thought while integrating expository information into narrative form, the child is helped to develop an integrated knowledge of the world. Expository information becomes usable for purposes of problem solving and thinking about the world, rather than becoming simply memorized lists of information and procedures.

Semantic Context

The situational and discourse contexts interact with the *semantic context,* or the level of abstraction at which the information is considered. The same concrete materials can be labeled, or described according to physical properties, or discussed according to actions performed, or evaluated for potential benefits and problems. Similarly, the same story can be understood and discussed on different levels of abstraction. A folk tale such as *Goldilocks and the Three Bears* (Moon, 1988a) can be understood as simply a description of a series of events, or as a moral lesson regarding other people's property.

Comparison of Whole-to-Part and Part-to-Whole Learning

Whole Language intervention facilitates learning by enabling children to explore and talk about meaningful information through the exploration of a complex topic. The adult assures that the learning is comprehensible, while at the same time challenging, by manipulating the situational, discourse, and semantic contexts of language. The adult provides scaffolding to help the child discover and organize more information within a context than the child would have noticed independently. By actively engaging in the meaning-making process at these higher levels, the child establishes new concepts and reorganizes existing knowledge, providing both the need and the social opportunity to learn the language used to talk about the information. Through this process, the language content, form, and use are simultaneously acquired.

Traditional Part-to-Whole Instruction

This whole-to-part learning is opposite in philosophy and instructional methods from more traditional part-to-whole learning paradigms. These language training strategies attempt to teach language by dividing it into a number of discrete rule systems. Each rule system is thought to be related to one or more aspect of language performance. These aspects of language performance become regarded as language skills that can be directly measured in testing and targeted in treatment. The professionals charged with facilitating the child's language development identify those language skills that the child does not possess and design systematic sequences of activities to directly teach or indirectly model those skills (Fey, 1986).

The part-to-whole strategy involves targeting and teaching specific aspects of language. This focus rests on the assumption that the emergence of language behaviors constitutes language development. Language development is viewed as the progressive addition of aspects of language form, content, and use. Goals are structured to add vocabulary, syntactic forms, or pragmatic uses of language that would usually emerge next relative to the child's current developmental accomplishments.

Having identified individual language components that are not fully developed, the adult then structures activities to model and elicit the targeted language behaviors with high frequency to establish and stabilize their production. The language behaviors are targeted individually or in small numbers. This practice is based on the belief that children are better able to learn one aspect of language at a time, rather than trying to simultaneously coordinate multiple aspects of language. It is also based on a belief that aspects of language are easiest to learn when they have been pulled out of context so that the child can be exposed to the most elemental forms of the aspect of language being targeted.

Problems with Part-to-Whole Instruction

One reason for limited identification of language problems among school-age children is that the superficial aspects of language appear to be mastered by these children when they are assessed in the simple contexts typically used in standardized testing procedures. By decontextualizing aspects of language function, content, and form into individual test items, the skills that are assessed may not be part of an integrated language system. This process of testing becomes doubly problematic when the test procedures are used as therapy techniques. For example, the child who is taught "vocabulary" by practice in naming individual objects and pictures may learn to pass standardized tests of vocabulary that use these tasks. However, that child may now exhibit "word finding" problems for the vocabulary that has been learned in this manner when the language context is more complex. Assessment of decontextualized skills does not assure that the child has integrated the skills into a flexible language system.

A classic problem with this approach to language intervention is that of limited generalization (Fey, 1988). Since the language to be learned is chosen by the adult, elicited in contrived situations, and established through repetitions in discrete contexts rather than within networks of integrated concepts, there is a large discrepancy between the manner in which the language was learned and the manner in which language is actually used for communication purposes.

A third problem is the time required to teach one language skill or behavior at a time. Few intervention programs are designed to continue to add skills through stages of acquiring multiply embedded sentences that incorporate both relative clauses and coordinating clauses with elaborated noun phrases, and yet this type of sentence structure is commonly encountered within third grade reading passages (Norris, 1989). It is neither practical nor time efficient to attempt to teach this level of complexity one skill at a time (Allington, 1989).

Whole-to-Part Instruction

The child with a less flexible language system lacks the internalized organization of language content, use, and form required for learning and use in a variety of contexts. Thus, Whole Language intervention seeks to assist the child to organize information to simultaneously integrate content, form, and use. The interventionist does this by providing the child with information while giving the child repeated opportunities to express that information using language. The adult informs the child about important aspects of the situation to consider and models language that can be used to talk about these insights. The adult then shares the responsibility with the child for communicating about and elaborating on this understanding.

The interventionist organizes the interaction so that the child has many opportunities to use language within the situation. She directs the overall discussion so that the children in the interaction remain on topic. Staying on topic ensures that the children will have numerous opportunities to use language to talk about the same concepts with greater specificity and refinement.

Consider the following interaction involving an 8-year-old boy telling a story about a picture from the Apricot I series (Arwood, 1985). The picture shows three boys playing basketball in a driveway with a car approaching. One boy has passed the ball over the head of the second boy who has his arms spread out to block the pass. The third boy is chasing the ball into the street, not noticing the approaching car.

"Kid . . . ball . . . car . . .
This boy try to grab his pants.
This boy put his hands like that

(continued)

> "And that car ran on the . . . the . . .
> the car . . . um . . . was was going and it
> . . . um . . . it it . . . um . . .
> and it . . . um . . . it hit the ball . . . um
> . . . the ball ran out the street."

This child's narrative exemplifies a number of the negative characteristics of less flexible language. It lacks narrative structure. This child has misinterpreted the action of the boy who is guarding another boy in the basketball game, not trying to pull his pants down. He uses gestures to compensate for his inability to structure the language needed to describe what the boy is doing. Nonfluencies mark the points where he is struggling to organize information. And, his language does not adequately express the meaning he does attempt to convey, for example, the ball is running **into** the street.

The facilitator first supplies information about the overall context and then provides the child with an opportunity to use some of that information in his story.

> "The boys were playing basketball. This boy, Andy,
> was trying to throw the ball to Chad (pointing
> between two boys as they are named). When Andy
> tried to throw a ball to Chad, Chad missed it. Now you
> explain what happened."

The child uses some of this information to start retelling the story. He establishes that the boy was trying to throw the ball, but becomes disfluent at the point where he tries to add more information about what happened next or why.

> "He tried to throw the ball and and um and um . . ."

The clinician restates the information expressed by the child using different language forms. This communicates to the child that the adult thinks his addition to the topic was important and provides models of alternative language forms that can be used to express the information.

This restatement also serves as a scaffold to the larger conjoined sentence that the child first attempted to produce. The clinician has produced the first part of the relationship and then she pauses to give the child the opportunity to structure the second part of the relationship.

> "Andy was trying . . ."

The child successfully finishes the first idea and then adds another, resulting in a sentence that coordinated the use of an infinitive verb phrase, coordination of a direct and indirect object, and a conjoined sentence. He additionally spontaneously revised his own false start.

> "to throw the ball to Chad and it um, he missed."

The clinician again accepts his addition to the story. She reexamines the same action, this time modeling a more elaborated statement of how one of the boys was trying to catch the ball, including an element of goal or motivation.

> "Right, Chad was supposed to catch the ball, but he missed it. What happened?"

The child recognizes the goal and attempts to incorporate it into his retelling. His resulting sentence lacks conventionality by adult standards, reflecting the process of inventive risks as he tries to use language to add an additional element.

> "Chad was supposed to catch it and he missed catch it."

By continuing in this manner with restatements and expansions of old information and introduction of new relationships among actors, actions, and objects depicted in the picture, the child is enabled to actively participate in creating a well structured narrative. The result is that he is better able to organize the information, including language forms, when he is asked to retell the story after 30 minutes of engaging in this process.

> "Andy wanted to throw the ball to Chad so he could make a point, and Tony blocked his hands like this so Chad couldn't get a point. And the ball went in the wrong place and rolled in the street, and a car was coming by, and if the car runned over the ball, the ball will get flat. And Chad didn't want the ball to get flat. Chad didn't want the ball to get flat so Chad can grab it and throw it in the goal."

The story now contains a number of statements about the characters' plans and motives that were not present in the first rendition. These are stated with complex sentence structure that also was not seen in the first story. Language also is used to code the relationships of time held between the actions. The scaffolded interactions provided a context for the content, use, and form of the language, including both sentence and discourse level structures, to be used and coordinated. With repeated opportunities to use language at complex levels, these aspects of content, use, and form become internalized and used independently.

Compare this approach for facilitating a change in language with that used in a part-to-whole approach. On the basis of the initial story, the production of simple, present progressive declarative sentences elicited in response to a picture might be targeted for intervention. The basketball picture might be used as one context for eliciting this targeted structure as follows:

The boys are playing basketball.

Chad is throwing the ball.

The car is running down the street.

The interventionist might point to a specific action and model the targeted sentence structure. The child would then be asked to describe the picture using the modeled form. Following the production of syntactically well formed sentences, the clinician might say something like "That was a nice sentence." Following an inappropriate sentence form such as "The boys playing basketball," she might provide corrective feedback such as, "That sentence did not have 'are' in it. You should say, 'The boys **are** playing basketball.' "

This approach has a number of negative consequences on language development. First, this interaction violates a basic premise of conversational discourse. The adult and the child are talking about different topics. The child is talking about the picture, while the adult is talking about the accuracy of the child's language forms. Normal discourse involves creating meaning about a single, meaningful topic shared by the discourse participants.

Second, by focusing on a particular sentence structure, the clinician is teaching the child to use a disjointed narrative style. To tell a coherent story, it is necessary to talk about actions across past, present, and future time frames. Each of these requires different syntactic structures and strategies for embedding and coordinating the ideas.

Third, narratives require insight into people's motives, plans, and emotional reactions to events. But such issues are not easily expressed in simple present progressive structures and so their introduction would have to wait until the child has advanced to embedded or conjoined sentences such as, "The boy was holding out his arms, so that he could stop the pass."

Fourth, language ceases to be real when it is artificially divided into pieces. Rather than a simultaneous expression of purpose, content, and form, divided language becomes an exercise in game playing. The child learns that successful participation in today's game consists of producing sentences that have a particular syntactic pattern. The adult takes the role of referee and tells the child whether he is violating the rules of the game. Meaning is merely incidental, and purpose is unrelated to communication.

Whole language intervention seeks to facilitate language learning and use within a meaningful context so that the language that is internalized is topic focused, coherent, variable in form and content, and purposeful. One way to create such a learning context while at the same time remaining systematic is to use written text as the learning context.

Using Written Language

Whole language views reading as a language acquisition process in which the patterns of written language must be internalized in much the same manner that oral language is learned. Written language is not merely mapped onto a well formed oral language system. Rather, experiences with reading refine the language system in the same manner that oral language experiences facilitate the learning of new content, forms, and uses. Thus, to facilitate the learning of written language, principles of Whole Language learning must be applied, including the presentation of integrated, meaningful text from which specific reading related knowledge is gradually parsed and refined. Similarly, written language provides a context for learning and refining language as content, form, and use of written language is explored. The print enables children to examine language in a concrete visual form, and to understand how word order and grammatical structures function to establish relationships of meaning between ideas. Consider the following text from *The Two Windmills* (Butterworth, 1988b)

The miller in the white mill was a kind and happy man. He had a wife and six children. When work was done, the miller and his wife played with the children in the fields. At night, after supper, they sang songs and told the children tales of long ago.
. . . the miller in the grey mill was just the opposite. He and his wife were mean and greedy and miserable. They never smiled or laughed, and all they ever thought about was money and how to get more money. They had no children. Each night, after supper, they took out their money to count it. That was the great joy in their lives.

This excerpt, taken from the beginning pages of the story, provides opportunities to explore complex grammatical structures including elaborated noun phrases, conjunction, direct and indirect objects, multiply embedded clauses in both subject and object positions, and a variety of strategies for marking temporal and spatial relationships between ideas. The manner in which these structures function to communicate meaning can be explored simultaneously with an awareness of their form. The text similarly provides opportunities to explore complex narrative structure, including character development, opposing goals and perspectives, and interactive sequences of goals, attempts, and consequences. The function of cohesive ties, including the use of pronouns and vocabulary to maintain the topic and referents can be physically pointed to and explained as they function within the meaningful context.

The narrative structure provides an overall theme that binds the events of the text together. The same content or events can be discussed at increasing levels of abstraction, beginning with simple descriptions of the actions and increasing to involve more interpretations of character motivation, evaluation of the attitudes and morals held by the characters, and an examination of the word choices and word order strategies that are used to communicate these explicit and implicit levels of meaning.

Events in the text can be generalized through comparisons to personal and world experience. On one day, the children might read the first few pages and discuss the physical scene of the story and the characteristics of the two millers as depicted in the text and pictures. On the next day, the children might identify things that people think will make them happy, and those things that actually do make people happy, by talking about the lifestyles of the two millers and relating examples of similar choices within their own experiences. Values and choices can then be discussed in relationship to societal and cultural values.

The adult scaffolds the interactions ongoing between the child and the author's words. As reading errors occur, the adult helps the child to establish the intended meaning of the passage and then examines the word metalinguistically for its representation of sounds and syllables. Thus, in this Whole Language approach to reading development, the experience of reading is used to develop all levels of language simultaneously. Reading behaviors, from letter-sound correspondences to narrative structures to metaphoric interpretations, are acquired in relationship to their role in the meaning-making process.

A more traditional view of the relationship between oral and written language is that it is a developmental progression from oral language to reading and finally writing. Reading is viewed as mapping onto established oral forms. This view leads some intervention approaches to separate instruction in oral language from instruction in written language and to teach relationships such as letter-sound correspondences as sequences of skills to be targeted and taught, first in isolation and gradually in longer contexts. Comprehension is viewed as a by-product of vocabulary knowledge, attention to main ideas, and other skills that can be targeted and taught.

■□ SUMMARY

Whole Language is a philosophy of language learning and use that involves the integration of multiple levels of information present within the social and physical context, as well as within the child's existing system of cognitive and linguistic knowledge. The principles of Whole Language philosophy are used to guide the curricula, methods, and interactions that are used to assess and to facilitate oral and written language acquisition and use. The principles include the presentation of information within unified, or whole, contexts, and the use of scaffolding techniques to assist the child to refine language by parsing the whole into gradually more specific and abstract parts.

When language intervention focuses simultaneously on a wide range of language abilities, it is important that the interventionist maintain organization within the interactions. The interventionist must provide the child with situational, discourse, and semantic contexts of learning that are comprehensible to guide the child toward the exploration and discovery of the many properties of language content, form, and use. A model for coordinating the situational compexity, discourse structure, and semantic level of abstraction will be discussed in Chapter 2. This model will be used to guide assessment and intervention for the school-age child across the continuum of development from early elementary through the upper grade levels.

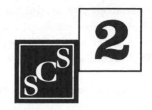

An Integrated Model of Language: The Situational, Discourse, and Semantic Dimensions

C onducting assessment and providing intervention using Whole Language does not mean that decisions are made in an unsystematic or random fashion. On the contrary, assessment and intervention strategies are carefully planned for specific purposes. The interactions take place within complex situations in which all aspects of language function in integration. The organization used to examine and plan the language within these situations must exist within the individual conducting the assessment or intervention. This chapter provides a cohesive model for understanding how to analyze and provide organization within complex, integrated situations. This chapter provides

- A model that can be used to examine language simultaneously in the Situational, Discourse, and Semantic Contexts
- Procedures for systematically using the model

- Examples of general uses of the model
- Examples of how goals and objectives can be formulated directly from the model
- A detailed description of the Situational Context
- A detailed description of the Discourse Context
- A detailed description of the Semantic Context

Over the past 20 years much has been learned about the structure, content, and uses of language within discourse patterns, such as conversations, and contexts of use, such as routine events or classrooms. Speech-language specialists have descriptions of the turn taking that occurs within conversations, the strategies used to initiate, maintain, and terminate interactions, the structures of narratives and the developmental sequence along which they emerge, and the types and purposes of different forms of expository discourse. Speech-language specialists are aware of the assumptions that speakers must make about their audience and the resulting language that is used to convey the message and communication breakdowns or failures that can occur when the speaker experiences difficulty coordinating all of the many levels of knowledge and patterns of convention that must be orchestrated during the production of speech (Damico, 1992; Gallagher, 1991; Gallagher & Prutting, 1983; Miller, 1991). However, while there is a greater description of language and its use within a context, to date we have no coherent model of language in which to integrate this information.

The absence of a coherent model is problematic on more than just a theoretical level. Without a coherent model to guide the decision-making process, it is difficult to determine exactly what is important to know about children and their language for purposes of assessment and intervention. The quest to attach norms to more objectively identify children exhibiting delays or disorders is elusive, because the language that is used in context depends on so many interacting factors, such as what is being talked about, to whom, and for what purpose. It is impossible to state how many conversational turns are "normal" for a child of a given age, or which purposes of language should be accomplished by children in a given context, because these factors are highly situation specific. However, our present state of knowledge *can* be used to impose some organization on our observations, assessments, and interventions. The information that is known can be used not only to describe *what* a child is doing within a meaningful context of language use, but also to make interpretations of *how* children are approaching a task and, therefore, *why* they may be responding in a particular manner. This explanatory power provides better insights into the level of refinement exhibited within a child's language system and, therefore, a better map of what can be done in intervention to facilitate higher levels of language organization and use.

■ THE SITUATIONAL-DISCOURSE-SEMANTIC (S-D-S) MODEL

This chapter presents a model for thinking about language and its use in an effort to impose some organization on the existing knowledge regarding language within a meaningful context. The model is applied in successive chapters to the assessment of language in the school-age child as it occurs in a variety of contexts of use and to intervention that can be provided to facilitate language in a manner consistent with the model. Among the uses of this model are

- Conducting naturalistic observation
- Conducting descriptive assessment
- Organizing learning in accordance with a multidimensional developmental sequence
- Curriculum development and modification
- Establishment of goals and objectives
- Planning and monitoring short-term development
- Planning and monitoring long-term development
- Program and curriculum development
- Coordinating collaborative efforts among educational team members
- Modifying activities to meet the needs of students with different abilities and learning styles
- Conducting task analyses
- Modifying adult behaviors to mediate learning within an event or activity

By using the same model for a range of purposes, an integrated view of children and their learning that encompasses short- and long-term language development and academic progress can be achieved. Individuals using the model can form a better understanding of the children with whom they interact, the curriculum that they are presenting, and the teaching strategies that they are using to facilitate learning among children.

Procedure for Using the Model

The model, outlined in Table 2–1 and detailed in Tables 2–3, 2–5, and 2–6, and throughout this chapter, can be used by considering each assess-

TABLE 2-1
The Situational-Discourse-Semantic Context Model used for assessment and intervention.

SITUATIONAL CONTEXT	DISCOURSE CONTEXT	SEMANTIC CONTEXT
Level X **LOGICAL** • hypothetical • mental objects • abstractions • principles	**Level VIII** **INTERACTIVE STRUCTURE** • multiple plots or topics • reciprocal • integrated	**Level VII** **METALANGUAGE** • knowledge of linguistic properties • separate form from meaning or function
Level IX **SYMBOLIC** • linguistically created • possible event	**Level VII** **COMPLEX STRUCTURE** • separate subtopics/episodes • each complete	**Level VI** **EVALUATION** • response to or reflection on event • judgment/value • significance
Level VIII **RELATIONAL** • relationships within event • scripts-schema	**Level VI** **COMPLETE STRUCTURE** • overall moral or objective • all elements	**Level V** **INFERENCE** • meaning beyond what is stated • meaning not present or suggested
Level VII **DECENTERED** • re-create event perspective of observer	**Level V** **ABBREVIATED STRUCTURE** • plans, intents • incomplete • most elements	**Level IV** **INTERPRETATION** • meaning not explicit but suggested in available cues • goals, states
Level VI **EGOCENTERED** • re-create event perspective of participant	**Level IV** **REACTIVE SEQUENCE** • cause-effect • no intent/plan • logical order	**Level III** **DESCRIPTION** • unify objects, events, agents • characteristic qualities • explicit
Level V **LOGICAL** • representation • logical reason • concrete	**Level III** **ORDERED SEQUENCE** • temporal order • no causality • arbitrary	**Level II** **LABELING** • name wholes • label parts within whole • categories • sensory input
Level IV **SYMBOLIC** • substituted objects • illustrations	**Level II** **DESCRIPTIVE LIST** • topic related • no unifying temporal frame	**Level I** **INDICATION** • nonlinguistic communication • meaning known in context
Level III **RELATIONAL** • relational actions, real functions	**Level I** **COLLECTION** • associations • no structure • change topics	
Level II **DECENTERED** • sensorimotor exploration • discovery		
Level I **EGOCENTERED** • sensorimotor stimulation • own body		

CONTEXTUALIZED — DECONTEXTUALIZED

TRANSACTIONAL FUNCTION — POETIC FUNCTION

EXPERIENTIAL — ERUDITE

EXPRESSIVE FUNCTION

ment, intervention, or accountability decision from three simultaneous and interacting perspectives. First, the characteristics of the event or activity should be examined, referred to in the model as the **Situational Context**. This examination involves two decisions: (1) decide whether the language that is being used within the event is related to the immediately present context, or must an imagined context be created through the use of language (i.e., a contextualized-to-decontextualized continuum); and (2) decide which of the 10 levels of cognitive organization (ranging from sensorimotor stimulation on the child's body, through the logical mental manipulation of abstract concepts) is most characteristic of the event or activity.

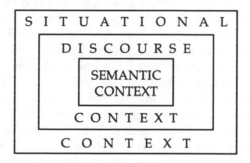

Second, the characteristics of the discourse used to talk about the event or activity should be ascertained, referred to in the model as the **Discourse Context**. Two decisions must be made regarding this dimension: (1) whether the function of the discourse is more narrative (i.e., termed "Poetic" in this model, following Britton's [1982] classification), more expository (i.e., termed "Transactional"), or more personal and responsive (i.e., termed "Expressive" in the model); and (2) which of the eight levels of discourse structure (ranging from a free expression of ideas to highly structured presentations of topics along the expressive-to-transactional versus expressive-to-poetic poles) is most characteristic of the discourse.

Finally, the characteristics of the language used to refer to concepts or ideas should be determined, referred to in the model as the **Semantic Context**. The two decisions to be made in this category are: (1) whether the meaning of the word or phrase is knowable from concrete actions and personal experience (i.e., Experiential meaning) or whether the meaning is embedded within scientific, cultural, world, or historical knowledge (i.e., Erudite meaning); and (2) at which of the seven levels of semantic complexity a word or phrase refers to an object, event, or concept, ranging from direct and explicit reference to a concrete or abstract concept (Indication or Labeling), to a highly indirect and implicit reference to concepts (i.e., Metalinguistic reference).

Example of the Model's Use

The S-D-S Contexts are simultaneously operating in each interaction within an event or activity. For example, a reading event using the storybook *The Gingerbread Man* (Young, 1988) involves a Situational Context in which the language refers to characters, actions, and entities present and visible in the immediate environment (i.e., contextualized to the book) and that are representational rather than real (i.e., pictures rather than real people or objects), thus placing the event at Level V: **Contextualized-Symbolic** level. The Discourse Context created by the author in the book involves a story (i.e., Poetic function) in which the characters are goal directed, with the Gingerbread Man successively chased by a man, a woman, a boy, a girl, and a fox who has a plan for tricking the Gingerbread Man, and an implied moral (i.e., a Complete Structure). The book reading event would thus be placed at Level VI: **Poetic-Complete** level of Discourse Context. Specific instances of language use can be examined using the Semantic Context, as well as general patterns of language use. For example, in the story the old woman announces that she has just made a delicious gingerbread man, to which the old man replies, "Good, I'm hungry and I love gingerbread men" (p. 2). The most explicit meaning requires an **Interpretation**, in that the words "hungry" and "love" do not refer to real world objects, but rather mental concepts that must be interpreted from perceptions or behaviors. A more implied meaning is also suggested, requiring an **Inference**, that is, the words suggest that the man intends to eat the gingerbread man. The interaction between the three contexts can be described as follows:

Contextualized-Symbolic × Poetic = Complete × Experiential-Interpretation and Inference

Any change in one or more dimension changes the dynamics between the three contexts and, thus, may increase, decrease, or modify the difficulty of the event. For example, a parent might read the book to a child without showing the pictures, thus requiring the child to mentally create the visual images from the words. Because the language would no longer be supported by context cues and all characters, their actions, and attitudes would have to be created through the language alone, the demands along the Situational Context would increase five levels on the model to that of Level IX: **Decontextualized-Symbolic**, while the demands within the Discourse Context would remain the same. An observation might reveal that without the benefit of the picture showing the man looking at and moving toward the gingerbread man, the child might fail to make the inference cited previously, and, therefore, not realize why the gingerbread man began to run, even though the same text could be understood when contextualized by the pictures. The change in the interaction is profiled below:

$$\textit{Decontextualized}\text{-Symbolic} \times \text{Poetic-Complete} \times \begin{matrix} \text{Experiential-Interpretation} \\ (\textit{No Inference}) \end{matrix}$$

Thus, the model provides both a descriptive and explanatory system for understanding events and interpreting behaviors or responses that may seem inconsistent or contradictory at first glance.

Nature of the Situational-Discourse-Semantic Continua

The S-D-S Contexts are distributed along their respective continua as shown in Table 2–1, with the least difficult aspect of each context positioned at the bottom of the chart and increasing complexity or abstraction represented as each continuum nears the top of the table. These continua are both *descriptive* of a wide range of contexts present within naturally occurring events within the environment, and *developmental* in nature, with children showing increasing competence at higher levels of the continua with age. For example, an adult might be able to provide the same information as either a **Descriptive List** (i.e., the kiwi is a bird, the kiwi has no wings, kiwis are found in New Zealand, New Zealand consists of a north and a south island, New Zealand originally had few carnivorous animals), or as a **Complete Text** (i.e., The kiwi is a type of bird that gradually lost its wings because it evolved on the north and south islands of New Zealand where few carnivorous animals lived. With no predators and an abundance of food, the bird had no need for wings, and thus today has only stubs and cannot fly). In contrast, young children might be capable of organizing the information only at the level of a Descriptive List, and would not be expected to coordinate all of the relationships into a Complete Text until middle childhood.

The remainder of this chapter presents a detailed description of the model, including the primary characteristics of the 10 levels of the Situational Context, the 8 levels of the Discourse Context, and the 7 levels of the Semantic Context as they are distributed along their respective continua. These characteristics are to be used to assist in descriptively identifying the levels at which an event is occurring along the S-D-S dimensions for purposes of assessment, intervention, and accountability.

Excerpts from children's literature and expository text are used to provide examples of the levels where appropriate.

In addition, a developmental discussion of each level within the continua is provided. This information provides guidelines for the types of expectations that might be held for children of different age and/or developmental levels, based on currently existing norms. These guidelines are far from comprehensive, since our knowledge of development is very incomplete, and even less is known about the influences of cultural or socioeconomic differences. However, understanding the developmental abilities of children can provide the means for making decisions regarding the activities or material to choose for specific purposes, the level of complexity or abstraction at which to focus the interaction, the expectations to hold for children, and the developmental characteristics displayed by a specific child. For example, while the Discourse level of *The Gingerbread Man* (Beasley, 1988) is written at the Poetic-Complete level, the book can be responded to at the Expressive-Personal level by a 1-year-old child (e.g., pointing to, naming and commenting on things noticed in the picture, such as "a man," "eyes, nose," "I like cookies"); at the Poetic-Ordered Sequence level with no Interpretation or Inference by a 2-year-old (e.g., talking about the events depicted in sequence, without recognizing the cause-effect relationships between them, as in "The old woman made the gingerbread man, the old man chased him, and the boy chased him, and the girl chased him, and the fox ate him"); at the Poetic-Reactive Sequence level with Interpretations by age 3 (e.g., interpreting the cause of a character's action, as in "The old woman made the gingerbread man cookie and the old man was going to eat him and he ran away. And a boy chased him, and a girl, and everyone chased him, and a fox ate him"); and at the Poetic-Abbreviated level including Inferences by age 5, where the goals of the characters, such as the trickery of the fox, are understood.

■□ ESTABLISHING GOALS AND OBJECTIVES

Knowing what to expect from children developmentally allows for observations or language samples to be examined from a developmentally appropriate perspective, for group intervention to be simultaneously conducted at different levels using the same materials or activities to meet individual children's needs, to use the same materials at higher or lower levels to achieve different goals, to establish developmentally appropriate goals and objectives, and to modify the level of explanation or mediation provided to children within an event or activity. It also allows for long-term planning. For example, a long-term goal might be to achieve age/grade level equivalence, while the successive stages out-lined on the model toward that target level might serve as a series of short-term objectives in approximation of that goal (see Table 2–2).

■□ SITUATIONAL CONTEXT

Using the model involves making a series of decisions. These decisions are made in a whole-to-part manner, with an analysis of the context as a whole occurring first, followed by decisions regarding progressively more specific parts. The Situational Context on this model refers to the analysis of the most global or whole view of the context. It involves analyzing what people within the event are *doing,* the materials that they are *using,* and the *manner* in which the language that occurs within the event serves to refer within this situation.

When examining the Situational Context, the event or activity should be compared to the 10 levels of organization profiled below to find the "best fit" or description. This will be guided, in part, by the pur-poses for making the observation. For example, if the reason for the observation is to find out why a child does not follow classroom rules, then aspects of the situation that might be focused on would be at Level VIII: Decontextualized-Relational in the model. However, if the reason for the observation is to determine in what manner a child participates in and learns from a situation, the level of focus will correspond to the ac-tivities that are occurring. The teacher may be conducting an oral lecture with no visual props, in which case the situation may be at Level IX (Decontextualized-Symbolic), or the teacher may be using objects to demonstrate a concept, in which case the situation may be rated at Level IV (Contextualized-Symbolic). To make this determination, the inter-ventionist must decide whether the language used within the situation is *Contextualized* or *Decontextualized,* and then decide the level of cognitive organization involved.

The levels profiled in Table 2–1 and detailed in Table 2–3 under the category of the Situational Context reflect the degree to which the infor-mation referred to through language is physically present (i.e., contex-tualized), and the degree of organization required to participate. The continuum, beginning at the bottom of the table and working upward, reflects (1) an increasing ability to use language rather than physically present objects to create the context, including all of the necessary peo-ple, objects, actions, or states (i.e., contextualization); and (2) an increas-ing ability to organize, understand, learn from, and communicate about the world at greater distances from the child's own body and physical manipulations (i.e., cognitive organization).

TABLE 2–2

Example of the use of the model for establishing long-term goals, measurable short-term objectives, and expected outcomes.

DATE OF GOAL IMPLEMENTATION: September 1, 19XX

EXPECTED DATE OF GOAL COMPLETION: June 1, 19XX

GOAL:

To exhibit age-appropriate narrative abilities (i.e., the Contextualized-Symbolic Situational level × the Poetic-Complex Discourse level × the Experiential-Inferential Semantic level).

CURRENT PERFORMANCE LEVEL:

Current narrative abilities are characterized by Contextual-Symbolic Situational level × Poetic-Collection Discourse level × Experiential-Labeling and Description Semantic levels.

Objective 1:

When given an illustrated book (i.e., a Contextualized-Symbolic Situational context) that depicts a story with Poetic-Complete structure, the child will generate a story characterized as a(n):

Approximation to Goal	Date Achieved
a. Descriptive List, with at least 90% of the comments made relating to the events depicted; few elements of story structure present.	October 15 (Criteria: three unfamiliar books)
b. Ordered Sequence, with at least 60% of the events linked with temporal terms, including "and," "and then," "when," "first," "next," "later," "last," and so forth; few elements of story structure present.	November 3
c. Reactive Sequence, with at least 60% of the events linked with temporal terms, and at least three references made to cause-effect relationships between events.	January 20
d. Abbreviated Story, where the goals of the characters are stated for specific events (or can be explained, if asked) for at least 80% of the goal-motivated actions.	March 30
e. Complete Story, where the overall lesson or moral of the story can be given, as well as the goals, attempts, and outcomes for specific events within the story.	_____

(continued)

TABLE 2-2 *(continued)*

Objective 2

When given an illustrated book (i.e., a Contextualized-Symbolic Situational context) that depicts a story with Poetic-Complete structure, the child will generate a story in which the ideas conveyed are characterized by:

Approximation to Goal	Date Achieved
a. Meaning at the Descriptive level or above for 90% of the sentences produced.	September 25
b. Inclusion of meaning at the Interpretive level or above for at least 20% of the sentences produced.	February 4
c. Inferences explicitly stated (or explained if asked) for at least 80% of the critical events in the story.	_____

If these objectives are met, the following outcomes can be expected and can be measured:

- longer sentences
- more complete sentences
- more sentences related to the main topic
- greater use of adjectives and adverbs
- greater use of temporal and spatial terms
- greater use of verb tense
- noun-verb agreement
- greater use of vocabulary related to motives, feelings
- greater variety of vocabulary words
- longer stories
- more specific language
- longer attention to task
- fewer off-topic comments
- fewer off-task behaviors
- fewer prompts or cues needed to complete task
- reference to events from the characters' perspectives
- more creative stories
- Ideas fit the content of the pictures
- more abstract vocabulary

◾️ CONTINUUM OF DECONTEXTUALIZATION

Contextualized or Decontextualized Language

The first decision to be made when examining the Situational Context is to determine whether the language in use is contextualized or decontextualized. All language learning and use occurs within a situation that exists at some level of physical reality. This may include reference to

TABLE 2-3
The ten levels of the Situational Context, distributed along the Contextualized to Decontextualized continuum.

SITUATIONAL CONTEXT

D E C	LEVEL X	LOGICAL	Language and logic are used to create a hypothetical context. The context created consists of mental objects that have no sensorimotor correlates. Topics deal with abstractions, principles.
O N T	LEVEL IX	SYMBOLIC	Factual or fictional experiences are created using language alone, as in learning about a different period in history or reading a novel. Language is not used to talk about the known world, but rather to create possible worlds
E T U	LEVEL VIII	RELATIONAL	Learning and functioning require an understanding of the overall structure of events and the relationships of the component parts. Includes scripts or schema for classroom or other conventional routines, self-monitoring to plan and complete a task.
A L I	LEVEL VII	DECENTERED	Language is used to create an event from the perspective of an observer. The child was present for the event, but not as an active participant. Language structures what was seen or heard.
Z E D	LEVEL VI	EGOCENTERED	Language is used to re-create an event from the perspective of a participant, or an experience that earlier was experienced on a sensorimotor level. The people, actions, and objects must be referenced through language.

Language refers to

objects, agents absent from immediate context

past and possible actions, states, or events

self-regulation including plans

primary responsibility for communication belongs to speaker

CONTEXTUALIZATION

Language refers to objects, agents present in the context; ongoing actions and states; social regulation of behavior of others; responsibility for communication shared

LEVEL V — LOGICAL	Objects are present but used in abstract, representational ways. Greater focus on mental concepts and language used to refer to them. Roles different from one's own are assumed. Logical reasoning about concrete objects. Social interaction facilitates learning *about* events.
LEVEL IV — SYMBOLIC	Language and learning are conceptualized to immediately present objects, events, and people, but objects can be miniatures, replicas, substituted objects, drawings, or other representations. Includes illustrated storybooks. Social interaction involves shared participation.
LEVEL III — RELATIONAL	Language and learning refer to objects used in sequences of relational activities. Actual objects are used for real functional purposes. Includes most self-help routines, such as eating, dressing, or bathing. Social interaction occurs for purposes of getting things done.
LEVEL II — DECENTERED	Language and learning occur in relationship to the sensorimotor exploration of individual objects for purposes of discovering the relationships of the parts to the whole, or the general function of the object. Social interaction occurs for the sake of interacting.
LEVEL I — EGOCENTERED	Language and learning are contextualized to immediately present sensory stimulation impacting directly on child's own body. Personal response to temperature, hunger, fatigue, as well as objects contacting child.

physical objects or ongoing actions that are present and can be seen and touched within the context, or only auditory signals (or in the case of reading, visual signs) that are received by a hearer as words, that must then be used to mentally re-create the references for the objects or events no longer present or observable. The level at which the things talked about are physically observable and manipulable determines the degree to which the accompanying language used within the situation is contextualized (Westby, 1986). The general characteristics of language used within a Contextualized versus Decontextualized situation are summarized in Table 2–4.

◼️⎵ LEVELS OF COGNITIVE ORGANIZATION

After making a determination of whether the situation in focus is contextualized or decontextualized, the event or activity can be more specifically described by also identifying the level of cognitive organization existing within the situation. The 10 levels of the Situational Context profiled in Table 2–1, detailed in Table 2–3, and described below reflect increasing levels of cognitive complexity. These levels are both descriptive and developmental, such that an adult would have the cognitive organizational abilities to use real objects in a functional way, such as opening doors with keys (Contextualized-Relational), but also would be able to think about keys in highly logical and abstract ways, such as viewing the neurotransmitters as keys to a neuron (Decontextualized-Logical). A young child, in contrast, might be capable only of thinking of keys as visible objects that open real doors and be unable to mentally create hypothetical objects through analogy until middle childhood (Piaget, 1952, 1970).

The 10 levels can be thought of as divisible into 5 levels that are within the contextualized end of the scale, requiring the physical presence and manipulation of objects versus five parallel levels that are decontextualized, where physical objects are not available, and words must be used to create the appropriate images of mental objects. For example, the words "Put the egg in the biggest bowl" while cooking requires relating the words to bowls, ingredients, and people present in the immediate situation, while these same variables are irrelevant to the words "Tomorrow I have to be at school by 8:00" spoken in the same context. A day, location, activity, and characters different from the ones immediately present in the kitchen must be mentally constructed to interpret the decontextualized statement.

For both the contextualized and the decontextualized dimensions of the continuum, understanding is easiest when the event is personally ex-

TABLE 2-4

A comparison of language used within a Contextualized versus Decontextualized situation.

Characteristics of Contextualized Language

Language frequently serves a social regulatory function
Information or objects are requested or commented on in context
Language is part of the actual ongoing experience
Interaction most often takes place as a dialogue
The responsibility for communication is shared
The persons involved in the communication are present
The same spatial location and temporal environment are shared
The language used is often informal, consisting of phrases instead of
  formal grammatical sentences
Nonspecific language such as "it," "that," or "thing" is accompanied by
  points used to establish reference
Spatial and temporal information are understood within the context and
  thus not specifically stated
Much of the communication is nonverbal, transmitted through
  intonation, body language, and gestures

Characteristics of Decontextualized Language

Language serves a more internal regulatory function
Language is used for purposes of thinking and planning, reflection
Language is used to seek information to integrate with existing knowledge
Concepts referred to through language are distanced from actual
  experience
Concepts are created through generalizations from other experiences
Language moves the child beyond his own experience and into pretend,
  imagined, and hypothetical events
Interaction increasingly is conducted in long periods of monologue
The speaker maintains most of the responsibility for presenting a
  coherent account of some event or concept
Language refers to people, objects, events, and entities not present in
  the immediate context
Roles, locations during the event, and the temporal frame must be
  established using language
Language requires highly specific word choices
Ideas must be organized in complete, multiply embedded grammatical
  structures
There is some reliance on intonation, gestures, and body language

perienced. Thus, objects are easier to understand if they are related to one's own actions or body (a hat is placed on the child = Contextual-ized-*Egocentered*) than if a cause-effect relationship between objects must be experimentally manipulated (the child places objects in water to discover what will float = Contextualized-*Logical*). Similarly, events are easier to re-create using language if they were originally personally experienced (the child reports how she hurt her knee on the playground = Decontextualized-Egocentered), compared to learning about hypothetical situations through lecture or discussion (the child hears a lecture about the particle versus wave-like properties of light = Decontextual-ized-Logical). The continuum represents this progressive increase in the cognitive organization from self outward in the parallel structure of the levels within the Contextualized and the Decontextualized ends of the continuum.

▪□ CONTEXTUALIZED LEVELS

The Situational Context is contextualized when the topic being considered corresponds to the physical and perceptual characteristics of the situation. Children can attend to people, objects, and actions present and ongoing in the environment to interpret and respond to the situation. Language refers to a topic that is related to the context, and so participants in the interaction need to rely less on specific language because much of the meaning can be understood or referred to by gesturing toward or indicating the intended objects and actions. Even at the highest contextualized level (i.e., contextualized-logical), the reasoning that is conducted is demonstrable with concrete objects, and thus children with less flexible language systems may understand many abstract or difficult concepts. The following discussion details the five levels of the Situational Context along the contextualized end of the continuum (see Table 2–3 for a quick reference to primary characteristics). Events from typical classroom activities are used to exemplify these levels.

Level I: Contextualized-Egocentered

At this level, learning and functioning are contextualized to immediately present sensory stimulation impacting directly on the child's own body. The child is centered on herself, with a lack of concern for objects in the environment or events occurring in the situation. Learning occurs in response to objects directly touched and manipulated. The child uses the sensory and motor systems to discover the physical properties of these entities. The child does not include others in this level of interaction, but is responsive to the initiation of others. In normal development, this level of contextualization is usually only observed during the first months of infancy, soon giving way to a more active and intentional exploration of the environment (Norris, 1992b; Piaget, 1954). Even older school-age children may exhibit remnants of this level when placed in situations that are too difficult for learning to occur. They may exhibit behaviors such as biting their nails, twirling their hair, scratching at sores or other behaviors that provide sensory stimulation to the child's own body and avoid processing information from the external environment.

Level II: Decontextualized-Decentered

At this level, learning and functioning are contextualized to immediately present objects, events, or people that the child actively seeks to examine through sensorimotor exploration. Learning occurs when the child is physically manipulating the objects for purposes of discovering the relationships of the parts to the whole, or the general function of the object. The object is used in isolation by the child, rather than in relationship to other objects or as part of a structured sequence of actions (even though the adults in the situation may view the object as part of a larger schema or event). In normal development, this type of exploration emerges within 3 months from birth, and becomes progressively more goal directed and intentional with age. Older school-age children may explore isolated objects at this level for purposes of curiosity, particularly with new or unknown objects. They also may manipulate familiar objects in nondirected ways when they are frustrated or bored. This level of exploration occurs for the sake of exploration, rather than to accomplish a goal within an event (Norris, 1992b; Piaget, 1954).

Other people may be observed when they are at a distance from the child. The child may use communication with others for purposes of maintaining social contact and sharing joint reference toward objects. This level of social interaction occurs for the sake of interacting, or entertainment, rather than to enlist others to provide assistance or to achieve other goals. Thus, learning and use of communication at this level is directed at exploring and maintaining contact with both the physical and social environment (Mahler, Pine, & Bergman, 1975).

Level III: Contextualized-Relational

At this level, learning and interacting are contextualized to immediately present objects and events, but the objects are used in sequences of relational actions. Objects are used for functional purposes, and the relationship of that object to others is meaningfully structured within the same event or routine (i.e., using spoons in relationship to bowls, cereal, milk, and the sink). The objects that are used at this level are real and life-size, rather than miniatures or toy replicas, and the actions are actually performed with the objects, rather than pretend actions with imaginary props. Many daily routines at home and at school could be described as fitting within this category, such as making a snack, school lunch routines, washing laundry, or yard work. Many play behaviors in young children also are at this level, as when children re-create familiar routines, such as eating, using the actual objects instead of toys. At this level, the objects are *part of* the events or routines in which they are used and are not used in any creative or imaginative ways. Their use indicates that the child has mentally constructed the object and its function so that it is no longer merely explored, but rather purposefully used to accomplish some goal (Norris, 1992b; Norris & Hoffman, 1990).

Level IV: Contextualized-Symbolic

At this level, learning and functioning are still contextualized to immediately present objects, events, and people, but the child's mental representation of the objects and events is more displaced. Thus, the objects no longer need to be the actual life-size objects, but rather can be miniatures (i.e., toy objects), replicas (i.e., models, figures), substituted objects (i.e., use of a yellow ball to represent the sun in a science demonstration), or drawings, including maps or illustrations of an event or story. From the symbolic object, the child is able to mentally re-create a corresponding real situation. Language is used to talk about the actions, events, cause-effect relationships, and so forth, but often the actions need to be done to understand what these events look like, or how the elements interact. In the science demonstration mentioned above, the children would hold balls to represent planets and physically walk around the "sun" to understand the concept of rotation.

Illustrated books in which the pictures closely parallel the text are at this level. The words in the book are contextualized to the picture so that both function to communicate the same information. The following text from *The Dandelion* (Cutting & Cutting, 1988b) accompanies an illustration of a backyard in winter, where a seed is partially visible in the snow.

> One dandelion seed
> landed in the garden.
> Winter came
> and covered it with snow.

The words are interpretable through an understanding of the context provided by the picture. The words and the text maintain a "near" relationship in Golden's (1990) words, where the information that the picture and the text provide overlap. Little information is provided by the words that is not also available from the pictured context. Many children with less flexible language systems rely on this pictured context when reading or listening and quickly lose comprehension when presented with text unaccompanied by closely related pictures.

Level V: Contextualized-Logical

At this level, the attention to objects within the environment is decreased, with a greater focus on mental concepts and the language used to refer to them. Often the objects that are present are used in abstract, representational ways, such as using a pencil to stand for a bone within a skeleton. Thus, the *words* "this is a bone" are more influential than the perception of the object in determining what meaning it will have in the context. While some objects and actions are present at this level, many others are created using words alone, such as "Let's pretend we have a skull bone too." Real people may be assigned roles that are different from their own, such as acting out a part in a dramatization, and characters or historical figures may be created by talking about them with no real person standing in.

This level is also characterized by logical reasoning about objects that can be physically manipulated. For example, science experiments may be conducted with real objects to make abstract concepts comprehensible. The book *What Will Float?* (Biddulph & Biddulph, 1992) discusses weight in relationship to floating. It depicts objects for children to consider, with the suggestion that similar real objects then be placed in water in order to discover the relationships between weight and buoyancy. The consequences of the actions demonstrated by the objects enable the child to extract the abstract, logical relationships that could not be understood by the words alone.

Illustrated books in which the pictures remotely parallel the text are at this level. The words in the book are distanced from the picture, so that each functions to communicate different information, or the illustration reflects only a general theme from the text. The following text from *The King's Jokes* (Mahy, 1987a) accompanies an illustration of a circus scene, where a king has just requested that his wife and son be called to see the clowns.

> "Ahem, your Majesty" said the butler. "I must point out that the Queen has been missing for at least a fortnight now, and Prince Tom has vanished with her."

The words are interpretable only through an understanding of the context created by the words, indirectly supported by the picture. Neither the Queen nor the Prince is depicted in the illustration, nor does anyone appear to be looking for them. The words and the text maintain a "distanced" relationship, in Golden's (1990) words, where the information that the picture and the text provide each contribute different information, both of which are important to understanding the situation. Many children with less flexible language systems who rely on this pictured context when reading will fail to understand the events that go beyond the picture.

■□ DECONTEXTUALIZED LEVELS

The situational context becomes decontextualized as the topic being considered becomes more abstract relative to the physical and perceptual characteristics of the situation. With increasing decontextualization, children must rely on information that they already possess, or mentally reconstructed representations, to understand and respond to the situation. As this occurs, the participants in the interaction rely more on language and less on the objects and actions in the environment to communicate. Unfortunately, as the context becomes more language based, children with less flexible language systems may understand less of what is occurring. The following discussion details the 5 levels of the Situational context along the decontextualized end of the continuum (see Table 2–3 for a quick reference to primary characteristics). Events from typical classroom activities are used to exemplify these levels.

Level VI: Decontextualized-Egocentered

At this level, learning and functioning is fully decontextualized. All of the referents, including people, their actions, and the objects involved in an event must be created through the use of language. When listening, the child must reconstruct the meaning and generate a mental image of an event from the words alone. Similarly, when speaking the child must use language to create the intended context and event for the listener. The immediate physical environment at this level must be disregarded in favor of locations and events that occurred in some past time frame or in some distanced location. Importantly, at this level the language is used to refer to the child's own experiences, rather than those merely observed or told about. Thus the images that are re-created or referred to were initially directly experienced by the child and thus are reconstructions of sensorimotor experience. This level of decontextualization is exhibited when children recount a personal experience, such as reporting on their weekend or a classroom experience. This task is more difficult than talking about activities in which the child is currently engaged because the child cannot rely on visual or other sensory input available in the current situation to help organize the language of the report. Thus, a child may not be able to explain what happened on the playground that caused him to get hurt, even though the accident happened minutes before.

Level VII: Decontextualized-Decentered

At this level, language must be used to create an event from the perspective of an observer or another participant. The child is present for the event, but is not an active participant within the activity. Instead, the action must be observed by the child, a mental image created, and then recounted by the child using words. The child must be able to use language to create a unified, whole event, while simultaneously specifying details, or parts of the events. These more displaced experiences are more difficult than personal experiences because they do not originally emerge from directly experienced events and thus have only indirect sensory sources of input (i.e., something that was seen or heard, but not acted or performed). At this level of situational context, children must consider the actions of others and view a situation from a perspective other than their own. For example, in the classroom, children are asked to comment on and write about science demonstrations that they have watched or to write about the behavior of animals that they saw on a field trip to the zoo. Their knowledge of these events is less perceptually based than experiments or dramatizations in which they played an active role, and the reporting of the event is distanced in time and space from its actual context of occurrence. Children with less flexible language systems may be able to use decontextualized language to recall a personal event, but exhibit greater difficulty when they attempt to use language at this level to describe events because of the increased linguistic demands.

Level VIII: Decontextualized-Relational

At this level, learning and functioning require the child to understand the overall structure of events and the relationships among components of the events. Understanding that events have component parts that exist in predictable and logical relationships allows the child to behave in a manner consistent with these mental representations, to make generalizations, and create new exemplars. These mental representations are referred to as *scripts*. Children at school age must develop many different types of mental representations to function within the school environment. One example is that of the *school script* (Creaghead, 1992; Nelson, 1986; Schank & Abelson, 1977), or knowledge of what is appropriate to do and say in a context such as a classroom. The script refers to a general pattern of what might occur in a generic classroom. The components within it could include elements of a classroom routine, such as when the class starts, where the child is to be located, when it is appropriate to talk versus to be quiet, how to ask questions, when instructions about assignments are given, what materials are supposed to be present, and so forth. The general script will hold for a variety of teachers, classrooms, and content areas. The specifics that fit the component elements need to be mentally filled for each specific class period. Children with inflexible language systems often do not develop these scripts or the cues that define the script in a specific classroom or other situational context (Creaghead, 1992; Nelson, 1986).

Level IX: Decontextualized-Symbolic

At this level, learning and functioning are not bound to any location, temporal frame, or events that the child has ever experienced. Rather, new worlds are created for the child through language. Through the processes of assimilation and accommodation of these new concepts to existing schemata, event representations, and other mental structures, the child must construct representations for this unfamiliar or unknown information. Much of school experience requires this type of high-level concept formation. In social studies, children are expected to learn about other parts of the world that are different from their own environment in geography, culture, politics, history, and commerce. In science, they must learn about microscopic worlds of plants and animals that are composed of single cells and behave in a manner different from those in the child's visible environment. At this level, language is not used to talk about the known world, but rather to create possible worlds.

Level X: Decontextualized-Logical

The highest level of decontextualization involves the use of logic and language to create a hypothetical context. The context created consists of mental objects that have no sensorimotor correlates. To function at this level, the child must use language to create constructs and consider what would happen if different aspects of those constructs were altered. This is the context of scientists who create language to symbolize unseen relationships of the physical and mental worlds and then imagine experiments whose results would confirm or disconfirm these hypothesized relationships.

Consider the scientific construct called "the life cycle" that appears in sixth grade science textbooks. This construct is applicable to all living things, including plants, animals, and single-cell creatures alike. It contains relationships among a sequence of constructs such as birth, growth, reproduction, and death. Each of these constructs can be exemplified, but each is more abstract than any of its exemplars. The construct "death" is more abstract than any single example. Human death has been defined with respect to brain activity. But such a definition cannot be applied to a plant. The construct is beyond the sensory motoric particulars of each case to which it can be applied. Teachers of creative writing are concerned with abstractions such as "the narrative." They analyze a wide variety of literary works using constructs such as "setting," "character," and "initiating event."

Having created a logically based model of abstractions, the scientist mentally manipulates the constructs to ask questions about what would happen to the model if one aspect or another were altered. These questions become hypotheses that can sometimes be tested by conducting experiments. If human death is the cessation of brain activity, then it might be hypothesized that a drug can be developed that increases brain activity, forestalling death. In literary analysis, the evaluation of competing views cannot be experimentally verified, but there is room for debate about the merits of an author's use of the various components of narrative structure. Children with less flexible language systems will experience difficulty establishing and then transforming all of the abstract concepts and the logical relationships held between them. By the end of the middle school years, much of what they are asked to do in all curriculum areas requires decontextualized logical thought.

Summary

The Situational Context refers to the degree to which language learning and use is contextualized to the objects and events present within the situation, and the level at which the information is cognitively organized. This must be viewed both from the perspective of the world external to the child (Nelson's "outside-in look," 1986), and from the perspective of the child's ability to meet the environmental demands (Nelson's "inside-out look," 1986), as well as the processes that serve to establish a link between them. The Situational Context may be thought of as existing along a continuum from the most contextualized (least abstract or displaced) to the most decontextualized. With decreasing contextualization, children are required to consider actions and objects that are farther removed from their own perceptual experiences within the situation. Children's abilities to deal with these situations are dependent on their development of higher levels of symbolic thought and the use of language to establish functional relationships between elements and to replace objects and actions present within the physical environment with conceptually created symbols.

When the less flexible learner encounters situations in which the information is more decontextualized and/or more logical, they are likely to fail to create appropriate meanings and associated language regarding the situation. The person facilitating learning must manipulate the Situational Context to include less decontextualized, more self-oriented information. Too often in school, the child is expected to change to meet the demands of the curriculum. This approach only leads to increased failure and frustration, because when the child cannot learn from the situation, the child's language system ceases to refine. If the language system ceases to refine, the higher levels of decontextualization and displacement cannot be attained, and so the child will not change to meet the demands of the curriculum. Rather than continuing to impose this cycle of failure on the child, the curriculum must change to teach children at a level and manner from which they can learn.

■□ DISCOURSE CONTEXT

If the Situational Context corresponds to the most global or whole view of the context, then the **Discourse Context** can be thought of as an analysis of a smaller part within the whole. From the global situation, a unit of interaction (i.e., a topic of conversation, the text of a storybook, a subtopic within a textbook, a segment from a lecture) can be examined for evidence of its complexity, structure, and purpose. While this dimension of the model is not limited to linguistic interactions and can also be applied to other symbolic behaviors, such as an analysis of the complexity, structure, and purpose exhibited in play, the discussion of the model in this book will involve only applications to language.

When examining the Discourse Context, the unit of interaction should be compared to the eight levels of organization exhibited on Table 2-1, detailed in Table 2-5, and profiled below to find the "best fit" or description. More than one judgment may be made, depending on how many participants are present in the interaction and what the observer needs to know about the interactions between them. For example, analysis of the discourse as it is printed in the storybook *Little Red Riding Hood* (Moon, 1988c) would reveal that the text is written at Level VIII (Poetic-Interactive), but the teacher might limit the discussion to individual episodes in an attempt to help children to become aware of goals and plans, or Level V (Poetic-Abbreviated). Observation of an individual child, however, might reveal that the child talks about only the actions within the events, without understanding the psychological goals or intentions underlying these actions, or Level III (Poetic-Ordered Sequence).

The levels profiled in Table 2-5 under the category of the Discourse Context reflect the *discourse functions* of the language (i.e., Poetic, Expressive, and Transactional), and the progressively increasing levels of *discourse structures* that are present in the language and used to develop a topic. The continuum, beginning at the bottom with unstructured, topically related comments, and working upward toward more complex and topic-centered presentations of information, reflects an increase within each discourse type of the use of language to organize the discourse in relationships of time, space, causality, conditionality, inclusion, exclusion, and so forth. The discourse at higher levels of the continuum reflects increasingly more conventional styles that conform to culturally determined patterns of Poetic and Transactional text.

■□ CONTINUUM OF DISCOURSE FUNCTIONS

The first decision to be made when examining the Discourse Context is to determine whether the function of the interaction is to talk about factual information using expository text structure (referred to as "Transactional" in this model following Britton's [1982] classification), or episodic information using narrative, poetic, or dramatic text structure (referred to as "Poetic," again from Britton's categories), or personal and responsive speech (referred to as "Expressive" in accord with Britton). Britton (1982) uses these terms somewhat differently than many linguists, who draw a comparison between "expressive versus receptive language," or "transactional versus private speech," for example. Therefore, when these terms are used in this book, they will refer to the *discourse function,* or type of information communicated unless otherwise stated.

TABLE 2-5
The eight levels of the Discourse Context, reflected across the continuum of Transactional to Expressive to Poetic functions.

DISCOURSE CONTEXT

TRANSACTIONAL	Transactional	Level	Poetic	POETIC
T R A N	Many dimensions of the same scientific, cultural, political, historical, etc., topic are presented in a manner that draws comparisons and contrasts within and among them. An integrated, rather than sequential, format.	LEVEL VIII — INTERACTIVE STRUCTURE	Two or more story lines develop separately within a complex story, each containing multiple problem episodes. The same set of events may be described from two or more perspectives, goals are reciprocal, and flashbacks reorder sequence.	P O
S A C	Each chapter or section within a chapter addresses a separate subtopic within a main topic, with little cross-referencing to the information discussed in preceding or following sections.	LEVEL VII — COMPLEX STRUCTURE	One story line develops but with a sequence of problems presented, each of which is resolved prior to encountering the next. The lessons learned in one episode are carried over to the next.	E
T I O	A complete and self-contained presentation of a topic is given. The information is unified by an overall objective, such as to explain a procedure, or present a problem and find a solution.	LEVEL VI — COMPLETE STRUCTURE	Exhibits all characteristics of a complete narrative, including an overall purpose or moral, told by establishing a setting, creating an initiating event, resolved by attempts, reactions, consequences.	T
N A L	A general but incomplete presentation of a topic is made with causal links between steps in a procedure and purpose or intent guiding actions or decisions. No higher-order goals unify topic.	LEVEL V — ABBREVIATED STRUCTURE	Story told for its own sake, with no overall purpose or moral. But characters have plans or *intents* that *precede* their actions. Story has initiating event, resolved by attempts, reactions, consequences.	I C

FUNCTION	Level	FUNCTION
A description of a logically sequenced event based on cause-effect relationships, but no plan or intent governing this order. Reporting on "what happens" in logical order but not "why."	LEVEL IV — REACTIVE SEQUENCE	Describe an event in which the actions of one character cause an unplanned effect on another in domino fashion. Order is important but not determined by intent. Has setting, problem, action, result.
Temporal sequences based on daily, weekly, monthly, seasonal, or yearly patterns, or spatial sequences based on actual location but not goal-directed planning. Arbitrary choice of details.	LEVEL III — ORDERED SEQUENCE	Recount the order in which events occurred, but no logic or cause-effect relationships necessitate that particular order. Order can be changed without affecting outcome. Setting, action, result.
Presentation of facts about a topic. All ideas relate to an overall general topic, but do not build on each other, no cause-effect or temporal relationships between them. Merely a list.	LEVEL II — DESCRIPTIVE LIST	Some elements of stories, such as action-based events organized around a central theme. No particular order in which events occur, no time frame unifies them, no reciprocal or causal relations.
Loosely organized presentation of a topic, where no single object, event, or activity remains in focus. Ideas may be linked through free association or general theme.	LEVEL I — COLLECTION	Response to immediate perceptions with no overall structure imposed. Focus of story shifts rapidly by free association. No setting, goal, attempts, consequences.

EXPRESSIVE FUNCTION

Britton's classifications also differ from many models that categorize discourse types as "conversational," "narrative," and "expository." Britton's (1982) model does not view *conversation* as a discourse function, but rather as an interaction that occurs as a dialogue. Conversation does not express a unique discourse function, but rather every conversation will entail one or more discourse functions. The speaker may converse in the Expressive mode, merely talking in an unstructured manner about wants, needs, ideas, impressions, or feelings. Or the conversation may recount to the listener a personal experience in the Poetic mode, told by chronologically recalling the sequence of events or by weaving a highly interactive account of all the participants and their roles. Or, the conversation may be used to impart some information, procedure, or explanation using discourse along the Transactional dimension. Thus, each topic within a conversation may serve as a unit of interaction that can be examined for its *discourse function*, which will be either Expressive, Transactional, or Poetic.

Discourse will vary in the degree to which it is conducted as a *dialogue* versus a *monologue*. In a dialogue, speakers have the support of other participants in organizing the structure and maintaining the topic of the discourse. Dialogue is highly interactive, with immediate feedback provided relative to the success of the communication. This shared responsibility and facilitative support enables young children to participate in complex storytelling, storybook reading, play, and other contexts of language use at a level beyond their independent abilities. Greater autonomy is required to produce monologues. Monologue requires that the speaker independently organize and maintain the discourse. Furthermore, the monologue often is structured in accord with higher levels of Transactional or Poetic discourse because of the need to communicate all of the necessary elements in a manner that maintains the theme and that structures the ideas with clarity and completeness (Sulzby, 1985; Westby, 1992). Much of what occurs in school, such as writing a report on a topic or taking notes in response to a lecture, requires considerable facility with monologue. This is difficult for many children with less integrated and flexible language systems who often resort to making Descriptive Lists instead of integrating information at higher levels of discourse function.

Britton (1982) noted that the Expressive, Transactional, and Poetic functions each are characterized by specific uses of language and relationships between the speaker, the audience, and the aspects of the real world that are referenced by the language used. Along the Transactional dimension of the continuum, the speaker uses language in the participant role to interact with people through informing, instructing, planning, explaining, or arguing. Along the Poetic dimension, the speaker uses language in the spectator role to present thoughts, often in the form of a story or poem as a means of contemplating what has happened or what could happen. In the middle, or Expressive function, the speaker functions in a role close to the self, where personal opinions, needs, wants, or reactions are stated. Each of these functions may be structured at any of the eight levels of the discourse continuum, although the Expressive function by its nature will primarily be less structured, and thus categorized at the lower levels of the model. The following descriptions detail the characteristics of the Expressive, Transactional, and Poetic functions to guide observations and decisions.

Expressive Function

The *Expressive function* of language is more private than social, described as being not very far removed from the speaker (Britton, 1982). It expresses more information about the speaker than it does about the outside world. An exclamation, such as "Ouch!," uttered after stubbing a toe is nearly pure expressive use of language. Listeners would be able to interpret the exclamation only if they knew enough about the context to know what had happened. The language of the exclamation expressed how the speaker felt about the circumstances, but did not refer explicitly to the aspects of the context, such as the door jamb that got in the way, to which the speaker is reacting. To fully appreciate the expression of feeling in this exclamation, a listener also would have to know the speaker well enough to judge the degree to which this expressive outburst differs from reactions to other life circumstances.

The expressive function of language thus is highly contextualized where it is assumed that the listener or reader shares common background knowledge and interest with the speaker or writer. It includes statements of needs and wants, such as "Would you hand me that ruler" or "I'm really thirsty," as well as personal reactions to or comments on things in context, as in "Isn't that cute!" or "I want to go there some day." Language within this function is spoken to serve personal needs rather than to provide others with information about the world or how to interpret an event or situation. Much of the language is spoken in first person, with a greater emphasis on self-expression and personal interest. The style of speaking and writing along the Expressive end of the continuum is informal and conversational, addressing the reader/listener directly and interspersed with personal opinions and comments.

On the model, the Expressive function exists on a continuum with the Transactional and Poetic functions. The same topic may be communicated in, for example, a more Transactional or more Expressive manner.

Many elements of the Expressive function thus are present in the speech and writing of children as they attempt to communicate Transactional or Poetic functions. A composition written about a topic, such as science, may contain much of the personal feelings and attitudes of the beginning writer, as in this composition written at Level III: Expressive-Ordered Sequence.

> I once turned a caterpillar into a butterfly. First I put him into a jar and then I had to make sure he had lots of fresh green leaves. I liked to watch him eat the leaves and he was cute. Be careful, cuz my brother shook the jar and it got upset. Then check the jar.

Expressive discourse is an easier function for many children and enables them to emerge into the more formal and structured functions of writing as a gradual process. Many classrooms currently use "dialogue journals" as a strategy for encouraging children to write. In this procedure, a dialogue is maintained in writing between the child and the teacher or other participant. Each person responds to the message that was written to him or her and then adds a message of his or her own. Response journals are often successful with children who are inexperienced with writing, or who have less flexible language systems, and who easily become overwhelmed when more sophisticated functions of writing are demanded (Staton, Shuy, Peyton, & Reed, 1988). A simple message saying, "I noticed you didn't write anything. Why not?" may prompt a nonwriter to respond with a one or two word reply and begin a written dialogue that can be expanded with time.

Transactional Function

The *Transactional function* of language is used to accomplish some goal, such as requesting information, giving information, or requesting that actions be executed (Britton, 1982). As discourse moves away from the Expressive function, it becomes more factual, public, and explicit. Because this language is goal-directed with respect to some aspect of the outside world, it must make specific reference to that world. For example, to compare two objects, the speaker must use language that is specific enough so that a listener understands the salient features. Similarly, to give directions, the speaker must specify all relevant objects or actions and sequence the information in appropriately ordered steps.

The form or structure of the discourse is important to the process of organizing and communicating content to achieve a purpose. The levels of discourse along the Transactional dimension of the model represent conventional form or structure found in Expository text to achieve purposes such as presenting a *description* or definition of key concepts or events, describing a *procedure* or sequence of steps for conducting some operation, *explaining* some phenomenon or concept by examining factors related to cause and effect, presenting information in a *problem/solution* format, where an issue is raised and possible solutions are explored, drawing *comparisons and contrasts* between concepts or events, and providing examples through *collection/enumeration* of things that are related to a topic (Flood, 1986; Flood, Lapp, & Farnan, 1986). For example, a *procedure* may be structured simply at Level III: Ordered Sequence (i.e., Put a plug in the sink, turn on the hot water, then the cold water, then wash dishes) or at a more complex level, such as Level VI: Complete (i.e., To make sure that water does not drain from the sink, a plug must be properly placed. The plug must be capable of creating a tight seal, so flexible materials such as cork or rubber work best.)

Expository text is a difficult form of discourse requiring a displacement from one's own personal perspective and an integration of multiple ideas into an orderly whole. The ideas are expressed objectively, without the inclusion of personal experience or response. The composition about the caterpillar written at Level III: Transactional-Ordered Sequence might read,

> To watch a caterpillar turn into a butterfly, place the insect in a jar. Provide it with food, including fresh green leaves. Leave the jar undisturbed, and wait for several weeks.

Many children with less flexible language systems have difficulty taking an objective and displaced perspective. They also experience difficulty abstracting the most relevant and important information from expository text when they read, and they struggle to organize facts into any logical expository format when they write or discuss (Raphael, 1982, 1986). Helping them to learn to use language in the Transactional function is an important part of intervention for the school-age child.

Poetic Function

The *Poetic function* of language refers to the use of language to make a "verbal object" that is organized in accordance with forms of drama, poetry, and narration. It is not created to get things done (i.e., language as an instrument or means), but rather for enjoyment or to create an attitude or belief in the listener, such as the morals expressed in Aesop's fables (i.e., language as an end in itself). As language moves away from the Expressive function and toward the Poetic, it becomes more public and implicit so that the real meaning must be derived, not from recognizing the events, but rather from recognizing the significance of the events.

Children who have internalized story structure expect characters to have goals, problems to have attempts to solve them, a situation to have a resolution, and a story to have a point or moral. Thus, the Poetic function relies on the *form* or the formal arrangement of sounds, words, images, ideas, events, and feelings, to give intensity and purpose to the ideas as much as it relies on the content. Knowing the conventions of the form of the language itself, such as poetic complete or complete story episodes, becomes as important as the message communicated when choosing the language.

Many stories are fictional, but throughout conversations and everyday activities people tell factual stories about events in their day, in their past, or in their dreams for the future. These differ from transactional accounts. The creator of Poetic discourse acts like an observer of reality, rather than an active participant in reality. Language is used to create something from experience rather than to merely represent it. The information given is not rigidly tied to an exact event or sequence of acts, but rather is rearranged, elaborated, or changed for purposes of analogy or to make a point. Many elements of form, such as flashback, embedding episodes, and coordinating parallel plots, allow meaning to be expressed in complex relationships. Thus, when telling a story about a real event, only the actions or states that serve to make a point or further the plot are recounted, often in a different order or with slightly different facts than those in the original event. Stories are told for purposes of creating an effect, not recounting the actions chronologically, as in this composition about the caterpillar written at Level III: Poetic-Ordered Sequence.

> Once there was a caterpillar who wanted to fly. One day a boy caught him and put him in a jar. He felt very sad. Then he ate some leaves, and then he went to sleep. After he woke up, the boy opened the jar. He started to climb out, and his wings started to flap. So then he flew away. The end.

A child who does not have an internalized understanding of Poetic form, such as narrative structure, will fail to understand the meaning and purpose of a story. Understanding stories is not just important to entertainment. Rather, the Poetic function is critical to a coherent understanding of experience. It serves the purpose of exploring and imposing order on experience to make sense of the world. Without such structure, events seem uncontrolled, unpredictable, and continuously changing. Use of the Poetic function reflects the individual's understanding of the physical and social world, and it is used to interpret everyday life, to give meaning to otherwise random events, to impart cultural values to others, and to make a point in a manner that entertains as much as it informs. School-age children require such structure to plan their daily schedule, deciding, for example, which books to collect from their locker depending on the anticipated school events and their role within them. They must possess an understanding of establishing goals to meet needs, formulating plans and attempts to reach those goals, and evaluating consequences or outcomes of actions to complete assignments. They must recognize the goals and attempts of others that they interact with to correctly interpret a social situation and react appropriately.

Many children with less flexible language systems lack this internalized structure and, as a result, exhibit a wide range of pragmatic disorders. Their lack of ability to impose structure on an event results in poor generalization of behavior from one situation to another, poor understanding of the interactions between goals and consequences, causes and effects. They produce narratives that are "impoverished" compared to those of their peers, containing fewer elements of story structure, fewer episodes, poor organization, fewer facts and details, limited use of language to mark temporal, causal, and spatial relationships, and less fluency of expression. Their stories more often function to describe events from the child's perspective as an observer or reporter, rather than to reflect on a problem or interpret an event for personal or cultural significance (Roth & Spekman, 1986). They may understand what happened within an event but not know how to organize and interpret the experience and thus fail to learn from it or to make generalizations to new events. Their behavior is seen as inappropriate or immature, because they fail to see the "big picture" or consider the perspectives and roles of others. Their interpretations of experience are organized according to lower levels of complexity, as described by the eight levels of discourse structure delineated below.

■□ LEVELS OF DISCOURSE STRUCTURE

The second decision to be made within the Discourse Context is the level of structure and complexity at which the text is organized. They are organized from the lowest level to the highest level of Discourse Context as profiled in Table 2–1 and detailed in Table 2–5, ranging from levels of loosely organized ideas that do not maintain a topic or theme and that lack any predictable order, to levels with highly and conventionally structured ideas that all serve to focus on and develop the same theme or topic. These levels may be used to order discourse according to the Expressive, Transactional, and Poetic functions of language.

Language is important to the capacity to organize experience or ideas in accord with themes or topics. Language provides the capability to classify, order, and coordinate objects and events at different levels of generality, and to interpret new events in relationship to familiar ones. The capacity of language to classify and order creates a verbally organized world, or mental schema, that weaves all of our experiences, feelings, ideas, and beliefs into unified and coherent wholes (Vygotsky, 1978). The degree of organization and complexity exhibited in discourse will vary depending on the demands imposed by the Situational Context and the ability of the speaker to establish and produce the appropriate level of organization required for a context.

The Discourse Context becomes more organized and complex as the discourse function moves outward from the private, personal orientation of the Expressive function, toward greater orientation to the listener and explicit reference to the outside world as it moves along the Transactional continuum, and greater social orientation and implicit interpretations of experiences and beliefs as it moves along the Poetic continuum. To interpret and/or produce informational text or conventional stories, children must have the internal mental schemata for the types and levels of Transactional and Poetic structures encountered in oral and written contexts of language use. Examples of these conventional structures are provided for each of the levels profiled below as they appear in expository and narrative books (i.e., a *descriptive* use of this model). Expectations that can be held for children of different ages also are given (i.e., a *developmental* use of this model).

Level I: Collection

At this level, located at the bottom of the Discourse Context continuum in Table 2–5, language is used to refer in random order to events or objects. Collections result as children talk about whatever catches their attention or whatever they remember about an event moment to moment. There may be a loosely organized topic, such as describing everything seen in a picture, or the topic may shift, as in free association where a disjointed train of thought may be followed. Collections often occur as language is used to make reference to things within an activity or event, including the expression of personal wants, actions, needs, or feelings. The information referred to can be more factual (i.e., Transactional), more personal (i.e., Expressive), or more reflective (i.e., Poetic), as shown in the examples below.

Transactional-Collections are produced in reference to factual topics. Text at this level consists of a loosely organized presentation of a topic, where no single object, event, or activity remains in focus, although a concept usually unifies the text. In the book *Water is My Friend* (Cowley, 1990q), pictures in the book shift from an outdoor tub, to an indoor sink, then a shower, a wading pool, an ocean, a waterfall, a swimming pool, and a hose. The accompanying text reads:

> I like playing with water . . . Water splishes and splashes . . . When water is little, it is my friend . . . But when water is big it can be dangerous . . . Big water can run fast . . . Big water can be deep . . . Can you see my friend in here?

In oral language these occur when a child attempts to provide information about a topic, but shifts between ideas or themes, as in the following explanation provided by a child in response to the request to explain how a baby chick hatches from its egg.

> Well, the baby chick is in the egg, and it starts to crack. And you can crack eggs and they're cooked you can eat them. And, like at Easter, eggs are dyed and then eaten. After Easter, another holiday is the Fourth of July.

The child attempted to talk on a factual topic, but engaged in free association rather than focusing on the main idea. Instead of developing a coherent topic, a recency effect was seen, as the child talked about the last idea expressed within the sentence instead of the subject.

Expressive-Collections are commonly produced in everyday activities, as individuals talk about whatever is within their focus. This may include reference to objects or actions present in the context, or to internal feelings such as sadness or hunger. The following excerpt of conversation exemplfies this.

Child	Adult	Comment
Can I have that?	Not before dinner	Referring to a cookie
Oh Oh, my shirt got dirty	I think you got too close to the tire in the garage.	Pointing to a black smudge on shirt
Oh, I left my drum in the garage. When is Jimmy gonna get home?	At 4:00, after band practice.	The garage reminds child of the drum, the drum reminds child of brother.

Poetic-Collections are produced in reference to events, including experiences, events pictured in a storybook, and dramatic play. The elements of the discourse are not related to a mental schema for narrative or poetic structure, but rather result from the child's immediate perception, so that attention is shifted from object to object with no overriding structure. There are few links among the elements. An example is found in the recounting of a dream in the story *Dreams* (Cutting & Cutting, 1988c).

> Everybody dreams. Mom dreams. Dad dreams. Do dogs dream? Do cats dream? I had a dream last night. There were monsters outside my window. There were lions and tigers in my room ... I could fly in my dream ... Tonight I will visit a magic land ...

In this passage the focus of the event changed repeatedly, from identifying who dreams, to describing scary characters in the dream, to flying, and finally a future dream in a loosely structured collection of ideas.

The following is an attempt to tell a story by a 6-year-old child with William's syndrome. It is told in response to a picture of a man crossing the street carrying groceries. The man has very narrowly escaped being hit by a passing truck.

Child	Adult	Comment
Runned over	What was run over?	Seeks clarification
Rocket		Points to another picture
	Tell me a story about this picture.	Points back to first picture
Get off the street! This is a snake. They say "hi."		Randomly points to different parts of the picture and comments

This story is composed of a random collection of comments, in which the child shifts from topic to topic, structuring his comments with respect to whatever has his attention at the moment. First he talks about the picture of the man in the street, then about a rocket on another page. When directed back to the original picture, he stays on topic for one comment and then focuses in turn on a series of unrelated pictures and objects.

The loose structure characteristic of Collections is appropriate for many Contextualized interactions, such as ongoing remarks produced within everyday activities. This level on the model can be used Descriptively to categorize instances of oral and written discourse encountered by or produced by a child. The levels of the model also can be used to suggest whether a child's performance is developmentally appropriate. For example, this level is characteristic of the writing attempts of kindergarten or beginning writers, where children focus on the act of writing with little attention to organization or purpose (Calkins, 1986). However, more sophisticated attempts at oral storytelling are achieved at a much younger age. Applebee (1978) found that even among 2-year-olds, fewer than 20% of the stories are told at this level, a developmental story structure type that he referred to as "Heaps."

Level II: Descriptive List

At this level, language is used to organize a group of objects or actions that all are related to some specific topic, often because of their physical presence within the same location or event (e.g., events in the same storybook), or because they are functionally related (e.g., all things that can be eaten, or that make one happy), or because they share some perceptual or categorical feature (e.g., types of plants). Thus, there is a central event or concept that serves as a coordinating topic. However, no relationships of time, space, cause-effect, or goal-attempt link ideas in any chronological or logical manner. The order in which objects and actions are presented is arbitrary.

Transactional-Descriptive List structures are produced to present a simple discussion of some factual information about a topic. The text is generally accompanied by illustrations that share the burden for unifying the text and explaining the concepts. Consider the following text *Underwater Journey* (Cutting & Cutting, 1988i):

> We are going to explore the sea.
> We see whales.
> We see sharks.
> We explore the coral reef.
> We dive to the bottom of the sea.

This Transactional text acts to describe aspects of the environment, serving as an introduction to the scientific stage of noticing events in the world outside of the child's direct experience. The first sentence sets the overall topic of exploring the sea. This topic is maintained throughout the book, as each sentence within the discourse provides an example of things that may be found in the sea. But there is no inherent time line or causal structure. Sharks could have been encountered before the whales. The bottom of the sea could have been explored prior to going to the coral reef, and no event in the series causes another to occur.

Expressive-Descriptive Lists consist of actions, experiences, beliefs, or events that are unified within a general topic. These are very common in books read to young children or by beginning readers, as in the text below, *To School* (Cutting, 1990), which describes actions from a personal perspective

> I am flying.   I am swimming.
> I am hang-gliding.   I am driving.
> I am skate-boarding.   I am surfing . . .
>   to school.

or a similar book, *I Love My Family* (Cowley, 1988c), expressing personal feelings

I love my father.	I love my mother.
I love my sister.	I love my brother
I love my grandma.	I love my grandpa.
But I don't love my grandpa's whiskers.	

Descriptive Lists are also commonly produced in conversation or for specific purposes, such as shopping, where individuals might list all of the things they intend to do, or things they saw on a trip, or items they intend to buy, and so forth.

Poetic Descriptive List structures have elements of stories, such as action-based events that are organized around a central theme. For example, the narrative text that follows, *Together* (Cutting & Cutting, 1988g), relates a list of activities that a young girl does with her family.

> This is my family. We do things together. We go to the game. We go ice skating. We go to the circus.

There is no particular ordering of these events, nor a specific time frame in which they occur. No reciprocal relationships exist between events, such that none causes the other, and none establishes a goal resolved by another.

The simple text structure of Descriptive lists is commonly found in science, health, social studies, and literature books presented to young children. They may be used to present the goals of expository text, such as defining key concepts or events, or providing exemplars of a collection or set. They also are appropriate for young school-aged children who are in the beginning stages of reading, where the repetitive text, minimal demands for processing discourse structure, and personal nature of the words enables a child to begin to understand how print represents meaning. They provide children with simple models for books that they can write themselves, using a combination of picture and print. This type of personal, unstructured discourse may appear in the writing of much older children with inflexible language systems who need to be helped to organize ideas at higher levels of discourse structure.

Simple books at this level, especially Expressive-Descriptive Lists that express personal needs, comments, wants, or feelings are appropriate to use for purposes of facilitating early oral languge development. They can be used with children who are chronologically or developmentally (as in children with mental retardation) as young as 6 months to 3 years of age, where the pictures and simple ideas can help them to learn to identify and provide names for common objects, actions, and feelings in the context of familiar events.

Level III: Ordered Sequence

An ordered sequence imposes a temporal or spatial sequence on the presentation of objects and actions. However, there are no causal relationships between events and no reciprocal effects between actions, objects, or events. Things are merely related because they bear a natural ordered relationship, such as the sequence that they happened to chronologically occur in or the order found in nature. The order of actions or events can be changed without altering the meaning or purpose of the story or discussion.

In a *Transactional-Ordered Sequence,* the temporal sequences may be based on daily, weekly, monthly, seasonal, or yearly patterns. Spatial sequences are based on principles, such as seriation, where objects are ordered from smallest to largest, for example. Consider the temporal sequence in the following Transactional text *Space* (Cutting & Cutting, 1988f):

> In the day, we can see the sun. Sometimes we can see the moon. The sun is the biggest thing in our sky. It is our star. Every morning, the sun rises. Every evening the sun sets.
>
> At night, we can see the moon.

The information about the sun and the moon is presented in a structure that follows the daily cycle of the rising and setting sun. However, the starting point of this discussion is arbitrary and could just as logically have begun by describing the moon at night.

Expressive-Ordered Sequences exist on the continuum between the Transactional and Poetic functions. They may refer to an experience, with frequent references to personal roles and responses within the event as shown by the example of the composition about the caterpillar discussed previously. They also can be found in books. For example, a personal response to an ordinary event such as making a sandwich is presented in the following text, *A Monster Sandwich* (Cowley, 1990l):

> Put some lettuce on it. Put some cheese on it. Put some pickles on it. Put some meat on it. Put some tomatoes on it. Put some bread on it. Now take a bite. Yum, yum!

The order in which the ingredients are added to the sandwich can be changed without altering the event. The sequence is arbitrary without changing the end result — the completed sandwich.

Poetic-Ordered Sequences are structured to recount the order in which events actually occurred (Stein & Glenn, 1979). In the following text, *Stop!* (Cowley, 1990p), a series of events occur in chronological order, but with no logical or necessary connections between episodes.

> "Stop!" said the milkman, but the truck went on.
> "Stop!" said the boy, but the truck went on.
> "Stop!" said the girl, but the truck went on.

The text refers to what a series of people do as a runaway milk truck heads down a hill. Each of the characters commands the truck to stop as it passes by, and they notice the truck. But there is no logic that guides the sequence, no reason why the girl could not have been introduced to the story before the boy, or the police officer before the postal carrier and so forth.

Text at the Ordered Sequence level provides a simple context for helping children to understand concepts such as "first," "next," "then," "before," and "after" in a much more natural and meaningful context than worksheets or other decontextualized activities. It also is the next level of Discourse structure to expect children to be able to read, write, and orally state once they can maintain a topic at the level of a Descriptive List. Children can easily add an episode at this level to an existing book by picking another character or event to add to the sequence then drawing and writing about it. Applebee (1978) developmentally refers to this level of story structure in oral narrative as "sequences" and found that this type of story is the most frequent structure produced by 2-year-olds, and its use continues in about 20% of the stories produced at ages 3 and 4 years.

Level IV: Reactive Sequence

Reactive sequences impose an order on presentation of objects and events that is based on cause-effect relationships. Each event in the sequence serves as a cause for a following event, but these causal links are not planned, nor are goals and purposeful attempts to attain those goals established. This causal sequence necessarily imposes a temporal order so that events cannot be moved around in sequence without changing the story, or resulting in illogical links. The underlying cause-effect relationships are usually implied rather than explicitly stated in the text. This type of structure, as is true of others, may occur alone or may be embedded within text structures at higher and lower levels (e.g., a reactive sequence with an ordered sequence comprising one of the episodes).

Transactional-Reactive Sequenced text provides a description of a logically sequenced event, without explaining why the sequence is necessarily so. The life cycle of a plant is tracked in the following text, *The Dandelion* (Cutting & Cutting, 1988b). Each stage in the life cycle sequence leads to the next with unplanned causal links, but with a necessary order so that the seed could not begin to grow before landing in the garden, and so forth.

The dandelion seeds floated on the wind . . .
One dandelion seed landed in the garden . . .
In spring . . . The dandelion seed began to grow

Expressive-Reactive Sequences can be found in personalized accounts (as opposed to objective descriptions) of experiences or events, such as "I once saw a dandelion seed blowing in the wind and it was really neat! I caught it and put it in some dirt." Examples of this level of discourse function may also be found in text that recounts personal experience, as in this logically sequenced series of everyday events from *Come On!* (Cutting, 1988):

"Come on. Wake up!"   "Come to breakfast."
"Come to school."   "Come to lunch."
"Come to play."   "Come to dinner."
"Come to bed."

Children telling personal accounts at this level describe *what* happened within an event, but not *why* at a level of either physical or psychological causality. For example, the child might describe that he went fast on his bike and that he fell, without recognizing or specifying that one caused the other. Since cause is not recognized, there is no reciprocal effect and so the child does not decide to ride the bike more slowly in the future (Applebee, 1978).

Poetic-Reactive Sequences describe an event in which the actions of one character cause an unplanned effect on another in a domino fashion. The action in the following text, *The Red Rose* (Cowley, 1990n), has each animal in a sequence taking notice of another animal. The order of appearance is important, but is not determined by a purposeful overriding goal (Stein & Glenn, 1979). For example, the caterpillar did not enter the garden *intending* to find a rose, but rather stayed *because* he saw one; similarly, the bird did not intend to find the caterpillar, nor the cat the bird and so forth. Each reacted to circumstances that arose without prior planning or goal-directed attempts to create those circumstances.

> "Ah," said a caterpillar, "I see a rose."
> "Ah," said a bird, "I see a caterpillar."
> "Ah," said a cat, "I see a bird."
> "Ah," said a dog, "I see a cat."

This sequence is unraveled at the midpoint of the story when the rose that attracted the caterpillar is picked by a human character. This provides a second reactive sequence among the characters.

> "Gone," said the caterpillar, and it went back home.
> "Gone," said the bird, and it went back home . . .

In an Ordered Sequence, characters do not plan the events, but, rather, the sequence occurs in a cause-effect chain. The cause-effect relationships are not reciprocal, so that, for example, none of the animals knew of the effect they were having on some other animal and thus did not change their behavior accordingly.

This level of text structure can be used to help children develop an understanding of simple cause and effect. It also develops inferential thinking, since comprehending the concepts or events must go beyond a simple description of the concrete properties or actions. It provides a context for meaningfully learning about scientific, historical, or social knowledge. In the example above, understanding cause and effect requires a degree of scientific knowledge, such as recognizing the predator-prey relationships in the food chain.

This type of Discourse structure is used by even young children, with about 20% of the stories told by 2-year-olds consistent with this level, and continuing to 10% of stories told at age 4. Older children generally include more direct reference to physical and psychological causality in their stories or discussions.

Level V: Abbreviated Structure

An abbreviated structure includes an order between objects and events that is based on cause-effect relationships and also *intent*, or psychological causality. Thus, causal links are not fortuitous, but are planned, with a statement of goal provided or at least implied. However, the *plan* for achieving the goal may not be explicitly explained, but often only described as it is implemented (Labov, 1972). The order of nearly all of the events is important to the text.

Transactional-Abbreviated Structures instruct or inform the listener/reader. The information may be only partial or incomplete, so that a procedure could not be carried out on the basis of this information alone. However, a general understanding of the procedure or event could be inferred from the description. In the following expository text, *The New Building* (Cutting & Cutting, 1988e), a sequence of stages for preparing a building site and erecting a new building are presented in sequence.

> The old building is coming down. The men smash the walls. The bulldozers push the bricks into a heap. The loaders load the bricks. The trucks carry them away.

The text does not explicitly explain why the old building is being knocked down, or that the bulldozers push the bricks in a heap so that the loaders can load them for the trucks to carry them away. The reader must infer the goals and derive the plan from the description that is given.

Expressive-Abbreviated Structures occur with high frequency in conversation, as students talk about things such as planning a party, scheduling a cycle of activities, preparing for vacation trips, planning the day's itinerary or other personal activities that require goals, planning, and ordered sequences of actions or events to achieve these goals. This same type of structure and function may appear in writing that is composed for personal expression, rather than for providing information to others, or for telling a story.

Poetic-Abbreviated Structures establish a setting, the characters, and the goals that guide actions within the story, thus including most of the major elements of story structure (see Poetic-Complete below). However, some elements of story structure are still missing, usually an internal response of a character or the overall moral or conclusion to the story (Stein & Glenn, 1979). In the following story, *Grumpy Elephant* (Cowley, 1990b), a sequence of characters seek to make the grumpy elephant happy. Each character who encounters the elephant establishes an intent to please him, and then engages in a purposeful attempt to make him laugh.

> Along came Parrot. "Poor old Elephant, I'll sing for
> you," she said. Along came Giraffe. "Poor old Elephant,
> I'll dance for you," he said.

Each attempt has a consequence, in that each animal failed to cheer the elephant. A crisis is reached when the elephant becomes bothered by their attempts and yells at the other animals, causing a series of pratfalls.

> Giraffe jumped and fell over Monkey. Monkey jumped
> and fell in his drum.

This turn of events results in achieving the goal established by the characters, but not in the manner they had planned.

> "Ha ha ha.
> I don't feel grumpy now," said Elephant.

The order of these events is determined by the relationship between one set of events and the other. The animals had to set the goal of making the elephant happy before they tried to entertain him. The elephant had to yell in annoyance before the giraffe and monkey could tumble. The pratfall sequence had to occur to cheer the grumpy elephant. Thus, the events are not only causal in this type of structure, but also reciprocal.

This type of Discourse structure is the most common form of narrative structure produced by children at age 5, accounting for over half the stories produced (Applebee, 1978). In writing, this type of structure may be present in the Expressive function, or compositions about personal experience. Children do not produce elaborated versions of this Discourse type in their writing until fourth grade. Any element of the Discourse structure can be presented simply, as in a single sentence used to establish the setting of a story or the topic of an exposition, or in an elaborated manner, such as a detailed description of a setting or topic that may include several paragraphs or even pages. This elaboration will, in general, increase to correspond with increasing grade or readability levels of the text.

For example, the setting in *Grumpy Elephant,* rated at an emergent level of reading, is established in one sentence, while the length of a setting for a beginning first-grade text is approximately a four-sentence paragraph, and by the beginning of second grade it increases to approximately four to six paragraphs. The length of the sentences within these paragraphs, and thus the amount of information given about each idea within the setting, simultaneously increases. Thus, when evaluating materials or the quality of oral or written discourse produced by a child, it is important to consider the readability level as well as the Discourse function and structure (see Chapter 3 for a discussion of readability).

Level VI: Complete Structure

This level of Discourse structure provides a complete and self-contained presentation of some sequence of events within a topic, including an overall objective or moral that unifies and gives purpose to the text. These events or concepts are related to one another in a complete temporal and causally linked sequence. Thus, there is a relatively elaborated discussion of a tightly organized event or topic that is produced to achieve some preplanned goal (Stein & Glenn, 1979).

Transactional-Complete Structure is planned to accomplish some informative function, such as explaining a procedure, presenting a problem and examining data for solutions, or drawing comparisons and contrasts between concepts or events. In the book *Look at an Ice Lolly* (Moon & Moon, 1986), the text describes the characteristics of an ice lolly (i.e., a frozen juice bar), states the procedure used in making one, and defines the underlying principle distinguishing solids and liquids.

First, the common characteristics of ice lollies are described:

> Ice lollies are cold and hard and smooth.

Then some potential differences among particular ice lollies are discussed:

> Ice lollies can be lots of different shapes and sizes.
> And they can taste different!

Next, the goal-directed sequence of making ice lollies is described:

> These children are mixing water and orange juice together. They are pouring the mixture into an ice-cube tray. Now they are cutting up straws and putting them into the tray for ice lolly sticks.

One of the differences between liquids and solids is described with respect to the process of making ice lollies:

> The mixture is liquid. It becomes the same shape as whatever you put it in. When the mixture comes out of the freezer, it is frozen into that shape. Now it is solid.

The description is complete, so that someone following such directions could successfully make the ice lollies.

Poetic-Complete structure exhibits all of the characteristics of a complete narrative. A complete narrative is structured according to an overall story schema which contains common elements, including a setting, a character, an initiating event, a goal, an attempt to reach the goal, a consequence of that attempt, and a resolution such as a lesson learned, an evaluation of the characters, or a moral (Stein & Glenn, 1979). The setting is the physical and social backdrop for the story. It is a description of the place and time of the story. It describes the typical actions or ordinary existence of the characters. The initiating event is something out of the ordinary. It can be a physical event that affects the usual routine of the characters, or it can be a psychological event experienced by one of the characters.

The initiating event often causes a problem for the main character. In response to this problem, the character establishes a goal to resolve the conflict. The characters then formulate a plan to achieve the goal, and they engage in a sequence of attempts to attain that goal. Each attempt will have some result, either a positive or negative consequence from the perspective of the characters. The author's overall purpose or reason for creating the story is often revealed in the closing statements or implied, as in "Don't touch other people's property" in *Goldilocks and the Three Bears* (Moon, 1988a) or "Hard work pays" in *The Little Red Hen* (Young, 1988b). An example of each of these elements can be seen in the story below.

In *The Fox and the Crow* (Biro, 1991), the setting, characters, and initiating event are established in a picture depicting a crow flying into a tree holding a piece of cheese in its beak, with a drooling fox looking on. The first sentence of text establishes the setting, or ordinary action.

> One day a crow found some cheese and flew into a tree.

Under normal circumstances, the happy crow would go about eating and enjoying his find. But stories must present a problem or something out of the ordinary. The second sentence establishes the initiating event, or an action that will lead to a problem or change from ordinary existence.

> A hungry fox saw him.

The feeling of hunger creates an internal response in the fox, which will result in the formulation of a goal.

> He wanted the cheese for himself.

The fox makes an attempt to achieve this goal.

> "You are a very beautiful bird and you have a very
> beautiful voice ... Sing to me," said the fox.

The crow, being easily flattered, sings for the fox. Of course, this action results in the cheese being dropped, or a positive consequence for the fox's attempt to reach his goal. An evaluation of the event, or point of reflection upon the experience is then provided.

> Clever fox!
> Silly crow!

This type of Complete structure emerges slowly in development, with little or no occurrence in the story types produced at age 2, and only 20% occurrence in the stories told orally by 5-year-olds. It is seen increasingly between the ages of 5 and 8 years, when more than 60% of the simple stories told orally by children are at this level (Peterson & McCabe, 1983). Written stories lag behind oral stories, so the structures that children produce orally may not show up in writing until one or two grade levels later.

This level of discourse structure is present in material presented to children from early childhood on, with most of the stories encountered within reading books by first grade exhibiting Complete structure or higher. In addition, each of the elements of discourse structure becomes increasingly more elaborated, as described under the discussion of Abbreviated structures.

Level VII: Complex Structure

Complex text structures are elaborations of basic complete structures that allow a larger number of related topics to be addressed. These elaborations can be achieved by conjoining other levels of Poetic or Transactional structures within the overall structure, such as Reactive Sequences or Abbreviated structures. The conjoining is done sequentially, but there is causality or reciprocity between the episodes or subtopics (Labov, 1972). That is, each subtopic or episode comes to a conclusion before the next topic in the sequence is introduced, but the order is important since information introduced in one is important to the events in those that follow (thus making this level more complex than a Complete structure with Ordered Sequences embedded).

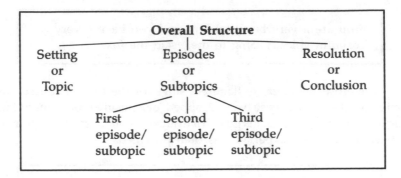

The subtopics or episodes may consist of any level of discourse structure. Thus, the first might be an Abbreviated structure, the second an Ordered Sequence, and the third a Descriptive List, or all may be of the same structure type.

Transactional-Complex structure is common in many expository texts. A typical form of this structure is found in textbooks where each chapter or section within a chapter addresses a separate subtopic within a main topic. Although the information builds, little or no cross-referencing to the topics discussed in preceding and following sections occurs.

Extremely Weird Frogs (Lovett, 1992) starts with an introductory chapter that describes characteristics that are common to all frogs. Then, each successive chapter provides a description of the physical characteristics and life styles of an individual frog species. Excerpts from the text describing two of the species of frogs follow.

SOUTH AMERICAN HORNED FROG (Ceratophrys ornata)
The South American horned frog has a powerful jaw and sharp, tooth-like fangs — the better to eat small mammals, snakes, birds, turtles, and other frogs. This frog likes to sit and wait for prey to pass by. Its colorful, armored skin provides great camouflage among leaves, dirt, and grasses ...
PAINTED REED FROG (Hyperolius marmoratus)
The South African painted reed frog and its 200 or so related species might be called quick change artists — they can change their colors without changing their skins. A painted reed frog could be black and pink one minute and yellow and black the next ... Reed frogs eager to attract a mate will sport their full colors.

In each of these excerpts, the author gives a description of the distinguishing anatomical characteristics of each species and one of its functional uses. However, the discussion of each frog is handled separately without cross-comparison or explicit statement of hypothetical generalizations such as: "Self-defense is a primary motivator of anatomical structure. The South African painted tree frog uses changing skin color to hide from predators, while the South American horned frog uses sharp fangs for defense."

Poetic-Complex structure is found in stories in which a sequence of problems is presented to the characters who resolve each problem prior to encountering the next. This type of sequential complexity is found in many stories, including classical fairy tales. In *The Three Pigs* (Moon, 1988d), the first pig meets a man with some straw, begs for some straw, builds a house, and is visited by the wolf who blows his house down and eats the pig. The second pig meets a man with wood, begs for some wood, builds a house, and again becomes lunch for the hungry wolf. Fortunately for the third pig, he finds a man with bricks, and his sturdier house withstands the wolf's blowing. The wolf reacts to this happening by adopting a less direct strategy in which he tries to lure the pig out of the house first to a turnip patch, then to an apple orchard, then to a fair in town. Each of these challenges is met in sequence by the pig who outfoxes the wolf. Finally, the wolf returns to the direct approach and enters the pig's house through the chimney. Well, the wolf only makes it into the house after being boiled and served on the pig's dinner table.

While each of these events builds on the other, and lessons learned in one episode are carried over to the next, the actions and events related to each episode are completed before the next is introduced. The embedding occurs within the overall structure, rather than within episodes. This level of narrative is also seen where repeated attempts to implement a plan occur because of some kind of complication in the pursuit of a goal (Stein & Glenn, 1979).

This level of text structure can be used to help children to learn to make comparisons of similarities and differences across concepts and within complex events. They also can be used to help older children learn how to take notes, by discussing what concepts are important in one chapter, and then looking for parallels in successive chapters. They provide opportunities to learn how two topics can be coordinated within a larger theme, or how solving one specific problem may not solve the overall problem. Structures at this level of difficulty are rarely produced by preschool-age children. They begin to emerge with greater frequency between 7 to 8 years of age, with 38% of children's stories produced in this structure, and become increasingly abundant with age. By 9 years of age, most children are capable of producing stories at this level of complexity and exhibit instances of embedded multiple levels of discourse structure under one theme. These embeddings result in long and highly sophisticated stories told by this age group (Peterson & McCabe, 1983).

Level VIII: Interactive Structure

At the interactive level of discourse, multiple topics are related to a common theme, but in an integrated rather than sequential format. Aspects of these topics are discussed as they relate to one another in a comparative manner, so that the same characteristic or problem or event is explored from multiple perspectives. Information introduced early in the text is integrated with events or topics that occur later. Some overall problem or main idea integrates aspects of these many topics into a unified whole (Labov, 1972; McCabe & Peterson, 1991; Peterson & McCabe, 1983).

Transactional-Interactive text presents an interactive discussion where many dimensions of the same scientific, cultural, political, geographic, or historical situation are discussed in a manner that draws comparisons and contrasts within and between them. For example, the book *Ecology — Plants and Animals* (Walker, 1992a) is an instance of an interactive Transactional text. The first section introduces the construct of a *biome,* a large area of the planet that has a particular combination of geography and climate. Nine different biomes, including tundra, deciduous forests, and deserts, are described. Each description includes information about where these biomes are found on the globe and which plants and animals are commonly found there.

The second section presents the concept of adaptation in which plants and animals have evolved to be better suited to their particular environment. Examples are presented for a variety of the biomes presented in the first chapter. The arctic fox's white coat is related to its snowy surroundings and the need for an animal to remain undetected by its predator. The heron's long legs and neck are described with respect to its need to hunt for fish in the shallow waters where it lives. The following excerpt from a discussion about the dandelion presented in *Ecology — Plants and Animals* (Walker, 1992a) is much more elaborate and is explicitly integrated with more general principles in comparison to the reactive sequence text cited earlier.

> Dandelions have adapted well to their environment: Their long roots can get moisture from deep in the soil. Their flat leaves keep the soil around them from drying out. The leaves also prevent other plants from growing next to them.

The third section presents the topic of communities. This discussion elaborates on the concepts of biome and adaptation to describe how different plants and animals live together. Two abstractions referred to as the food chain and food web are explained and exemplified with instances from specific species in biomes that were described in the earlier sections. The concept of adaptation is expanded on within the concept of community. It is explained that different animals in a community undergo different adaptations so that the animals in a community will not all be competing for the same resources.

Poetic-Interactive. In an interactive narrrative, like a complex narrative, there are usually multiple problem episodes. However, the story may develop for awhile along two or more separate story lines, or the same set of events may be described from two or more perspectives, where each character has goals that influence the others. Unlike the complex narrative, the problems are viewed in an overlapping fashion as the action within the same event first follows one character and then shifts to another. The temporal sequence of the presentation of events may be modified through flashbacks that relate a crucial piece of history at just the right time to provide the reader with important background, a literary strategy used to highlight a point or to to build suspense. The reader uses a knowledge of basic story structure to re-create the underlying flow of events from the order in which they are presented by the author. Interactive episodes may be found in combination with other narrative structures, so that there can be interactive texts with multiple plot lines, one of which is structured as a Reactive sequence, for example (Stein & Glenn, 1979).

The Man Who Enjoyed Grumbling (Mahy, 1986) provides a simplified example of interactive narrative structure. The story starts by describing the background of the story from the perspective of the main character.

> Scratchy Mr. Ratchett enjoyed a good grumble. He got plenty of practice because he lived next door to the Goat family. The Goat family liked making trouble. They bunted and bleated. They nibbled his hedge.

The initiating event is described from Mr. Ratchett's perspective.

> Mr. Ratchett looked over the hedge. He saw a moving van.

Mr. Ratchett asks what is happening and is told that the Goat family has moved because they wanted more room to run around. Mr. Ratchett's response is rather unexpected.

> "What nonsense! They can jump around here!"

The story describes how Mr. Ratchett goes on with his gardening, complaining to himself that it is too quiet without the Goat family next door.

The scene shifts abruptly to Goat family's new home in the hills where the discussion is about their new surroundings.

> "It's very quiet up here," said Father Goat. He
> sounded rather sad. "It's too quiet," said Mother Goat.
> "There is no one to tease," said the little Goats sadly."

Another abrupt scene shift and the reader is back in the garden with Mr. Ratchett, who hears a moving van going into the next yard. Of course, the Goat family is moving back.

Interactive discourse structure is difficult for children to comprehend and produce. While many storybooks for young children are written at this level, such as books from the *Clifford* (the big red dog) series by Bridwell, children may not follow the complex plot, but rather only understand the events as an Ordered Sequence, or recognize the goals within specific episodes. Texts written at this discourse level are found in many textbooks by third grade, and increase in complexity, number of ideas coordinated within a sentence, and elaboration of a topic with succeeding grades. Children do not truly produce interactive episodes in their own oral stories or discussions until 8 to 9 years of age (McCabe & Peterson, 1991; Peterson & McCabe, 1983), or in their writing until the middle school years except for some comparisons and contrasts that appear in isolated segments (Calkins, 1986).

Summary

The Discourse Context refers to the functions of the discourse used within a Situational Context, falling along a continuum from expressing personal opinions or reactions to events, or stating personal needs and wants (i.e., the Expressive function), outward toward instrumental use of language to accomplish goals, such as informing, persuading, or questioning (i.e., Transactional), or toward the reflective, entertaining use of language for purposes of making sense out of experience or imparting cultural values to others (i.e., Poetic).

With increasing Situational demands, the language used to accomplish Transactional, Expressive, or Poetic functions must become more precise in its reference to the people, actions, objects, and the relationships held between them. The structures for accomplishing this organization exist along a continuum, from simple and loosely organized, to complex and interactively organized. This continuum is seen in different types of literature, personal response, and expository text, as well as developmentally as children begin to acquire the mental structures of schemas underlying text structure. This continuum thus can be used both *descriptively* and *developmentally*. Descriptively, it can be used to evaluate the discourse demands placed on the child in a classroom or other setting, as well as the level of discourse structure exhibited by the child for each type of discourse function. A mismatch between the external demands and the child's internal schemata for text structures would indicate that a greater level of dialogue must be used when interacting with the child to bridge this gap.

Developmentally, the model can be used to help make decisions on what is developmentally appropriate to expect from a child. For example, even though a story might be written at the *Poetic-Complex* level of discourse, it may be developmentally appropriate for a child to understand only simple cause-effect relationships occurring within a single episode and not all of the interactions across episodes. Thus, the teacher can discuss the story primarily at a level of *Poetic-Reactive Sequence*, but include increasing reference to other, more advanced, relationships within the story. The use of scaffolded dialogue, or shared responsibility for both interpreting the text produced by others and producing text to accomplish the child's own goals, will enable the child to successfully use higher level discourse structures than can be independently produced, and thus to begin to internalize these more complex structures.

■□ SEMANTIC CONTEXT

The most specific decisions to be made when using the model involve the **Semantic Context**, summarized in Table 2–6. In this observation, the meaning expressed by individual sentences or sequences of sentences is examined. For example, it may be found that in the context of an oral dis-

TABLE 2-6

The seven levels of the Semantic Context, reflected across the continua in both Experiential and Erudite Knowledge.

SEMANTIC CONTEXT

EXPERIENCE	LEVEL	ERUDITE
Unconscious knowledge of the properties of language. Can use and invent metaphors, rhymes. Can state when a sentence is ungrammatical, name letters, has concepts of wordness. Interprets metaphors by personal experience.	LEVEL VII METALANGUAGE	Conscious knowledge of the properties of language. Can explain metaphors, rhymes, grammatical rules, orthographic rules. Interpet metaphors, etc., through world, academic knowledge.
Personal evaluation of an event or situation. Indicates attitudes, likes, and beliefs. Often more closely aligned to opinion than to fact.	LEVEL VI EVALUATION	Culturally valued responses, world significance, or lesson considered. Value judgments, justification of behavior, moral standards, principles.
Meaning goes beyond what is stated to include information derived from personal experience or common knowledge. Inferred information not present or suggested by context.	LEVEL V INFERENCE	Meaning goes beyond what is stated to include information related to world, scientific, academic knowledge. Inferred meaning not present or suggested by context.
Cues for interpretation present in context but not explicitly stated or depicted. Predicted from personal experience. Includes goals, states, qualities, changes.	LEVEL IV INTERPRETATION	Cues for interpretation present in context but not explicitly stated or observable. Requires specific scientific, historical, or world knowledge.

Descriptions of the relationships of action or state between two unrelated objects, agents, events; or characteristics of objects such as color, size, shape, height, etc.	LEVEL III DESCRIPTION	Descriptions of historical, world, scientific events that include actions, characteristics, qualities. Information explicitly stated or observable.
Names for concrete, observable objects or agents, including the whole object and labels for parts within the whole. Little distance from sensory perception.	LEVEL II LABELING	Names for abstract, mentally created objects or agents. Categories or classes refer to groups of objects having similar semantic properties. Distanced from perception.
Nonlinguistic communications used to share reference to information existing external to the speaker, such as pointing to something that is noticed.	LEVEL I INDICATION	Nonlinguistic communication that exists or originates within the speaker. Communicates implied information, although the form is nonspecific (wink, shrug).

N T I A L

I T E

cussion in science class (i.e., Situational Context), a child produces a Transactional-Complete discussion of a topic (i.e., Discourse Context), but 80% of the ideas expressed merely explicitly describe or interpret personally experienced aspects of that topic (i.e., Semantic Context), compared to a presentation at a comparable Discourse level that includes inferences and evaluations that incorporate world or scientific knowledge. This analysis of the child's discussion would suggest that the child's ability to structure discourse is adequate, but the ideas expressed are concrete and do not go beyond literal meaning to incorporate world, scientific, or social knowledge.

When examining the Semantic Context, the ideas expressed within sentences should be compared to the seven levels of semantic complexity exhibited on Tables 2–1 and 2–6, and profiled below to find the "best fit" or description. A sentence may have characteristics of more than one level, in which case the utterance should generally be rated at the highest level of meaning. For example, the sentence might state "The dog was small and plain brown (i.e., description) but the boy thought he looked like a champion (i.e., interpretation) = Level IV: Interpretation.

The levels profiled in Table 2–1 and detailed in Table 2–6 under the category of the Semantic Context reflect the depth of meaning (i.e., Experiential versus Erudite), and the progressively increasing levels of semantic abstraction and complexity expressed by the language. The continuum, beginning at the bottom with gestures and other forms of indication and working upward toward abstract, metalinguistic analysis of language, reflects an increase at each level in the distance between the perception of an action, object, or event and the language used to talk about it (Blank, Rose, & Berlin, 1978; Monroe, 1951). As with any other context on the model, analysis of the Semantic Context can be applied to the language of any participants, including the written text, the teacher, and the child for evidence of the degree of difficulty exhibited, and any mismatch between participants.

■□ CONTINUUM OF DEPTH OF MEANING

Experiential and Erudite Meaning

The first decision to be made when examining the Semantic Context is to determine whether the meaning of the message is knowable from concrete actions and personal experiences (referred to as "Experiential" meaning), or whether the meaning reflects knowledge of largely academically acquired knowledge, such as scientific facts, historical events, and cultural patterns (referred to as "Erudite" meaning). Experiential meaning can be based on the perception of what something "looks like" rather than its function or what it is "used for." For example, the child might look at the picture in Table 2–7 and interpret that the ball is falling out of the tree and the girl is catching it, because that interpretation matches the perception as well as the belief that the girl is throwing the ball at the tree. Only by recognizing a function (i.e., throwing the ball to knock leaves off) does the interpretation become clear. In general, with increasing grade levels, children should have a greater background of experience and academic knowledge to draw on when interpreting a situation, and this greater sophistication should be reflected in both understanding and use of language (Rosenblatt, 1985; Straw, 1990; Wells, 1986). For example, consider the following text from *The Wonderhair Hair Restorer* (Jackson, 1990):

> No one was allowed to mention it, but there was a big shiny patch on the top of Dad's head where he was going bald. Dad went on and on about it. "I'm getting old! Losing all my hair!" he wailed every morning, standing in front of the mirror. Poor Dad got very upset. So Mom bought Dad a very expensive bottle of Wonderhair Hair Restorer for Father's Day.

Several ideas within the passage may be understood either at the Experiential or the Erudite depth of meaning. Dad's wailing might be understood to mean that he believes his appearance is lessened by baldness (Experiential), or that baldness is a culturally undesirable quality that may cause Dad to lose business because people are more likely to buy products from young, attractive people (Erudite). The bottle of Hair Restorer can be understood simply as a present for Dad (Experiential), or interpreted relative to drugs such as Menoxydil that are currently medically available for such purposes.

Depth of meaning is integrally related to the knowledge domain associated with a topic (Graesser, Magliano, & Tidwell, 1992; Smith, 1990). Thus, the same individual may demonstrate primarily Experiential understanding for one topic (e.g., food and nutrition) but a highly sophisticated, Erudite understanding for another (e.g., marine biology), because of prior exposure, interest in the topic, or previous extensive study. One way of determining what understanding children should be able to bring to a topic is to look at the curriculum, including the content covered at given grade levels and the books used to teach this content.

TABLE 2-7

Examples of Experiential and Erudite meaning along the Semantic continuum.

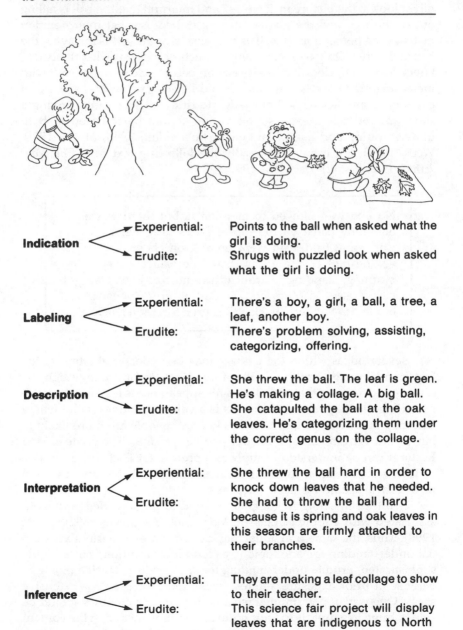

Indication

Experiential: Points to the ball when asked what the girl is doing.

Erudite: Shrugs with puzzled look when asked what the girl is doing.

Labeling

Experiential: There's a boy, a girl, a ball, a tree, a leaf, another boy.

Erudite: There's problem solving, assisting, categorizing, offering.

Description

Experiential: She threw the ball. The leaf is green. He's making a collage. A big ball.

Erudite: She catapulted the ball at the oak leaves. He's categorizing them under the correct genus on the collage.

Interpretation

Experiential: She threw the ball hard in order to knock down leaves that he needed.

Erudite: She had to throw the ball hard because it is spring and oak leaves in this season are firmly attached to their branches.

Inference

Experiential: They are making a leaf collage to show to their teacher.

Erudite: This science fair project will display leaves that are indigenous to North America.

Evaluation	Experiential:	Trees are interesting and important to study.
	Erudite:	Failure to protect the trees in our environment will result in increased pollution and loss of important natural resources.
Metalanguage	Experiential:	The word "fall" is a noun, "boy" and "ball" start with /B/, "tree" rhymes with "she."
	Erudite:	The alphabet bears an indirect relationship to sound; the /ea/ in "leaf" may have the same pronunciation as the /e/ in "she," or may be pronounced as in "head."

Children with less flexible language systems often interpret meaning with more perceptual and Experiential understanding, since their reading, listening, and learning problems typically interfere with the learning of academic information, and because they typically display poor generalization of known information to new contexts.

■ LEVELS OF SEMANTIC COMPLEXITY

Along with making a determination regarding the depth of meaning conveyed or understood in a message, a second decision must be made about the level at which the words refer to something, ranging from concrete noticing and identifying the object or entity through engaging in high levels of reasoning about it (see examples in Table 2–7).

Blank, Rose, and Berlin (1978) refer to this continuum as the Perceptual-Language Distance. In their model, the term *perceptual* refers to the appearance or characteristics of the material presented or discussed. The term *language* refers to the instructional language used to direct the child's analysis of the material. The term *distance* refers to the relationship between the material and the language, ranging from a close relationship where language labels or names the material or object to a distanced relationship where perceptions must be evaluated, judged, and mentally manipulated to determine what may, might, could, or would happen to materials. As the distance between the material and language widens, the focus must change from recognition of the material to recognition of properties or information that can be abstracted from the material.

The seven levels of Semantic complexity of this model are profiled below, classified in accord with an adaptation of a continuum first proposed by Monroe in 1951. Meaning at the lower levels of the model, located at the bottom of the continuum, maintains a close perceptual-language distance, where the information needed for interpretation is explicitly stated. At higher levels, the distance between the perception and the language is far, and much of the meaning is implied. Children with less flexible language systems have difficulty deriving meaning at more abstract semantic levels, and often when they do attempt to communicate information at higher levels, a high number of word-mapping problems are exhibited such as false starts, linguistic nonfluencies, fillers such as "um" or "er," and inappropriate word choice (Damico, 1992; Loban, 1976).

Level I: Indication

The level of Indication refers to gestures, vocalizations, imitations of animal or environmental sounds, and other nonlinguistic communications that may occur independent of or accompany language. They may be produced intentionally, such as a direct point to an object or event for purposes of getting another person to attend, or unintentionally, such as a head turn and eye gaze toward a noise or change in the environment.

Indication-Experiential reference is externalized, where the meaning is pointed to or indicated by identifying the physically present object or event with a point, vocalization, or other sign.

Indication-Erudite, in contrast, refers to an idea that exists or originates within the speaker. This level of Indication implies that the individual has an internalized idea, or symbolically created concept, that is referred to. This might be a wink to indicate "We'll talk about this later" or "I'm just teasing." The meaning is not specific, and this level of indication must be embedded within a context for an interpretation to be made.

Indications of an unintentional nature are present from infancy and continue to be produced throughout adulthood. Intentional Indications are produced by 10 months of age and become increasingly more conventional and purposeful with age. Older children and adults typically accompany their language with a variety of Indications that may emphasize, enhance, or extend the verbal message. Many children with inflexible language systems resort to this level when they are unable to map language to the meaning they are attempting to communicate, as in the following excerpt produced by a 12-year-old child attempting to describe his model train:

> You make little — make tracks that go to it — with it, the engine, and then um just put them, um, the engine onto the um um thing (pretends to do so with an imaginary engine). And then there's a little box, a thing that you flip back and forth (pantomimes the motion), and there's a little button that goes like this (pantomimes) . . .

In this example, the Indications are used to replace or support the language that the child has struggled to retrieve and organize, rather than to enhance and extend the verbal message.

Level II: Labeling

At the level of labeling, language is used to refer to an object (e.g., "car") or to parts of objects (e.g., "tires," "window," "door"). There is very little distance between the perception of the object and the word used; the word essentially re-creates an image or the thing to which it refers.

Labeling-Experiential refers to concepts of objects, properties, or events that have physical correlates. That is, the word "chair" refers to the concept of a real chair. The concept is general and can include a wooden chair, rocking chair, overstuffed chair, or a stool so that the label can be used to refer to a wide variety of chairs in an infinite number of different contexts.

Labeling-Erudite refers to concepts that are mentally created abstractions, rather than representations of physical objects. Labeling at this depth of meaning refers to categories or classes that are named, such as kinds of animals = birds, mammals, fish.

A wide variety of children's books are written at this level and can serve a wide variety of purposes. Many are designed for young children and help to facilitate language development and vocabulary acquisition by depicting one large single picture on each page (a book of farm animals, or body parts, for example). Others have many unrelated pictures on a page that are labeled, such as a picture dictionary. Still others depict examples of items within a unified topic and appear in books designed for beginning readers. The following texts are examples of books that label objects (*Huggle's Breakfast,* Cowley, 1990e):

> A carrot   A cake
> A fish   A bone
> A banana   A sausage
> A telephone.

and parts of objects (*In the Mirror*, Cowley, 1990i):

> See my fingers.
> See my toes.
> See my tongue.
> See my nose.

Children can recognize written language at the level of Labeling at a very young age, including printed words for their own names, names of familiar stores, and brand names for toys and household products. In the context of storybook reading, they are able to identify printed words for characters or objects (e.g., point to Little Pig's name on the page) and their actions (e.g., "huffed and puffed"). This is a common activity conducted between parents and their children during book reading when parents encourage Labeling by asking "Who is this?" and "Where is his name?" (Ninio & Bruner, 1978). It is an appropriate level of reading and writing to present to school-age children at the emergent stages of literacy development. It is also commonly used throughout the advanced grade levels with teaching tools such as maps, where countries, rivers, cities, and landmarks are labeled and with charts or figures, such as those depicting the bones and muscles of the human body.

Labeling is common in the language of young children or children with less flexible language systems. Instead of telling a story, they may point to and name objects depicted, as in "There's a straw house and there's a wood house and there's the little pig and, oh look! The Big Bad Wolf!" They have also been shown to have greater difficulty than their peers retrieving the names or labels for pictures in isolation or in context.

Level III: Description

At the level of Description, language is used to refer to either qualities (e.g., the car is red) or actions and states (e.g., the car hit the post) attributed to objects. Descriptions require selective attention to different aspects or features of the situation rather than global perceptions of objects or events (Blank, Rose, & Berlin, 1978). Selective attention allows for a focus on perceptually available features, such as the color, shape, and size of objects. It also allows for the integration of different elements into unified ideas, such as establishing the relationship between *who* does and *what* receives the *action,* as in "The cat chased the ball of yarn."

While more abstract than labeling, the cognitive distance between the material being talked about and the language remains close. Children at this level are able to identify and describe objects by their function, name characteristics of an object, describe an event, recognize differences, and simultaneously attend to two characteristics (Blank, Rose, & Berlin, 1978).

Description-Experiential describes characteristics or unified ideas between objects, events, or states present in concrete, physical materials. The information that is needed to make these analyses remains perceptually available and can be seen, heard, touched, smelled, or tasted. This can include descriptions of characters such as color, size, shape, location, distance, weight, volume, height, and so forth, or actions between people and objects.

Description-Erudite refers to descriptions of historical, scientific, or world objects and events. Many of these components are hypothetical, or at least unobservable, such as "Many galaxies are so far away that they look like stars" or "The earth has a crust that is cool, thin, and solid except for a few large cracks."

Description provides a simple level of discussion or presentation of a topic or event. Often it is used to establish basic facts within a text or story prior to the introduction of more complex ideas. Text for younger children or beginning readers and writers is often produced almost exclusively at this level. These descriptions may relate a sequence of actions, as in the following description of a temper tantrum from *I Want Ice Cream* (Cowley, 1990g):

I cry.	I stamp.
I pound.	I kick.
I smash.	I yell.

An example of Description communicated in syntactically more complex sentences is found in *Little Brother* (Cowley, 1990k). This simple level of text can be used to introduce a wider variety of words in slightly more complex sentences for beginning or poor readers.

> Grandma made a dress.
> Grandpa made a chair.
> Uncle made a blanket . . .
> Mommy had a baby.

The descriptive level also involves attributes of objects. Books of this type can be used to introduce a variety of adjectives, adverbs, and prepositions into a child's reading and writing vocabulary, as in *Houses* (Cowley, 1990d):

> By the red house there is a blue house.
> And by the blue house there is a pink house.
> And by the pink house there is a yellow house.

as well as concepts of number as in *On a Chair* (Cowley, 1990m):

> Look! Where? Over there. One little monkey on a chair.
> Look! Where? Over there. Two little monkeys on a chair.
> Look! Where? Over there. Three little monkeys off a chair.

Books at the Descriptive level can be used to develop problem solving and critical thinking skills, as in *What Am I?* (Cutting & Cutting, 1988j):

> I am long and live in the river.
> I have a big mouth and terrible teeth.
> What am I?

Adults and older children may bring multiple levels of meaning to the same language, including that of Description and, for example, Inference. In the sentence "Three little monkeys off a chair" from *On a Chair* above, the adult might interpret the explicit meaning (i.e., the monkeys are no longer on the chair), but also the implicit meaning (i.e., too many monkeys tried to sit in the chair, so they all fell off). Young children or children with inflexible language systems may only interpret the most explicit level of meaning and thus know that the monkeys are off, but not why. When asked comprehension questions about information read or heard, they may appear to understand the message, but really only comprehend what the words *say* and not what they *mean*. It is important to probe understanding at all of the relevant levels of meaning when evaluating comprehension. Similarly, when children with less flexible language systems attempt to tell a story, they often merely describe things that they are able to perceptually see, as in "The man is holding the straw. The pig is standing there. The pig has a pink face. And he's wearing a hat. And the man is wearing a farmer's hat." The level of Description is often a necessary level of language interpretation and use, but not always a sufficient level for true understanding.

Level IV: Interpretation

At the level of Interpretation, language is used to refer to internal states, motivations, or underlying qualities of agents, objects, or actions (i.e., psychological causality or response) rather than perceptual qualities. Information that *suggests* these qualities is observable (i.e., it can be Interpreted that the pig is *scared* because the pig has wide eyes), but the perception of wide eyes must be combined with personal experience, world, cultural, or other knowledge to derive an interpretation of "scared." Thus, at this level the distance between the perception and the language is increasing. Interpretations may attribute feelings, motives, or internal states to people, objects, or actions, or impose a temporal or spatial frame on the event (e.g., carrying the straw suggests that the pig will build the house). Meanings at this level are increasingly implicit.

Interpretation-Experiential refers to interpretations that could be predicted from personal experience. They are goals, motivations, states, or qualities that are generalized from similar events or situations, such as Interpreting that a boy is sick because he has spots on his face. The interpretation of illness could be made because that was a reason for the blemishes in some previous experience.

Interpretation-Erudite refers to interpretations that require specific scientific, historical, or world knowledge. For example, knowing that the rash occurred as an allergic reaction to a particular medication taken for a stomach problem requires knowledge of the drug and its side effects.

Interpretations are required to understand a variety of language found in children's texts. In *Grumpy Elephant* (Cowley, 1990b), the main character makes a statement about his internal feelings:

"I feel grumpy," said the Elephant.

This statement can be interpreted with respect to attributes of the elephant's facial expression, such as narrowed eyes and downturned mouth. Emotional states cannot be observed directly, but are interpreted with respect to observable characteristics of others and their actions. Our own emotional reactions can be described with respect to sensations regarding internal states, such as feeling nervous.

Interpretations are made regarding the motives that underlie people's actions. Sensing that the elephant is grumpy, the monkey character promises to play some music for the elephant.

> Along came Monkey. "Poor old Elephant. I'll play for you."

The reader interprets the monkey's action as stemming from a motive, or a wish to cheer up the elephant. The text does not explicitly state this motive with a sentence like, "I will play for you so that you will not be grumpy." Rather, the implicit meaning must be derived by associating the monkey's actions with the reader's personal or cultural knowledge.

Interpretations also are made with regard to common knowledge about events within the culture. In *Hairy Bear* (Cowley, 1990c), the bear's wife hears a noise downstairs in the middle of the night and interprets these noises.

> "Hairy Bear, Hairy Bear. I can hear robbers."

She also states her emotional reaction to this situation.

> "Hairy Bear, Hairy Bear. I'm frightened of the robbers."

When Hairy Bear opts to stay in bed, rather than go downstairs, she interprets his actions.

> "You're just a scaredy bear."

Interpretations are related to an understanding of cause-effect, as well as transformations across time, location, and perspective. Children with less flexible language systems often fail to interpret meaning at this level of perceptual-language distance, and they omit these markers from their language. Instead, the ideas are connected with simple conjunctions that result in elaborated Descriptions, as in "The pig made a house and he made it out of straw and then the wolf came and he huffed and puffed and the pig said 'Not by the hair of my chinny-chin-chin,' and then he ran away," which primarily lists events in chronological order with no interpretation of why any action occurred or the effects on other events.

Level V: Inference

At the level of Inference, language is used to go beyond the information that is either present in or suggested by the perception. From given information, a probable or possible past or future event must be inferred, or meaning generated that goes beyond the words themselves. For example, knowing that one pig made his house of straw, and inferring that the straw and string used to tie it together were not strong enough to protect the house from the wolf, can lead to the Inference that strong bricks and the mortar will be more difficult for the wolf to destroy and the pig will be saved. The meanings derived at this level are highly *implicit*, with the child creating a context for the events and actions that are not explicitly stated in the words themselves.

Inference-Experiential meaning is derived from relatively common experiences or background knowledge. Meaning at this level is related to event knowledge. For example, to infer that the sick boy will go to the doctor, knowledge of the types and sequences of activities within the event must be known.

Inference-Erudite meaning is derived from cultural and world knowledge. Meaning at this level requires predicting not only what will happen, but also why from a scientific or historical perspective, as in "The sick boy will go to the doctor who will recognize the problem because the rash is distinctive."

School-age children often are called on to understand information at this Inferential level of meaning to comprehend the curriculum. For example, in *Hairy Bear* (Cowley, 1990c), cultural knowledge of robbers and what they might be doing in a house is needed to understand Mrs. Bear's comment:

"Hairy Bear, Hairy Bear. They might get all our money."

The picture that accompanies this text contains no money. Under-standing this statement requires that the reader know that it is the role of robbers to steal valuables and that the family is likely to have at least some money in the house.

In a similar fashion, background information regarding the food chain is necessary to understand what is happening in the following story *The Red Rose* (Cowley, 1990n):

> "Ah," said the caterpillar, "I see a red rose."
> "Ah," said the bird, I see a caterpillar."
> "Ah," said the cat, "I see a bird."

These statements infer that each of these animals is interested in the preceding character as something to be eaten. However this information must come from the reader, for it is never explicitly written in the text, nor do any of the pictures show anything being eaten. Many children with less flexible language systems do not have expectations that there should be a level of meaning beyond that which is explicitly stated, and do not have a broad network of information from which to generate an Inference.

Level VI: Evaluation

At the level of Evaluation, inferences are not only made but also justified, evaluated for strengths and weaknesses, compared to alternatives for good and bad points, judged in terms of moral or social appropriateness, explained in relationship to precipitating causes or probable outcomes, or summarized in terms of the functionally most important features. All of these meanings are completely separate from the perception of the ac-tual object or action, which in itself is neither good or bad. Rather, these value judgments reside completely within the individual who has inter-nalized them from personal experience, world, scientific, cultural, and linguistic knowledge. This level of meaning gives purpose to experience.

Evaluation-Experiential relates to a personal evaluation, including a self-concept and personal identity. These are produced by even young children, who indicate likes and dislikes, as in "He's funny" or "I like that." Often they are more closely aligned to opinion than to fact.

Evaluation-Erudite considers the cultural and world significance or evaluation, as well as personal reaction. This level of meaning is central to most cultural institutions, such as the legal system, politics, religion, and education, as well as to self-concept and personal identity. Humans are constantly evaluating the phenomena that they encounter with respect to their previous experience. They seek to make sense out of their social situations and their personal roles within those situations. They use language to summarize events, make value judgments, justify their own behavior, and set abstract moral standards to guide behavior.

One of the primary purposes of literature, in both the Expressive and Poetic functions, is to reflect on language and to contemplate the meaning of some real or imagined experience. One outcome of this reflection is to impose a value judgment or moral on an event, as exemplified in the book *Road Robber* (Cowley, 1988d). In this fanciful story, a giant sneaks into town at night and steals the main street. On discovering this problem, one of the townspeople makes an explicit moral judgment.

> "It's that wicked Road Robber."

The people from the town find their road being used as the Road Robber's airstrip, and they steal it back. Not having an airstrip, the now unhappy Road Robber must land in the sea. The moral of the story is summed up in an explicit story coda.

> "Served him right!"

Authors of both transactional and narrative works seek to teach cultural values at a variety of degrees of explicitness. *Oceans of Fish* (Walker, 1992c) ends with an explicit appeal for concern about the plight of the oceans.

> The one great ocean we have must be nurtured and cared for.

Support for this appeal is provided in the form of discussions of a sequence of topics, the collective oceans as a single environment, the nature of communities of plants and animals in the oceans, and people's uses and abuses of the ocean.

Similarly, Aesop's fables make explicit statements about the cultural value, or moral, of each story. In an adaptation of one of these fables, *The Farmer and His Sons* (Biro, 1990), a hard-working farmer tells his three lazy sons that there is treasure in the grape fields. Motivated by greed, the sons dig up the fields after the father dies. Their hard work cultivates the fields so that there is a good harvest. The moral of the story is stated on the last page.

"The grapes are the treasure," they said. "Hard work brings treasure." And they have worked hard in the vineyard from that day to this.

A similar theme is expressed in the story of *The Little Red Hen* (Young, 1988b). Each time the hen seeks help in doing work, none of the other animals is interested. However, when it comes time to eat the cake, everyone is willing to take the time to help. The hen takes on society's role and shows that only those who do hard work get rewards. While the moral of this story is not explicitly stated, few primary-grade children would not personally react with a judgment that the other animals did not deserve the cake since they did not help to make it.

Language is critical to the ability to impose evaluations on a situation or state. Language is used to reflect on the nature of the human experience in the studies of psychology, sociology, and philosophy. Language is used within institutions such as government and religion to convince people to adhere to culturally determined mores and to behave and even think in socially consistent manners. Psychoanalysts use language to help people examine their thoughts and actions to increase their abilities to function within their cultures. Businesses use advertising to convince people that their lives are less complete without a product. Politicians use language to convince voters that their lives are less complete without them. All of these actions require language to create a contrast of objects and principles that are not visible in the real world. Often children with less flexible language systems have difficulty generating Evaluations at levels beyond simple personal reactions or opinions.

Level VII: Metalanguage

The level of reasoning with language that is most removed from perception of the object or event is Metalanguage, or the use of language to reflect on language itself. At this level, language is separable into arbitrary parts, such as content versus form versus use, or letters versus sounds. Comparisons can be made between words or concepts based on partial features of meaning, form, or function. With language itself as the topic, the meaning of the words must be deferred in favor of a focus on its structural or functional components. Metalinguistic uses of language include using language to define words, sorting language into grammatical or semantic categories such as nouns versus verbs or agents versus actions, abstracting rules that describe allowable combinations of sound sequences, letter sequences, word sequences, or story grammars, or assigning metaphoric or figurative meanings to words (van Kleeck, 1984; Yaden & Templeton, 1986).

Metalanguage-Experiential refers to the **use** of metalanguage or the ability to apply knowledge of words and their structure without explicit awareness of the rules or patterns underlying this application. It includes such things as rhyming words, telling a joke, or identifying letters within words. It also includes the ability to interpret metaphors or figurative language that is understood through personal experience.

Metlanguage-Erudite refers to the understanding of **why** words rhyme, have double meanings, or are synonymous, as well as explictly knowing the rules governing patterns of language. It also includes the ability to interpret metaphors or figurative language that is understood through world, scientific, cultural, or historical knowledge.

Use of Metalanguage requires that certain properties or characteristic of a word or concept be abstracted from the whole. An example is found in the story *Something Strange for Sale* (Candappa, 1988b), where a man tenses his muscles in anticipation of picking up an obese ghost, only to find out that ghosts are quite light. This lightness is expressed in the simile:

> "So a ghost can be as light as a butterfly."

Later in the story, a mule who is actively resisting attempts to control his behavior is described "as if the very devil is in him." The use of simile is Metalinguistic, requiring that only key aspects of a concept be abstracted, such as the weight of the butterfly or the behavior of the devil, while all other features of the concept are ignored.

Metalanguage also relates to the ability to create an image or impression by using language to conjoin two concepts in a way that transfers the meaning of one over to the other, as in the metaphor "John has ice water in his veins." Metaphors often have connotations that require Erudite meaning, as in *The Secret of Spooky House* (Cowley, 1990o), where Mr. Monster, tired of listening to his children cry, yells,

> "Stop! You're making my blood curdle."

Understanding this metaphor requires understanding the process of curdling when a liquid boils. Metaphoric language is used in literary writing to enliven the language forms used.

While similes and metaphors abstract aspects of meaning or semantics from the whole, other Metalinguistic abilities require the segmentation of aspects of form from the whole. Alliteration is one example, where words are used in combination because their initial phonemes are alike, as in the following report of final sports scores:

> "Braves bounce Buffalo. Tigers top Tampa."

The creation of rhymes involves another example of segmentation of form. Rhyming requires determining that the codas of the last syllables of words contain the same sequence of phonemes. Young children demonstrate the ability to rhyme at the Experiential level when they playfully rhyme words. Poems require coordination of the form of the Discourse structures with the form of the word syllables along a continuum of complexity. Children's literature is filled with examples of rhyming at a wide variety of levels of complexity.

At a Poetic-Ordered Sequence level there are texts like *One, One, Is the Sun* (Melser, 1985):

> One, one is the sun.
> Two, two are the shoes.
> Three, three are the trees.
> Four, four are the doors.

Not only is the pattern of rhyming within each line maintained throughout, but also the meter. A more complex rhyming pattern is found in *Captain B's Boat* (Cutting & Cutting, 1988a), where the rhyming pattern is built across couplets.

> The animals went in two by two.
> The tigers and the kangaroos.
> The animals went in three by three.
> The zebras and the chimpanzees.

An even greater coordination of the Discourse context and the syllable structure is found in the Poetic-Reactive sequence of *A Wizard Came to Visit* (Vickers, 1987), which tells a story about a boy's adventures with a wizard using a four-line rhyming pattern.

> A wizard came to visit
> one cold and rainy day,
> Riding on a shooting star
> that came from far away.

School-age children are repeatedly asked to perform metalinguistic tasks in school. From kindergarten onward, they are expected to isolate letters from words, words from sentences, identify all of the words that are nouns versus verbs, punctuate sentences in accord with categories such as "interrogative" versus "declarative," distinguish between common and proper nouns, and use capitalization accordingly, diagram the grammatical structures of sentences, evaluate the noun-verb agreement between words, and learn the orthographic rules or "phonics" that describe patterns of written words. They are asked to explicitly identify elements of Poetic Discourse, such as the characters, setting, and goals, and recognize properties of Transactional Discourse, such as the topic sentences and supporting ideas.

Children with less flexible language systems have been shown to have difficulty with almost all types of metalinguistic abilities (Bryan, 1986; Roth & Spekman, 1989; van Kleeck, 1984; Wiig & Semel, 1984; Wren, 1983; Yaden & Templeton, 1986). Often, instruction is presented at this level, as in asking a beginning reader to learn letters and their corresponding sounds in isolation, while the child has at best only a vague understanding of what reading is and how these Metalinguistic aspects of words might fit within the complex act of reading. The teacher might believe that it is easy to understand how a letter makes a sound, while to the child this concept is abstract. Looking at the inanimate and meaningless configuration of lines and curves, the child cannot imagine how it can produce a sound. Similarly, the teacher might ask how rhyming words such as "fog" and "dog" sound alike, because she can easily separate semantics from form. The child who cannot easily separate these aspects of language might become increasingly confused, acknowledging that the dog can make a sound (i.e., "woof") but believing that fog as a weather condition is silent. The teacher's question thus appears to violate the child's understanding of reality and seems impossible to answer. Sometimes in an effort to make things "easier" for children by teaching small concepts in isolation, teachers make them more difficult. Teaching these same concepts in ways that are consistent with the Semantic Continuum, first at levels of Description where the words, letters, and print are seen as unified wholes and then parsing them into aspects of wholes, helps the child to first view reading as an act in which language is *integrated*. Teaching reading from the Descriptive level upward on the continuum toward Metalanguage allows the child the time and the necessary foundation to develop an understanding of the Metalinguistic separation of content, form, and use.

■□ SUMMARY

The model of increasing levels of linguistic complexity within the Situational, Discourse, and Semantic contexts can be used to impose some organization on the existing knowledge regarding language and its use within a context. It enables the interventionist to go beyond describing what a child is doing with language within a context and to make some interpretations about how the child is using language to think about and to organize experience. Understanding how a child is using language provides explanatory power to observations so that judgments can be made regarding the level of task difficulty presented to the child, the level of strategies that the child is using to approach the task, and the effectiveness of instructional strategies used to help the child attain success in the classroom.

The model demonstrates that the Situational, Discourse, and Semantic contexts provide varying levels of support for the child's organization of language. Children with less flexible language systems might be able to use language productively under certain conditions, such as when the Situation context supplies much of the information, the Discourse context is at a low level of complexity, the level of Semantic interpretation is concrete and explicit, and the responsibility for the communication is shared. However, it might be found that as the topic becomes more distant from the Situation, or as the Discourse demanded becomes more structured, or as the meaning becomes more dependent on language, the child with a less flexible internal system of language understands and organizes less of the information.

The interventionist uses a knowledge of these contexts to evaluate and to facilitate the child's language development and use. In assessment, the contexts are manipulated to determine the degree of organization the child can apply as the Situation, Discourse, and Semantic contexts become more difficult. An example of this type of descriptive assessment is provided in Chapter 3. In intervention, the adult may manipulate the interaction between the Situational, Discourse, and Semantic contexts to facilitate development within and across the three domains. By engaging the child in language experiences that are structured to be within the child's level of comprehensibility and providing the child with assistance to perform at levels higher than her or his independent level of language use (i.e., Vygotsky's Zone of Proximal Development), the child is enabled to refine language and to function more competently in a variety of settings. Chapters 4 and 5 will apply this model to intervention and present examples of its use in the context of oral and written language intervention.

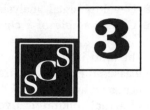

An Integrated View of Assessment, Intervention, and Accountability

The model for examining the Situational, Discourse, and Semantic contexts of language presented in Chapter 2 can be used to capture many of the dynamic interrelationships between the context, the participants, and the language used within a communicative situation. The flexibility of the model enables the same criteria to be used for many different assessment purposes, including naturalistic observation of a complex setting such as the classroom, descriptive analyses of language samples, and the written language of reading and writing. The child's performance can be compared to locally derived norms, or to existing norms for oral and written discourse. The model also allows for the establishment of goals and objectives, including those directly related to changes expected in the child as a result of intervention, and those related to changes in the interactions used by teachers or others to improve the child's classroom performance. This chapter discusses:

- Assessment of language in naturalistic environments
- Assessment of oral language

■ Assessment of reading
■ Assessment of writing
■ Developmental analysis of spelling
■ Case example of a child diagnosed as exhibiting dyslexia

The shift in the last decade away from a syntactic model of language assessment and toward a more pragmatic, contextualized model has increased awareness of the importance of obtaining language samples of actual communicative behavior. At first consideration, this appears to be a fairly straightforward task in which a language sample is obtained and then analyzed according to a set of behaviors, such as the number of utterances produced on a topic, types of turn-taking strategies used to maintain interaction, or types of intentions expressed through speech acts. But actual communication does not fit into a discrete dichotomy of behaviors that can be performed by the child versus those that cannot. Rather, what is produced and how successfully it is expressed depends on the complex interaction between the amount of contextual support provided by the communicative Situation, including the familiarity of the topic to the child, and the degree of responsibility for the communication shared between the child and other conversational participants; the type of Discourse structure that is used by the participants within the interaction to impose organization on experience for purposes of making sense of it; and the Semantic context, or level of meaning at which the information is interpreted.

The model for examining the Situational, Discourse, and Semantic contexts of language presented in Chapter 2 can be used to capture many of the dynamic interrelationships among the context, the participants, and the language used within the communicative situation. This flexibility enables the same model (and therefore the same criteria) to be used for many different assessment purposes, including naturalistic observation of a complex setting, such as a classroom or an interaction on the playground; descriptive assessment of the actual language used in a setting for the characteristics of its Situational, Discourse, and Semantic complexity; and assessment of the difficulty of the curriculum that the child encounters for insights into the demands placed on the child from the "outside-in," as well as the child's current level of development, or the "inside-out" (Nelson, 1992), and any characteristics within the environment that widen or lessen the distance between the two. The model allows statements to be made about the child's development relative to the existing norms for elements such as story structure, or more preferably, relative to local norms made by comparing the child's performance to that of peers. Thus, the flexibility of the model allows it to simultaneously be used both *descriptively* and *developmentally* for any instance of use.

From this assessment, the model allows for the establishment of goals and objectives, including those that are directly related to changes expected in the child as a result of intervention, and those related to changes in the behaviors of teachers and others who interact with the child. Changes in the interactions used by others can serve to enable the child to perform at his highest potential given his present level of language (i.e., the expected short-term changes) and, therefore, to refine his language system so that future learning will be more independent and organized (i.e., the expected long-term changes).

This assessment also can enable educational team members from different disciplines to understand the interaction of language with other aspects of learning and performance. Thus, it can be used to facilitate better coordination of collaborative efforts among educational team members, more integrated program planning and implementation, and better monitoring for changes in performance and development across short- and long-term periods. The assessment using the model can lead to insights for modifying an activity to meet the needs of students with different abilities and learning styles and for modifying adult behaviors in order to mediate learning within an event or activity. By using the same model for a range of purposes, a more integrated view of children and their learning that encompasses short- and long-term language development and academic progress can be achieved. Individuals using the model can form a better understanding of the children with whom they interact, the curriculum which they are presenting, and the teaching strategies they are using to facilitate learning among children.

This chapter explores the interactions among contextual variables and the language produced by children as they are exhibited in general contexts, such as patterns of behavior within the classroom, and in specific contexts, such as samples of oral language, reading, and writing elicited under a specified condition. The Situational-Discourse-Semantic (S-D-S) model developed in Chapter 2 will be used to conduct each of these analyses. This chapter will provide explanations of and examples from a case analysis for each of the following areas of language assessment:

- Assessment of naturalistic environments using the S-D-S model
- Assessment of oral language using the S-D-S model
- Assessment of reading using the S-D-S model
- Assessment of writing using the S-D-S model

Analyses of each of these language uses will be exemplified with language used by a child with a poorly integrated and less flexible language system. These analyses will be used to demonstrate what makes language difficult for a child to learn and use as an instrument for further learning.

They will provide a means of viewing the child as exhibiting developmental patterns of oral and written language that represent qualitative differences rather than deficiencies. The analyses also will lead to a recognition that an understanding of what is difficult and what is not difficult can result in the development of an appropriate intervention program that will simultaneously teach language and make use of language as a tool for learning (Vygotsky, 1962; Wells, 1986).

An assessment of a child should involve at least three types of information gathering. The first should include information about the child's current and past family, medical, educational, and speech and language history. This should be obtained through traditional procedures, such as reviewing existing reports, completing case history forms, and interviewing parents, teachers, and others integrally involved in the child's educational planning. The second should include observation of the child in the environment(s) where expressed concerns exist, such as in a specific class or on the playground or lunchroom. The interactions between the child and others should be examined for characteristics of the setting that either facilitate or inhibit learning and functioning. The model presented in Chapter 2 can be used to guide these observations. The third should include an individualized language assessment where representative samples of language at different levels along the Situational-Discourse-Semantic continua can be obtained.

■□ ASSESSMENT OF NATURALISTIC ENVIRONMENTS USING THE S-D-S MODEL

The contextualized nature of language obtained through observations in naturalistic environments and through language sampling provides a more realistic view of a child's language than standardized tests can. In the "real world," language use never occurs in isolated sentences or tasks that separate syntax from semantics from pragmatics from phonology. Rather, the speaker must coordinate all aspects of the speech act to decide what to talk about, how much information is needed by the listener, and to express this information using language that is sufficiently organized, clear in reference, and appropriate to the age and abilities of the listener. The dynamics between these variables enable the evaluator to determine the conditions under which the child can successfully use language to communicate and learn and those where the child has greater difficulty. Once a contextualized sample of language is obtained, it can be subjected to any type of analysis, from a syntactic or phonological description to a holistic description, depending on the needs and purposes of the assessment.

■ ASSESSING LANGUAGE WITHIN A NATURALLY OCCURRING CONTEXT

When assessing the language abilities of children, it is critically important to examine language in actual contexts of use, particularly those contexts in which the child is expected to function on a recurring basis, such as the classroom. Only in a meaningful context can all of the dynamics that interact to make the child a successful or unsuccessful communicator be observed and a realistic view of communicative expectations, needs, and abilities be derived. A language sample obtained in context is far more meaningful than information gleaned about a child's language from discrete tasks that attempt to assess the semantic, syntactic, morphological, phonological, and pragmatic components separately. In context, these components of language must function in integration so that word order or syntax is used to establish the intended relationships of meaning between agents, their actions, and the objects with which they interact. Multiple goals, such as informing, persuading, and seeking information occur as an inherent part of utterances used in a context, with the same sentence often expressing multiple levels of meaning and intent. The use of linguistic strategies, or form, to express relationships of meaning and purpose within and across sentences, as well as between and across conversational participants, are observable only when language is examined in context (ASHA, 1989; Damico, 1986, 1992; Lahey, 1988).

Classroom observation provides the opportunity to examine the actual language demands that the child encounters in the curriculum, or the "outside-in look," in comparison to the language used by the child when attempting to meet the classroom demands, or the "inside-out look" (Nelson, 1992). In addition, the factors that facilitate or impede learning within the situation can be ascertained by examining the dynamics that occur within the interaction ongoing in the classroom. Understanding the very high linguistic demands placed on children in the classroom can help educational team members develop the most appropriate program to meet the child's current learning needs and to plan for the future.

Language in the Classroom

The classroom is a contextually complex environment with the potential for Situational, Discourse, and Semantic demands to outstrip the capabilities of the child with less integrated and flexible language organization. The child participating within an elementary school classroom encounters an environment that becomes increasingly language based and decontextualized with each passing grade. Even at the kindergarten and first-grade levels, the child encounters an environment that is qualitatively very different from the sensorimotor, action-based milieu of preschool. The focus away from learning concrete, personal knowledge and toward learning historical, scientific, and cultural knowledge results in many activities where **Situationally**, the child is expected to be able to create the entire context for an experience, event, or hypothetical concept using language, with little or no additional support from pictures, props, or environmental cues. Information, ranging from classroom rules to procedures for completing assignments to the discussions about far away places and invisible scientific concepts, is continuously presented in the classroom, with the expectation that the words themselves can be used by the child to create meaning (Cazden, 1988; Creaghead, 1992; Wells, 1986).

In **Discourse**, the child is expected to be able to impose some structure on experiences to make sense out of them, to use this structure to communicate and share this knowledge with others, and to understand the information presented by others, such as the teacher or peers. The child must have the flexibility to impose organization consistent with the requirements of a specific situation or task. With increasing grade levels, the discourse participants become increasingly removed in actual time and space, as the child reads for content from a textbook written by an author who is never seen and cannot make adjustments, clarifications, or provide feedback if the child fails to understand the meaning of the language. The teacher expects that the discourse structures within and across sentences in the story are understood by the child, so that when the words are successfully read, comprehension will be a natural outcome. Thus, in reading instruction, a primary focus is often placed on learning how to decode. Similarly, in writing, a primary focus is on form, with the expectation that the child will be able to compose once the mechanics have been mastered. In lectures and discussions, it is expected that the child will recognize what information is important and whether comparisons are drawn or reasons for an event are explained (Applebee, 1978; Calfee & Curley, 1984; Roth & Spekman, 1989; Scott & Erwin, 1992; van Kleeck, 1984).

Semantically, the child is expected to be able to form hierarchies of interrelated categories and concepts, where abstract ideas are recombined to form new concepts such as animals + gone = "extinction," birth + growth = "life cycles," motion + unchanging = "inertia," or particle + atom = "molecule." These Erudite concepts, unlike ones learned through personal experience, have no concrete, visible referent and can only be imagined through language. Through reading, writing, and classroom lectures and discussions, 3,000 new words are added to the average child's vocabulary each year, many of these referring to scientific concepts or abstract mental constructs. Furthermore, with increasing grade levels, fewer of the words within a sentence have a concrete referent, and more are composed of grammatical structures that set up meaningful relationships of time, space, state, causality, number, and so forth between elements. A progressive understanding of metalinguistic concepts also is developed during the school-age years, including metaphors and other figurative language, moving from those that are concrete-descriptive (e.g., as big as an elephant) to those that are more psychological-poetic (e.g., the ground was as dry as Joe's humor) (Graves, 1988; McKeown & Beck, 1988; Nelson, 1985).

The child increasingly is expected to use language Metalinguistically to consciously reason about language itself, such as learning to differentiate nouns from adjectives or adverbs, identify and produce orthographic patterns common to English spelling, and realize the pragmatic function of a sentence as it is expressed through punctuation. The child is expected to interrelate the ideas expressed within and across sentences, maintaining the appropriate temporal, spatial, additive, causative, adversative, conditional, categorical, inclusive, exclusive, or other relationships between the elements (Bowey, 1986; Downing & Valtin, 1984; Roth & Spekman, 1989; van Kleeck, 1982).

To meet the many school expectations encountered every day in the classroom, sufficient flexibility must be present in a child's language system to understand the complex Discourse structures used by the teacher and the textbooks to provide an organized account of abstract events, to create a Situational context that is far removed from personal experience using language, and to understand the linguistically created concepts that compose the content or the discussion or text. Sufficient flexibility also must be present to use an appropriate Discourse structure to meet rapidly changing Situational needs, expressed with clarity and specificity at the appropriate level of Semantic abstraction for the audience with whom the information is to be shared. For children with less flexible language systems, many of these expectations are not realistic. Difficulties in school are often present in kindergarten or first grade, and by the third grade academic failure, social problems, and low self-esteem are an everyday school experience (Bryan, 1986; Maxwell & Wallach, 1984; Nelson, 1982).

Children with language systems that lack the flexibility needed for school achievement have been labeled many things, including language delayed, language disordered, learning disabled, language and learning disabled, dyslexic, attention deficit disordered, low achievers, behaviorally disordered, unmotivated students, and lazy. Analysis of language samples across the dimensions of Situational, Discourse, and Semantic contexts will usually reveal that these children are not able to use language at the levels required by the situation in which the problems that led to the label are showing up. For children with very inflexible language systems, the problems are apparent in almost all situations typically found in school and many outside of school. For those with greater flexibility, the problems are not noticeable except in situations where all factors along the Situational-Discourse-Semantic dimensions are near the upper ends of the continua, or where the child lacks sufficient background knowledge for the topic under consideration (Roth & Spekman, 1989; Spekman, 1983). For children with less integrated and flexible language systems, assessment must seek to discover the levels of Situational, Discourse, and Semantic complexity at which a child can learn. Independent work then must be presented near the lower level of the child's Zone of Proximal Development (ZPD) so that the child can use her present language system to successfully learn and intervention near the upper end of the ZPD to increase the organization and complexity within the child's language.

Situations and Questions to Guide the Analysis Procedure

The Situational-Discourse-Semantic model can be used to make observations of the use of language for learning and communication in naturalistic environments such as the classroom. The six decisions profiled in Chapter 2 should be used to guide these observations. The first two decisions involve the Situational context, and include (1) deciding whether the language used referred to information present within the ongoing setting, or whether language was used to create a displaced location, event, or context (i.e., contextualized to decontextualized continuum); and (2) deciding which of the 10 levels of cognitive organization is most characteristic of the event or activity. Table 3–1 provides examples of different types of activities that are characteristic of each level along the Situational continuum.

After the level of Situational context is determined, then the discourse used within that situation should be examined, referred to in the model as the **Discourse Context**. The interactions occurring within any of the example activities specified in Table 3–1 can be structured at any level of discourse, so that, for example, the response to a picture may be organized as a Descriptive List, an Ordered Sequence, or a Complete structure (see Chapter 2 for descriptions of these levels). Furthermore, in any naturalistic setting, there will typically be at least two participants, that is, the child and the person interacting with the child, such as the

TABLE 3-1

Examples of activities and the language used to refer to events or states at different levels of the Situational context.

Contextualized Egocentered

Play: imitate environmental sounds, actions
Talk: refer to personal feelings, moods
Write: doodling, marking without purpose
Read: available but ignored
Research: observe objects without anticipating or causing change
Math: related to own body (toes, fingers, eyes, etc.)

Contextualized Decentered

Play: explore toys for purpose of exploration, no goal
Talk: in order to get others to notice things, share focus
Write: experiment with writing instruments for their own sake
Read: regard book as an object, inattentive to the pictures/words
Research: talk about objects, explore to see what happens
Math: experiences without awareness (climb steps but do not count)

Contextualized Relational

Play: take role in play with life-size objects
Talk: as part of a real event, such as cooking, dressing
Write: alphabet letters or notes, copied words
Read: talk about books with photographs, realistic pictures
Research: talk about events, relationships between objects
Math: talk about objects by number, size, shape, other perceptions

Contextualized Symbolic

Play: take role in familiar event using miniature objects
Talk: talk about a picture or ongoing events
Write: about a picture depicting event or ongoing event
Read: talk about a story or text in which the words and picture match
Research: talk about world, historical, cultural information supported by text
    and pictures or miniature objects (farm set)
Math: use math (counting, measurement) for goals with present objects

Contextualized Logical

Play: take role in imaginary event using substituted objects
Talk: about topic only suggested by pictures or objects
Write: about a topic only suggested by pictures or present objects
Read: organize sequential cards and tell the story
Research: talk about problems-solutions depicted in pictures
Math: talk about math operations with objects present

(continued)

115

TABLE 3-1 *(continued)*

Decontextualized Egocentric
  Play: take role in familiar event, no props
  Talk: talk about an event from child's own experience
  Write: about personal experience
  Read: letters written to child, dictated stories
  Research: report on experiment conducted by child
  Math: use math to solve a problem related to real objects

Decontextualized Decentered

  Play: take role within imaginary events with no props
  Talk: talk about an event observed by the child
  Write: about an event observed
  Read: about observable events or topics, no pictures
  Research: report on teacher or peer demonstration
  Math: convert between a story problem and equation

Decontextualized Relational

  Play: play and explain the rules of a game (Monopoly)
  Talk: explain the rules of a situation or event (ordering food)
  Write: take notes, agendas, schedules
  Read: reference books, tables, an index
  Research: report on the procedures used in some process
  Math: solve and explain the operation of fractions

Decontextualized Symbolic

  Play: play a game with symbols (rebus pictures in Concentration)
  Talk: explain an unexperienced event or retell a fictional story
  Write: for specific purposes (letter vs. story vs. exposition)
  Read: creative stories or unfamiliar topics, places, people
  Research: use one book to explore many topics or events
  Math: solve and explain steps in problems with multiple steps

Decontextualized Logical

  Play: explain team games where roles change and rules interact
    (baseball, basketball)
  Talk: explain an abstract concept, such as photosynthesis
  Write: write outlines, grammatically analyze sentences
  Read: explain the narrative structure of a story
  Research: use many sources to explore one topic
  Math: explain the derivation of a mathematical formula

classroom teacher or the author of a book read by the child. Therefore, the discourse of both participants should be analyzed. Two decisions must be made regarding the evaluation of the discourse: (1) whether the function of the discourse is more narrative (i.e., termed "Poetic" in this model), more expository (i.e., termed "Transactional"), or more personal and responsive (i.e., termed "Expressive" in the model); and (2) which of the nine levels of Discourse structure (ranging from a free expression of ideas to highly structured presentations of topics along the Expressive-Transactional-Poetic poles) is most characteristic of the discourse.

Once the general structure of the discourse is ascertained, specific sentences or ideas should then be examined for the degree of abstraction in the language used to refer to the events, referred to in the model as the **Semantic Context**. The same unit of discourse (a lecture, a conversation, a story read, etc.) will contain ideas at many different levels from sentence to sentence depending on what is being referred to at any particular moment. Therefore, for each sentence within the discourse, the two decisions to be made are: (1) whether the meaning of the word or phrase is knowable from concrete actions and personal experience (i.e., Experiential meaning) or whether the meaning is embedded within scientific, cultural, world, or historical knowledge (i.e., Erudite meaning); and (2) at which of the seven levels of semantic complexity a word or phrase refers to an object, event, or concept, ranging from direct and explicit reference to a concrete or abstract concept (Indication or Labeling), to a highly indirect and implicit reference to concepts (i.e., Metalinguistic reference).

The questions specified in Table 3–2 can be used to guide the decisions and analysis of observations along the Situational-Discourse-Semantic contexts. They help the examiner to focus on the dynamics between the setting, child, and the other participants within the interaction.

▪️ EXAMPLE CLASSROOM OBSERVATION

The following observations were conducted in a third-grade classroom and focused on the interactions involving an 8½-year-old child, diagnosed as exhibiting dyslexia by a multidisciplinary team. The child had been participating in a resource program in his school, but was mainstreamed into the regular classroom for all but 3 hours of small group instruction in the resource room. Classroom teachers reported increasingly poor performance and distractibility.

The first classroom observation involved the child's participation in a whole group lecture with some discussion. The conversation provided

Table 3-2
Questions that can be used to guide the analysis of language along the Situational-Discourse-Semantic dimension.

Situational Context

Are the objects and actions being talked about present (Contextualized) or absent (Decontextualized)?

How much distance from the child's own perspective does the situation require (Egocentered, Decentered, Relational, Symbolic, Logical)?

How well is contextual support used by the child?

Does the teacher provide more contextual support when the child fails to respond appropriately?

Does the teacher associate the information with the child's own experiences or perspective if the child fails to respond?

Discourse Context

What type of discourse structure is presented by the task or situation (Transactional, Poetic, Expressive)?

What level of discourse structure is presented by the task or situation (Collections, Descriptive Lists, Ordered Sequences, Reactive Sequence, Abbreviated, Complete, Complex, Interactive)?

Does the teacher typically use a particular level or type of discourse during discussions?

What type and level of discourse structure is used by the child to respond to the task or the situation?

How much social support or mediation is given to the child within the situation?

Semantic Context

How familiar is the topic that is under consideration?

What type and level of meaning is the language used by the person interacting with the child exhibiting?

What type and level of meaning is the language used by the child exhibiting?

Is there a discrepancy between the level at which the teacher is discussing a topic ("Every plant has a life cycle" = Erudite construct) and the contributions that the child makes ("I planted flowers in the garden and they died" = personal experience)?

What level of questioning is the child most able to respond to?

What type and how much assistance is required to increase a child's level of responding?

Does the child show evidence of difficulty talking at the level of Semantic complexity required by the interaction (i.e., linguistic nonfluencies, hesitations, fillers, false starts, word-finding problems, repetitions, mispronunciations)?

many insights about the dynamics ongoing between the curriculum and the child. The analysis revealed that the **Situational Context** involved primarily an oral discussion on the rotation of planets around the sun, or a *Decontextualized-Logical* level of context. In this discussion, the **Discourse** level at which the teacher presented the information was largely *Expository-Complex*, where each of the nine planets was discussed in sequence, including details about its size, distance from the sun, temperature, and the time required to rotate around the sun. **Semantically**, almost 40% of the teacher's remarks were Metalinguistic, involving definitions of concepts, and 30% were at the level of Description. When questions were asked, they were frequently at the level of Inference, such as "Why is Mercury hotter than Pluto?" or "Why is the Earth's rotation shorter than that of Saturn?"

Observations of the child within this context revealed that the **Situational Context** attended to by the child was at a *Contextualized-Symbolic* level for over 60% of the time observed. That is, the child looked at pictures in his textbook, pretended that his pencil was a rocket ship or other object tangentially related to the topic, or watched the actions of others. When called on, the **Discourse** level used by the child most typically involved either *Expressive-Collection* comments such as:

> I like the planet Mars.
> I saw a movie about traveling in outer space.

or *Expository-Descriptive Lists* such as:

> Earth is in the middle and Pluto is tiny and they go around the sun.

The child was unable to respond at the Inferential level to questions, instead recalling a Descriptive fact.

> **Adult:** Why is the Earth's rotation shorter than Saturn?
> **Child:** Saturn is the planet that has rings.

These observations revealed that the child attended to the topic and used strategies to remain an active participant, but consistently reduced the level of complexity along the Situation, Discourse, and Semantic contexts relative to that of the curriculum. Behaviors that might initially be perceived as off-task (i.e., playing with the pencil) or related to failure to listen (i.e., answering a "Why" question with a "What" response) are shown to, in fact, be productive strategies that the child uses to make sense of the discussion at his level of understanding.

The child exhibited several responses that were more consistent with the level of classroom discussion. Analysis of these instances revealed the factors that facilitated more successful participation included the teacher providing greater contextualization, such as a diagram showing the distance of each planet from the sun, or a *Contextualized-Symbolic* level of Situational Context. With this visual support, the child was able to relate some facts at the level of an *Expository-Reactive Sequence.*

> First is Mercury and it goes fast and it's real close to the sun, and then next is Venus and it's a little further away but still close, and then Earth.

With this visual context and leading questions, the child also was able to generate the inference missed earlier.

> **Adult:** Look at the picture, and compare the distance of Saturn from the sun versus Earth. Why does Saturn make it around the sun in less time than the 365 days that it takes the Earth to go around?
>
> **Child:** [pointing to the diagram] Cuz the circle around the sun is smaller, cuz its closer to the sun and that makes it smaller.

Similar observations could be made for other classroom activities, or similar activities involving different topics. These would reveal whether the child's performance was typical, or whether the topic was in some way uniquely difficult or familiar to the child. Using this procedure across several observations, a systematic profile of the classroom dynamics begins to emerge. Objectives derived from this observation might focus on how the Situation should be established to meet the learning needs of the child and behaviors that the child can engage in to function more successfully within the setting.

Objective 1

Given a topic that is at a Decontextualized-Logical level of Situational Complexity, the teacher will accompany the discussion with visual support for the ideas presented (incuding diagrams, charts, pictures, demonstrations with objects, or main ideas displayed on a graphic organizer). She will facilitate the development of higher level language abilities by asking scaffolded questions or providing information at lower levels of Semantic complexity that will enable the child to reason about the information and draw conclusions at least five times during a group discussion.

Objective 2

Given an oral discussion or lecture, the child will write down key words or ideas highlighted by the teacher.

Approximation Toward Objective   **Date Achieved**

Writes key words of answers
    that are given following a question.
Writes key words from both the
    questions and the answers.
Writes key words related to each topic
    developed after a question.
Writes key words to topics developed
    throughout a discussion or lecture.

■□ EXAMPLE CONVERSATIONAL ANALYSIS

The second observation involved a conversation between the child and his friend. The language used within a conversation will depend on who the participants are, including their relative status and familiarity; what the purposes of the conversation are, ranging from nondirected social interactions to goal-specific exchanges; what the topic is, ranging from here-and-now events to highly displaced hypothetical ideas; and the context in which the conversation occurs, including casual encounters to formal meetings that adhere to rules governing who speaks, when, and about what (Brown & Yule, 1983). Analysis of conversation provides the opportunity to examine the degree to which the child can successfully initiate, maintain, and terminate a conversation; develop a topic to include relevant information with sufficient specificity for the situational requirements; structure discourse to coherently establish the intended relationships of meaning between ideas; and accomplish goals such as affecting the behaviors, beliefs, or attitudes of others.

Analysis of the interaction with the classmate revealed that two different topics were developed during the exchange. The first topic involved the child's recounting of a car accident that he had witnessed. Thus, the **Situational** context involved a *Decontextualized-Decentered* level event, the recounting would require a **Discourse** context along the *Poetic* dimension, and the **Semantic** context would minimally demand *Descriptions* of the scene, participants, and events. Analysis of the child's language revealed that the actual level of discourse used was that of *Poetic-Reactive Sequence*, where the child recounted causally related actions about the event from his own perspective in simple linear order.

> "There was a red light and this car didn't stop. And the other one didn't stop, and they crashed. And someone called the police and they were there, and then the ambulance and then they took the guy, um the people, away in the police car or the ambulance and one guy in the tow truck."

While most of the information recalled was descriptive of what the child saw, some inferences were drawn, such as the fact that someone must have called the police for them to appear. The language used became more dysfluent, characterized by false starts and awkward use of word order when he had to talk about multiple events that were happening simultaneously (e.g., how various people left the scene), and he could not use his strategy of sequentially describing single ideas.

A second topic involved the child negotiating to borrow a pencil from his friend. Thus, the **Situational** context was primarily at the *Contextualized-Relational* level, the **Discourse** context required *Expressive-Collective* use of language, and the **Semantic** context demanded an expression of needs, or a level of *Interpretation*. The exchange took place as a dialogue, in contrast to the monologue used to describe the car accident. Analysis of the exchange revealed higher levels of reasoning occurring frequently along the **Semantic** dimension, including explaining, predicting, and specifying objects, locations, and needs.

> **Child:** Can I borrow that pencil?
> **Friend:** I just gave you one yesterday, what did you do with it?
> **Child:** I don't know, but I need one for math.
> **Friend:** This is my last pencil. See if you can borrow one from him (pointing).
> **Child:** Don't you have another one in your desk I can borrow?
> **Friend:** Just ask him, he has two on his desk.

These observations revealed that the child was capable of making some inferences and predictions if the information was concrete and Experiential, but that he was limited in this regard when the topic was Erudite. He was able to use language to accomplish personal goals, and was fairly specific in the language used when there was little displacement in the topic. As he was required to coordinate more information within an utterance, the number of linguistic nonfluencies increased, indicating that he was nearing the upper limits of his Zone of Proximal Development.

■□ ASSESSMENT OF ORAL LANGUAGE USING THE S-D-S MODEL

The Situational-Discourse-Semantic model also can be used to elicit individual language samples. Individual language assessment allows for representative samples of language to be obtained at different levels along the Situational-Discourse-Semantic continua. The context of one-to-one interaction, opportunities to talk about personally relevant topics, the setting uncomplicated by competing distractions, and the flexibility afforded to the examiner to increase or decrease the level of difficulty along any contextual dimension, or to provide verbal mediation, enables a sufficiently lengthy and coherent sample to be obtained at different levels of complexity for analysis and comparison. It also increases the probability that samples of the child's best language performance will be obtained, without interference from classroom distractions, noise, interruptions by peers, or other factors.

■□ ELICITING REPRESENTATIVE SAMPLES

To conduct a comparative analysis, the child's use of language must be observed in a number of Situational contexts that vary in the degree of support for language performance and that provide for the use of complex levels of discourse structure. Table 3–1 can be used to either select a type of activity to use or to provide guidance for judging the level of complexity of a sample spontaneously obtained. The materials selected can have an effect on the organization and complexity displayed in a language sample, so the examiner must be aware of these influences. For example, elicitation at a Contextualized-Symbolic level refers to the use of representations, such as drawings or pictures, instead of real objects. However, not all pictures are equally difficult, and the one chosen can greatly influence the quality of the language used by the child. For example, a picture of a single object in isolation (e.g., an apple) or a single agent performing an action (e.g., a cat sleeping) will require a high degree of language competence if the task is to generate a story. An adult might be able to look at such an unelaborated picture and say "Once there was a cat who lived in a big house all alone. He didn't sleep very well, because he always had to watch out for the dangers of the neighborhood dogs who would climb through a broken window in the house to try to catch him while he was sleeping . . . " and so forth. Thus, although a picture is provided, the task is highly Decontextualized, requiring most of the ideas and referents to be created by the child using language. This type of picture will be likely to elicit discourse Collections from children, consisting of a few Labels and Descriptions, and will not provide a representative view of the child's language abilities.

Similarly, many pictures that look like they might be more conducive to telling a story because they have many agents engaged in many different actions (a scene of visitors at a zoo, people playing and picnicking at a park) may have the same inherent problem. Each person or animal in the picture may be doing something that is essentially unconnected to anything that anyone else is doing, and so a high level of language competence would be needed to unify the events in a meaningful way. For example, an adult might say "July Fourth was the annual company picnic. Every employee was invited to bring his or her family for the big celebration. Once they arrived, families found many interesting things to do for children of all ages. The older boys and many of their fathers had started a game of baseball, wearing the team t-shirts supplied by the company . . ." and so forth. Thus, while many of these events were depicted in the picture, the minimum level of the Semantic context at which an integrated story could be generated was the level of Inference. This type of picture will be more likely to elicit Collections or Descriptive Lists from children, as they move around from scene to scene in the picture describing what is seen, as in "They are having a picnic. And they are roasting hot dogs. And they are swinging. And the boys are playing baseball." Once again, a sample that is misrepresentative of the child's language abilities might be obtained primarily because of the materials chosen.

Therefore, pictures in which all of the characters are doing things that focus on the same goal are most conducive to eliciting a story at the child's highest level. Goal-directed activity in the picture will provide the opportunity to talk about the temporal order of actions, the cause-effect relationships between attempts and outcomes to solve the problem or accomplish the goal, and the psychological planning or intention to achieve the goal — that is, the elements of a Complete level of story structure or expository text. Many illustrated children's books will have pictures that satisfy this criterion. For example, one page from *Clifford Takes a Trip* (Bridwell, 1966) shows Emily hugging two bear cubs, while the angry mother bear is charging her from behind. Another two-page plate from this book shows Clifford blocked by the toll booth attendant from crossing over the river on the bridge because he has no money, followed by Clifford jumping in the river to swim across. Another source of pictures designed to meet this criterion is the Apricot I picture set (Arwood, 1985).

Similarly, if objects are chosen to provide a context for talk, they must be selected to be conducive to eliciting the type of discourse that the examiner is interested in observing. For example, blocks might keep a child actively engaged and even talking for an extended period, but the level that they are most conducive to talking at is Contextualized-Relational ("I'm gonna put the red one on top. Oh no, it fell down"), or if Contextualized-Symbolic, the talk might be limited to simple Labels and Descriptions ("I'm making a building. It's gonna have ten floors, and it will need an elevator"). In contrast, blocks accompanied by a set of farm animals and vehicles would be more likely to elicit talk at higher levels of Disourse structure.

■ EXAMPLES OF ORAL LANGUAGE SAMPLES

The following series of language samples and their analyses were obtained from the 8½-year-old child exhibiting dyslexia described previously. The activities used to elicit samples of language at different levels along the Situational continua were to tell a story about events depicted in a picture (Contextualized-Symbolic), to tell about a personal experience (Decontextualized-Egocentered), to tell about an imagined event (Decontextualized-Symbolic), and to tell about a movie that the child had recently seen (Decontextualized-Decentered and Interactive level of Discourse required). Each of the samples is contrasted with language generated by an age-matched peer with normal language abilities. The language samples are analyzed for their level of Discourse structure and Semantic complexity. Finally, the language abilities of the child with dyslexia are summarized.

Example of Oral Language at the Contextualized-Symbolic Level

The first elicited language sample was obtained by presenting the child with a picture depicting a sequence of interrelated events, selected from the Apricot I picture set (Arwood, 1985). The picture provides visual representations of people, actions, and objects, therefore presenting a Situational context that is **Contextualized-Symbolic**. The instructions provided to the child were to tell a story about the events in the picture, or a requirement for a discourse context that falls along the **Poetic** continuum. Analysis of the child's actual story provides evidence of the level along the Poetic dimension at which he is able to generate and communicate a story from pictured stimuli, and the **Semantic** context he creates indicates the level of abstraction at which he is using language to interpret the information depicted.

> **Child:** Uh, they gonna play ball . . . They probably can't 'cause all the stuff is falling out. And (6-second pause) that kid doesn't have the right pants. That's all.
>
> **Adult:** Tell me more.
>
> **Child:** And that kid doesn't have the right sleeves.
>
> **Adult:** Is he a kid?
>
> **Child:** Uh huh. And it looks kinda dark in the sky so it's probably gonna be raining. That's all I know.

The child's description is highly dependent on the context provided by the picture. A listener would have difficulty visualizing the scene from the child's words alone. Nonspecific referents, such as "they," "stuff," or "right pants" are used that only have interpretations through reference to the picture (i.e., two baseball players, balls and bats in a bag with a hole, baseball jersey). While the child uses discourse along the Poetic dimension, it is a simple story that is told by marking the beginning and endpoint — what the picture suggests the characters were going to do and then why they probably cannot, or the frame for a simple Abbreviated Episode. After stating these two elements, he is unable to organize any additional actions into relationships of time, causality, or intentionality, as reflected by the drop in the level of discourse to that of Descriptive Lists. The child talks about things that he notices in the picture without establishing any relevance for this information. These things are perceptually based, or what the pants, sleeves, and sky *look* like, with no reference to function or what relationships these things might hold to playing the game.

There is no elaboration along dimensions of story structure such as characters' goals, responses, plans, or reactions; roles are not defined, so that the bat boy is not differentiated from the baseball players nor the coach (who is referred to as "that kid," even when this interpretation is challenged). The story is told from the child's perspective, with no differential comments from the players', bat boy's, or coach's viewpoints, some of whom can see the torn bag and some who cannot. Thus, the linguistic context is primarily a description of what is visually perceptible to the child.

Therefore, even though the information is available in the picture, the child cannot use language to organize and make sense out of the events. He is more reactive to the external perception of what things look like than to an internal representation of how those perceptions can be recombined and coordinated to create a complex event.

Comparison to Local Norms

The best way to determine what is appropriate language organization and complexity for a child at a given age or grade level is to establish local norms. Local norms involve presenting the same task to peers with no suspected language disorder and average to high average achievement in school. Local norms enable nonbiased assessment to be conducted, so that the child's performance can be shown to be related to an underlying disorder rather than factors such as socioeconomic level, gender, or dialect. Many norms are available in the reserach literatuare for connected discourse, particularly narratives, including a longitudinal study by Loban (1976), and studies by Liles (1987), Merritt and Liles (1987), Norris and Bruning (1988), Ripich and Griffith (1988), and Roth and Spekman (1986, 1989).

For example, the story told by the child with dyslexia was compared to the story told by a comparably aged peer with no language or learning disorder:

> "Well, there's three boys and an adult, and the adult is the coach of a baseball team. And they're about to play a game. And the bat, and all the bats and the balls and the gloves are in a bag, but there's a hole in the bag and everything is falling out. They might get lost and they won't be able to play. That's all."

This story is told in a much more decontextualized manner. All of the referents are well established, the vocabulary is highly specific, and the relationships between the ideas are clearly stated. The story begins with the establishment of a setting, clearly states the characters, their roles, and intentions, introduces an initiating event that causes the problem and the potential consequences, and ends with a conclusion and a coda (i.e., "That's all). The story is at the level of an Abbreviated Structure, with eight ideas that develop the plot, compared to three produced by the child with dyslexia. The number of plot-irrelevant ideas, nonspecific referents, linguistic nonfluencies, and ideas at the Descriptive level or below are other outcomes that can be quantified in establishing local norms. These outcomes should reflect the quality of the Discourse and Semantic contexts. The differences between the local norms and the child's performance can be used to establish objectives.

Objective 3

Given a picture depicting characters, a goal, and a problem that interferes with achieving that goal, the child will tell a story at the level of an Abbreviated Structure, including 6 to 8 ideas that develop the plot and include at least 4 elements of story structure.

  Baseline: Descriptive List   3 out of 7 story related

Approximation Toward Objective   **Date Achieved**

Descriptive List of related ideas
Ordered Sequence of related events
Reactive Sequence including causality
Abbreviated Structure, intentionality

Example of Oral Language at the Decontextualized-Egocentered Level

A second topic was discussed during the language sampling, this time requiring the linguistic re-creation of an event from the child's own experience. The experience could be structured using any discourse function along the continuum from a Poetic organization of the event into a story through an organization of facts about the experience in an informative manner within the Transactional function. The discourse function actually used was the personalized and more private Expressive function.

Adult: Have you ever been to the aquarium?
Child: Yeah, and I *love* New Orleans.
Adult: Tell me about the aquarium or why you love New Orleans.
Child: Oh, I love New Orleans because they have this good, humongous mall. I think it is the best one in the universe I've ever been to.
Adult: What is its name?
Child: Riverwalk. It's called Riverwalk.
Adult: What does Riverwalk have?
Child: They have this mask shop there and that's where I got my George Washington mask. And also the aquarium. I like it because they have sharks and stuff. And also you can walk through this tunnel of water. And stuff like that.

When asked to tell about the aquarium, the child's discourse function is Expressive, with no attempt to generate a specific story about a trip (Poetic function) or to provide facts or information about the aquarium (Transactional function). Instead, personal reactions are stated in one or two comments with no supporting details. The interaction occurs as a scaffolded dialogue in which the adult structures the discourse with more specific questions, such as asking for the name and contents of the mall. Even then, the child responds with a description of the store where he personally bought something, rather than a more general description of the mall. General reference is established by using the word "stuff." The child lists things within the broad topic of the mall and aquarium that were perceptually salient to him, such as the mask shop, sharks, and tunnel of water with no temporal connections (*first* we went to . . .) or elaborations (sharks that you could see up close; sharks that you could watch as you walked through the tunnel of water). His listing strategy continues when the adult asks him about going on the trip with his family; he ignores the question and attempts to recall other concrete things that he saw. Although the aquarium was an experience designed to increase a visitor's scientific and world knowledge, none of the information reported by him was Erudite, but rather focused on his own concrete actions or perceptions. The discourse was structured as Expressive-Collections and the Semantic context primarily Experiential Labeling with some Description and personal Interpretaton.

Again, compare his account to one told by the child with no learning problems, referring to a shopping trip. The account is organized at a Complete level, with setting, characters, roles, initiating events, intentions or goals, attempts, and consequences for three related problems. Semantically, the recounting provides numerous Interpretations and justifications for events, all expressed using specific vocabulary and clearly designated relational terms.

> "Well, yesterday I was at work with my mom and I was getting bored so I called my grandmother. She said she would come pick me up today, and we went shopping. And I asked her if we could look in my department, and I saw this (pointing to a new outfit she was wearing) and she got it for me because it was on sale. And I begged her to buy me a swimsuit that I wanted, but she had to call my mom, she's gonna call my mom and ask her."

Her re-creation was told using the Expressive function, structured as monologue, unsupported by questions or prompts from the adult. The text contains 10 ideas that develop the same topic in detail, specifying appropriate relationships of time, location, causality, conditionality, intentionality, and adversity with clarity and complexity. This can be compared to the maximum of 2 ideas used to talk about any one topic in the experience recounted by the child with dyslexia, none of which expressed supporting details or relationships that linked anything beyond personal response to an event.

> **Objective 4**
>
> When recounting a story or event at a Decontextualized level, the child will establish a topic and develop it with a minimum of 6 ideas structured at the level of at least a Reactive Sequence (i.e., time sequence, location, and cause-effect established).
>
> Baseline: Collection   2 ideas per topic
>
> **Objective 5**
>
> When recounting a story or event at a Decontextualized level, the child will include information beyond labeling and personal response, including other people's roles, action sequences, and Erudite meaning, when appropriate.
>
> Baseline: 95% Labeling things observed or describing personal response

Example of Oral Language at the Decontextualized-Symbolic Level

Later in his discussion of the mall, the child with dyslexia described a sighting of a ghost who is purported to live in the Riverwalk. This is a decontextualized experience, or one that he only heard about but did not actually see, and for which there are no visual referents.

> "They had all these people who were working and they all went home and the boss of the um, working thing went down in it and um, he heard a bunch of tables and stuff movin' around and laughing whenever he turned around. So he went back in, he looked, and nothin' was there, turned around again and it was all laughing and stuff again. And then he turned back around and it was still doing it and looked around the room and it was lookin'. And this ghost, and this girl started walkin' up these stairs and it started laughing her head off and just walked right by."

This story had been linguistically structured by someone for the child and was told from one perspective, or that of the boss. It is more elaborated than the pictured story, which required the child to interpret, infer, structure, and word the story himself. While the story is sequential and has causal ties between actions (i.e., a Reactive Sequence), he continues to establish reference with nonspecific or unidentified markers (i.e., they, working things, it, stuff, went in, there), with most of the links established additively (and . . .). Thus, the point where the ghost is spotted is not highlighted, but rather only presented as another element in the sequence. The significance of most events is not stated, but rather only recalled, so that the child indicated that most of the people went home, but not that this caused the boss to be alone in the building; that the boss went down in something to someplace, but not where or why that place was significant. The information given by the child is presented Descriptively, with no indication that the child was drawing appropriate Inferences from those facts given to him by the original storyteller.

By comparing the narratives spontaneously generated by the child to the retelling of a narrative structured by others, an indication of the child's Zone of Proximal Development is obtained. Unlike the previous two samples, the topic is maintained throughout a sequence of events, the information is action based and less Expressive, and the temporal order is present. He was able to displace from his own perspective to talk about the experiences of another, unfamiliar character. The story was relatively simple, told from one perspective, with all events told in simple, linear order. Even then, the child struggled to establish referents. This simple story thus nears the upper end of the child's ZPD, as reflected by the retelling of the more complex one that follows.

Example of Oral Language at Decontextualized-Decentered Level

When this child was asked to structure a story himself from a plot that was not organized linguistically by someone else, but was observed and therefore experienced visually (i.e., watching a movie), there is far less cohesiveness or structure even though the Situational context is at a lower level of Decontextualized-Decentered. The retelling is not supported by any visual reference, and an accurate account required the coordination of many characters and their respective roles and perspectives (Poetic-Interactive).

Adult: Did you see *Robin Hood*?

Child: Yeah, it was the best movie I ever saw.

Adult: Tell me about the movie *Robin Hood.*

Child: Um, the uh, bad guy Sheriff, the Sheriff of Nottingham, got stitches in his face and he had these statues of him. And whenever he got stitches in his face, this, this guy had to go around to every statue like that and carve stitches in the statue (laughing) like that.

Adult: Why did he have to do that?

Child: I think because Robin Hood um did like that with the sword (demonstrates charging with a sword), probably a bow and arrow came down from a tree from somebody who went (demonstrates shooting the bow and made sound effects), like that.

Adult: What else happened?

Child: He was, um, he took — coulda took three bow and arrows and shoot 'em in the tree at one time. And he also um lit fire in the bow and arrow and shot it in the sky and burnt and blew the guy up. He blew him up.

> **Adult:** Well, how did the story start? What happened at the beginning?
>
> **Child:** Um, it started like. I can't remember if it started like whenever he was a little kid or whenever um, you saw these three bow bow and arrows fly up in the tree and then it started, you know, showin' the movie.
>
> **Adult:** How did the movie end?
>
> **Child:** Robin Hood and Maid Marion got um married and stuff like that. And there's this real funny part in it, and um, this guy he said, he said somethin' about his grandpa or his father or someone he knew. And he said about that guy teacher that, um, something only about a beard.

No concept of plot is evident in this retelling of the story. There is only a description of some perceptually salient events such as the stitches in the statue, or the bows and arrows, resulting in discourse that is Poetic (events from the story rather than his personal response) but at a level of Descriptive Lists with a few episodes of Reactive Sequences present. Even these events required the coordination of multiple perspectives, so that one had to understand the relationship of the sheriff to the statues, the sheriff to Robin Hood, and Robin Hood to the statues. As he tried to express these relationships, the child's speech exhibited numerous nonfluencies, fillers, and false starts (um, the uh, bad guy sheriff of Nottingham) and extensive use of nonspecific language and unclear references. Semantically, he described the stitches on the statue, but when asked a more abstract question of why the stitches were made, he responded with a concrete description of how it was done and not a judgment or explanation of why. Even in his description of "how," he resorted to gestures and physical demonstration of the actions to support the nonspecific language used to express these acts, and he never did relate them to the statues. Similarly, no reasons are given for shooting, lighting, or using arrows to blow up some unspecified person, and this event was not embedded within any recognizable plot or surrounding context.

When asked for a beginning and ending to the story, the child reported the perceptual events that occurred at the beginning of the movie that indicated it had started, rather than any reference to plot. At the end, the child tried to explain some dialogue that he perceived to be humor, or *Metalinguistic* meaning. At this level of language use, where the Situational, Discourse, and Semantic context are all very difficult, he was unable to express the ideas related to the funny statement and only vaguely referred to information needed by the listener.

Compare an excerpt from the beginning of the retelling of the movie *Home Alone* by the second child. This story coordinated multiple perspectives, and used discourse strategies such as flashback to create Interactive Episodes.

> "Well, in *Home Alone*, see, Kevin's dad has been transferred to work in Paris, so they take a Christmas vacation to Paris. And all his brothers, and Kevin's cousins and everything, everyone's there and they're all going to leave, but they are in such a rush they forget Kevin. And it happened because the night before he got in trouble with his brother, 'cause his brother ate all of his plain cheese pizza. And he got mad at him for it, and he hit him, and he knocked over all the coke and everything, and he got sent up to the third floor. And he said that he hopes he will never see his family again and he hoped they would all just disappear. And then the next morning when he woke up, he thought he had made his family disappear because they had forgot him!"

The comparison of the language used by the child with dyslexia to that of peers suggests that Interactive structure is a level that other children are using to organize and structure their experiences. Since the level of discourse is so complex and the child's organization so limited, the initial objective might be to acquire experiences using this level of discourse in a Contextualized situation first.

> **Objective 6**
>
> Given a story in which multiple subplots must be coordinated from multiple perspectives (i.e., an Interactive discourse structure), the child will tell a story that develops three interacting subplots at the level of Reactive Sequences and unify them within a common theme or plot line.

Approximations Toward Objective	Date Achieved
The three Interactive subplots are each depicted in illustrations within a story.	
The three Interactive subplots are each displayed on a Graphic Organizer.	
The three Interactive subplots are first presented visually and then retold.	
The three interactive subplots are told from a story in which several subplots are embedded within an overall plot.	

■□ ANALYZING LANGUAGE BEYOND THE SCOPE OF FORM

The problems exhibited by the language samples from the child with dyslexia are typical of those experienced by children with learning problems in school. The problems are far more complicated than merely ascertaining whether the child has mastered appropriate syntactic forms or elements of vocabulary. In fact, on the *Test of Language Development — Primary: 2* (Newcomer & Hammill, 1988) administered during the same week, this child had tested in the very superior range for picture vocabulary, above average for word discrimination, and average for oral vocabulary, grammatical understanding, sentence imitation, grammatical completion, and word articulation. Indeed, analysis of the structure of the sentences he produced, such as "They probably can't 'cause all the stuff is falling out" or "They have this mask shop there and that's where I got my George Washington mask," reveal the use of complex sentences incorporating conjoined clauses, participle movement, prepositional phrases, and relative clauses, often combined within the same sentence.

Rather, the problem exists in the complex interaction between (1) the Situational requirements, including the level of Decontextualization, or the degree to which the communication is dependent on language alone to establish reference, as well as the complexity, or the distance from the child's own perspective that must be taken; (2) the Discourse requirements, or the degree to which the sentences and ideas can be organized in accord with principles of narrative or expository structure, and the degree to which the child can independently achieve this organization within a monologue as opposed to a dialogue where this responsibility is shared by both speakers; and (3) the Semantic requirements, or the degree to which the child considers the information at a level beyond what is perceptually available to the sensory system, and reorganizes those perceptions with past experiences and academically acquired knowledge to evaluate, analyze, and draw inferences from them. All of these considerations must be put into words that specify the intended meaning and that suit the purposes and needs of the speaker, the listener, and the situation.

The whole language analysis of the child with dyslexia revealed important insights about how he uses language to interpret events and impose organization on the environment. This analysis revealed that the structure that he imposes is limited and not well elaborated or networked. He generally does not activate appropriate background knowledge needed to create the overall scene, but rather attends to small events within the whole. These tend to be the more concrete and perceptually salient actions or features of objects, particularly things that are visually salient. He depends on the organization provided by other discourse participants and thus expresses his ideas with greater clarity and elaboration when the responsibility for maintaining the topic and deciding what is relevant is shared conversationally, or when he is repeating what has been told to him by others.

The child is able to infer causality in closely related events or actions, but fails to consider how these fit into overall goals; thus he focuses on perceptions or concrete action rather than motives, reasons, evaluations, or intentions. This visual/action-based processing is seen in his reliance on giving specific instances of something to explain a concept rather than generalizations. It also is seen in his strategy of listing events sequentially, with little or no use of language to reorder them to make a point or to integrate the specific event within the whole scene. Thus, main points or high points are treated as just another event, with no differentiation from background or supporting actions.

When the child attempts to use language to express changing perspectives, the poor flexibility of his language is evident in an increase in linguistic nonfluency, fillers, and false starts. He finds it difficult to specify a referent, and the problem appears to go beyond difficulty with rapid word finding in that he also misinterprets roles (i.e., perceives the coach to be a "kid"; listed a range of possible roles for the character in his joke). When the task requires an interpretation at the more critical-creative end of the Semantic continuum, his interpretation and response are more concrete and literal.

By analyzing the complex, integrated context, individuals working with children with less flexible language systems can begin to understand how they are perceiving and organizing a situation or task and, therefore, make changes in the situation that will enable the child to learn and, at the same time, to work toward developing a more decontextualized, organized, and displaced system of whole language processing.

■□ ASSESSMENT OF READING USING THE S-D-S MODEL

Many contexts of language that the child encounters are organized and structured by others and must be actively reconstructed by the child. Listening to directions or attending to classroom lectures are examples of such contexts. Reading is another such context. Speech-language pathologists must become actively involved in dealing with the reading problems exhibited by school-age children. Many of the reading problems are language-based — if the child cannot understand or use language to impose organization on an experience, then much of the language used by the authors of literature and expository textbooks will be too difficult for the child to reconstruct, and reading will become increasingly more difficult. Many of the remedial reading strategies used are Metalinguistic, a level that may be beyond the child's Zone of Proximal Development and which does not address the language processing and comprehension problems of the child. Another reason for becoming involved in reading is that written language provides a visual medium whereby the child can examine the complexities of language, including the Discourse structure and the words and word order used to express different levels of Semantic information. The permanent, stable input from the print allows the child to view language repeatedly and to see how it can be broken into parts and reconstructed to learn how it works. Thus children with auditory processing difficulties can begin to understand the complexities of language and to refine their own language systems.

The following discussion provides an overview regarding the nature of the reading process, including the variety of levels of information that must be attended to during reading, the nature of disordered reading, and a method for analyzing children's reading abilities.

■□ THE NATURE OF READING

In reading, the person in the author's role generates a Situational context that falls somewhere along the Contextualized to Decontextualized continuum, ranging from text that may label actual objects (i.e., cereal or other product boxes, street and store signs, or other environmental print), to text that is accompanied by representations of almost all of the words (i.e., illustrated storybooks or illustrated nonfiction), to text that requires most of the context to be created from words, either primarily (i.e., books with only a few pictures or graphs in a chapter or episode) or entirely (i.e., a text with no pictures). The author selects an appropriate discourse structure along the Transactional-Expressive-Poetic dimensions for the information to be presented, and for the purposes of communicating this information, the author selects words and sentence structures that the author believes will best express the intended ideas and organizes these ideas within the discourses, establishing a Semantic context (Bruce, 1981).

The reader's task is every bit as complex as the author's, and makes similar demands on organizational and linguistic processes. The reader must integrate his own language and concepts with those of the author (Rosenblatt, 1985; Smith, 1985). To accurately interpret the author's message as intended, the reader's language must be consistent with the level of language at which the author wrote the text (just as we talk in different registers to people of various ages and at different levels of sophistication, so does an author write differentially for an intended audience). If the Situational context is too Decontextualized, or the Discourse context is too complex, or the Semantic context is too abstract, then the reader's interpretation will reflect a simplification along one or all of these dimensions.

Facility with Language Structure

Reading is a meaning-making process. The meaning that is constructed by the reader depends on the reader's beliefs about the purposes of the text, or the reasons for reading it, and understanding of the information that is communicated through the words and other context (Bruce, 1981). One level of this understanding involves comprehension of the vocabulary used by the author and facility with the grammar in which the words are embedded. If the child has difficulty with either of these components of language, then errors and misinterpretations in reading will occur. Numerous studies have established that school-age children with learning disorders have difficulty with all aspects of language that work to organize and communicate meaning, including abstract vocabulary, figurative or metaphoric expressions, complex grammatical structures such as relative clauses, inflectional and derivational morphological markers, subject-verb agreement, complex sentences with multiply embedded clauses, and phonological awareness (Gibbs & Cooper, 1988; Stanovich, 1988; Wiig & Semel, 1984).

As a reader, the child must acquire new concepts and vocabulary by interpreting unfamiliar words in a manner that makes sense within the context, and the child must learn to combine a greater number of ideas in a manner consistent with the relationships established through such grammatical strategies as conjunction, embedded clauses, and morphological markers. When a child is experiencing difficulty learning to read or reading fluently, then it is important to initially present reading material that does not contain difficult vocabulary or grammatical structures (Nagy, 1988; Nagy & Herman, 1987). During intervention, it is important to continuously assist the child to use context to provide an interpretation to unfamiliar words and to parse complex sentences into their constituent ideas so that the child can begin to see how the language works to establish the integrated relationships of meaning.

Facility with Discourse Structure

Reading is not an act that is conducted one word or one sentence at a time, but rather within a Discourse context. The ideas expressed in the first sentence of a story or expository text establish a frame for interpreting the meaning of successive sentences. For example, in the book *Cousin Kira* (Cowley, 1988a), the first sentence establishes the primary character and an important feature about her:

> "Our cousin Kira was clever, but she was bossy."

The knowledge that she was bossy establishes the frame for the next sentence in which she ordered the other children to:

> "Do this! Do that! Get this! Get that!"

which in turn sets the frame for the next page in which all of the other children had to watch her scary video instead of their preferred funny film. If processed one sentence at a time, instead of as overlapping discourse, a reader would have no interpretation of why the children had to watch the scary video (Halliday & Hasan, 1976). Many comprehension problems and reading miscues are related to a child's inability to reorganize old or prior information with new information in relationships of overlapping meaning within discourse.

Text that is written with good discourse structure is easier to read and comprehend than text with poor structure (Mandler & Johnson, 1977). It has been shown that good readers have internalized patterns of text structure and read with expectations consistent with these patterns. Poor readers are not as affected by poor text structure, indicating that they have not internalized these patterns of language structure and/or do not access them during the process of reading. If a reader has facility with discourse structure, the patterns can facilitate reading by enabling the child to establish frames for interpreting successive text relative to previous events or information about characters. If the reader lacks this facility, the reading task will be more difficult because of the failure to establish a frame and the effort required to recognize words and reconstruct meaning when relevant background information is not activated.

It is important to provide reading material that is at an appropriate level of discourse structure for the purposes designated (Clay, 1991; Jalongo, 1988). If the purpose is to enable a child to begin to coordinate the multiple levels of language required for fluent reading, then simple discourse types comprised of patterned language where the same or parallel events are repeated with different characters or objects are most facilitative. An example is provided by *The Jigaree* (Cowley, 1990j):

I can see a Jigaree. It is jumping after me.
Jumping here, jumping there. Jigarees jump everywhere.
I can see a Jigaree. It is *dancing* after me.
Dancing here, dancing there. Jigarees dance everywhere.

---

and so forth through the actions of swimming, riding, skating, climbing, and flying. Once facility with reading a simple text has been established, then priorities would change to a focus on acquiring more advanced discourse types by reading and talking about stories with more elaborated story structure, such as the Abbreviated Episode from *Dragon with a Cold* (Cowley, 1988b):

When our dragon got a cold, we had a big problem.
Every time the dragon coughed, he burned the
wallpaper. When he sneezed, he cooked the apples on
the apple tree. The dragon couldn't sniff without

> burning himself. Dozens of handkerchiefs and paper tissues went up in flames.

For further discussion of different purposes for different levels of Discourse structure and function, see the examples provided in Chapter 2.

Activating Background Knowledge

While comprehension involves an understanding of vocabulary, grammatical, and discourse structures used by the author, or logical systems of language, the ability to understand also is influenced by content knowledge, or knowledge of the physical, social, and cultural environment (Smith, 1985, 1990; van Dijk & Kintsch, 1983). Much background knowledge can be acquired from the exploration of concrete objects and through personal experience (Experiential meaning), while other knowledge must be learned through academic endeavors (Erudite meaning). For example, the amount of prior knowledge about a topic will greatly influence understanding. Consider two books, one on the topic of pets and the other about microscopic organisms. The grammatical and discourse structures and even much of the vocabulary used in the two texts might be identical, but the book about pets would be more comprehensible to most because the concepts referred to through the language would activate a broader network of familiar, integrated ideas that already existed as background knowledge (Experiential knowledge) compared to the Erudite knowledge required for understanding microorganisms. The reader thus brings as much or more information to the interpretation of the language as the author provides.

In contrast, if the concepts referred to have only unelaborated meanings and limited networks of previous knowledge to activate, then the reader has to depend primarily on the information provided by the author for an interpretation. This will result in interpretations that are much closer to the concrete, literal end of the **semantic** continua, often causing misinterpretations or limited interpretations of the author's meaning. Many of the problems exhibited by school-age children occur because they lack sufficient information, or the words do not function to activate existing background information, or the information is not organized into interrelated networks of easily accessed concepts needed to guide interpretation and thus simplify the reading process (Smith, 1990).

As a reader, the child must use information provided by the pictures and the written language and integrate existing knowledge with new information to form an interpretation of the author's message. When a child is having difficulty learning to read or to read fluently, then it is important to present reading material on topics that are interesting to the child and for which considerable background knowledge already is possessed. During intervention, it is important to continuously assist the child to activate the appropriate background knowledge and to network the new information encountered in the text with related existing knowledge.

Processing Orthographic Cues

Print constitutes one mode of processing language that in many ways parallels the auditory mode. Both refer to the same abstract phonetic representation of words possessed by speakers of a language, both are used to refer to meaningful concepts, and both have a similarity of form, in that words that are pronounced as CVC syllables have letters that correspond to consonant-vowel-consonant (CVC) structure. However, the English spelling system does not directly map a printed letter to a sound in one-to-one correspondence. Rather, the system is closely related to morphophonemic aspects of language, or a balance between the representation of a sound and the representation of meaning (Chomsky, 1979, 1980; Read, 1971, 1986). The integral link between the orthographic cues of reading and the morphophonemic characteristics of language make this system an important part of the whole language system that must be integrated for the child with a less flexible language system.

The speech-language pathologist, with the background of knowledge in speech perception, acoustics, phonetics, and phonology, is prepared to understand the orthographic system underlying spelling and reading better than any other professional in the schools. For example, an understanding of speech perception and acoustics enables the speech-language pathologist to see that vowel letters correspond to more than one sound in English in a manner that is more directly related to meaning than to pronunciation. The tongue and lip position for the /ai/ (long a) is almost identical (i.e., tense/lax cognate pairs) to that of the /ɛ/ (short e) and different in tongue and lip position from the /æ/ (short a) which actually shares the same letter "A" in spelling. In fact, young children and poor spellers will spell words such as "peg" with the letter "A," as in "pag" because of the acoustic and production similarity of /ai/ to /ɛ/ (Read, 1971, 1986). Instead, the conventional vowel spellings are as closely related to meaningful representations of words as to their phonetic representations. A word such as *sane,* pronounced with a long a, does not shift in pronunciation to the lax cognate pair /ε/ when a morpheme is added (which would result in a pronunciation of "senity"), but rather to the /æ/ sound, as in *sanity.* Thus, conventional spelling uses the alphabetical letter "A" to represent the /ai/ and /æ/ sounds in order to maintain the spelling similarity between the root word and its derivations created by the addition of prefixes and suffixes. The reader shifts pronunciations in accord with an understanding of the language, rather than phonetic correspondence (Chomsky, 1979, 1980).

Other alphabetical representations of vowel pairs bear similar morphophonemic relationships. While long e (i.e., /i/) is a cognate pair to short i, the letter "E" is used to represent the /i/ and /ε/ sounds because of the morphophonemic relationship of words such as *extreme-extremity.* Long o is paired with /a/ as in "got" rather than the acoustic pair /ω/ as in "good"; long u is paired with /ω/ as in "good" rather than the acoustic pair /ʌ/ as in "gun." Many children are thus confused by the vowels when attempting to sound out words because they are operating on acoustic and production cues, while the spelling system is based on morphophonemic relationships.

The spelling system also is based on words borrowed from many different languages and dialects. The pronunciation of many of these words has undergone historical changes, but the old spellings have been retained. The word "been" in the previous sentence is one good example, in that it used to be pronounced more like "bean" and thus the spelling still captures the long e historical derivation. Thus, many of the phonic "rules" governing vowels have limited applicability. For example, the generalization that when there are two vowels together, the first is long and the second silent only holds true for 45% of high-frequency words; the silent e rule at the ends of words only holds for 63% of high-frequency words; the letters *wa* are pronounced as in "watch" for 32%; the letters *ow* are pronounced as in "own" for 59%; the letters *ew* are pronounced as in "grew" for 35% of high-frequency words, and so forth (Clymer, 1963). Since many different rules can apply to the same word, each with equal predictability, the reader must make decisions about the correct pronunciation based on meaning in the context of the sentence.

As a reader, the child must use information provided by the context of the sentence and surrounding text, knowledge of the meaningful relationships between root words and their derivations, awareness of the acoustic and production correlations between many consonants and their letter representations, and familiarity with patterns of spelling found in written language as an *integrated system of cues* used to interpret the representation of words in print. When a child is having difficulty learning to read or reading fluently, then it is important to facilitate this integration by maintaining a focus on meaning first and then to examine patterns in word structure that are important cues to the reader. During intervention, it is important to assist the child to activate words that would make sense in the context when miscues occur so that the child learns to read for a balance between the representation of sound and the representation of meaning (Chomsky, 1971). Thus, as the patterns of spelling are examined within these words, the meaning remains simultaneously attached.

■□ PATTERNS OF NONFLUENT READING

Nonfluent or poor reading is characterized either by attention to only one aspect of language when difficult words are encountered, such as the phonetic representation, or an imbalance between all of the cuing systems that must be coordinated, often caused by lack of facility with some of those systems (i.e., the semantic relationships expressed through grammatical structures, morphological derivations, vocabulary, background knowledge, discourse structure, phonetic structure, and semantic displacement). Fluent reading requires *multilevel processing,* or the simultaneous coordination of all levels of language that inform each other during the process of reading (Clay, 1991; Downing, 1984; Forester & Mickelson, 1979; Sulzby, 1985).

From studies of both oral and written language, we know that their are both bottom-up and top-down effects occurring simultaneously during language processing (Rumelhart, 1977). An example of the top-down effect is seen when the sentence "The girl dropped the hot ____" is considered. From the range of all possible words in English, only a few will predictably fit this context. Grammatically, the word must be able to function as a noun, thus eliminating all words that cannot fit this role. Semantically, the object must be capable of being held by a girl, dropped, and hot. Background knowledge makes some possibilities more likely, such as water, soup, coffee, pan, wire, iron, or ember because these are familiar mishaps within commonly experienced routines. Information from the surrounding discourse context, such as knowing that she was getting dressed but found her clothes to be wrinkled further limit probabilities of word choices (Goodman, 1986).

At the same time, bottom-up effects are occurring. The length of the printed word will provide indications of the syllable and morphological structure of the word, so that if the word is represented by only four or five letters, it is more likely to be "iron" than "appliance." Orthographic features provide additional cues so that the appearance of the letter at the beginning of the word eliminates the majority of all possible choices that fit the semantic, syntactic, and syllabic criteria and increases the probability of words such as "water" and "wire." A cursory processing of additional orthographic information, such as the letter at the end of the word, is all that is needed to recognize the actual word (Vellutino & Scanlon, 1987). In fact, research in reading demonstrates that word recognition does not occur by a systematic left-to-right processing of each letter in sequence, but rather in patterns that the reader has organized as drawing meaningful distinctions between words. For example, it takes a fluent reader the same amount of time to read a column of four-letter words that adhere to patterns of English spelling as it does to a column of isolated letters, but not four times as long as a left-to-right processing model would predict (Huey, 1968). Bottom-up effects also influence comprehension so that depending on whether the word is recognized as "water" or "wire," you might infer that the girl was either burned or shocked (Goodman, 1985).

Ignoring either top-down or bottom-up cues results in making the reading process more artificial and difficult than natural language processing, which is simultaneous and integrated. All levels of information are necessary to the process of reconstructing the author's message, and a disruption of any one level will have reciprocal effects on all levels. Listening to children read can provide us with important insights into why they are failing to process information in a simultaneous and integrated manner and, as a result, suggest intervention strategies that can facilitate multilevel processing.

■ ANALYSIS OF ORAL READING

The Situational-Discourse-Semantic model can be used to examine the variables that affect reading fluency and comprehension, including oral reading. Text that differs in the amount of contextual support provided by pictures, ranging from a close relationship where the illustrations and text provide overlapping information, to a distanced relationship where the illustrations and text provide different information (Golden, 1990), through text that is unsupported by pictures, can be presented to determine if reading fluency and comprehension differ under these increasing levels of decontextualization. Similarly, text that varies in the level of Discourse Structure and Discourse Function can be presented to determine if increasing complexity affects reading performance. Text that requires higher levels of Semantic interpretation for understanding also may be provided for insights into the language and reading relationship. An analysis of the patterns of reading exhibited by a child during oral reading can provide insights into the strategies used and the difficulties experienced by the child in the reading reconstruction process.

Descriptive Assessment of Reading

One method for assessing reading is through the use of an informal reading inventory. These inventories provide lists of single words, each list designated to be at a specific grade level of difficulty from pre-primer through grade eight or above, depending on the specific instrument. Following the word lists are graded passages, ranging in length from a few simple sentences at the pre-primer level, to 200–300 word excerpts from adult literature that contain long, multiply embedded sentences and abstract vocabulary. The examiner records errors, called *miscues,* as the child reads, and then asks a series of six to eight comprehension questions that are designed to be at different levels of semantic complexity, from a literal recall of facts to critical evaluations of events. More than one passage is provided at each grade level so that the comprehension of text read silently or read to the child can be compared to text read orally by the child, or different passages can be administered across time as measures of change.

The inventories are informal, meaning that the word lists and passages are designed to represent specific grade levels of difficulty, but the child's performance does not yield norms such as percentile scores, quotients, standard deviations, or other standardized scores. Rather, general guidelines are provided for interpreting the child's performance to be at the independent, instructional, or frustration level. The *independent* level is the level at which material is read with little difficulty and without instruction, or a level where the child can read for enjoyment and learn content area information without assistance (the lower level of the ZPD). The *instructional* level is the level at which material is read with understanding when assistance is provided. With appropriate assistance, the child should have little difficulty understanding the information. At this level, the child learns considerable new vocabulary, complex grammatical structures, and other elements of language, as well as the content area information. The *frustration* level is the level at which material is sufficiently difficult that the reader is unable to benefit from the material, or above the child's ZPD. Reading at this level is often slow, laborious, nonfluent, and stressful to the reader. So much information is difficult or unknown at this level that learning will not occur, even when assistance is provided (Pikulski, 1990).

The results indicating the grade levels at which material is independent, instructional, and frustating to a child can be used to select reading material for different purposes, such as classroom activities, free reading, and intervention. In addition, qualitative information can be obtained by analyzing the patterns of errors produced by the child during oral reading, termed *miscues*. Miscues consist of

> substitutions of a nonword for a word in the passage
> substitution of another real word for a word in the passage
> omission of a word in the passage
> ■ insertion of a word into the passage
> reversal of the order of the words read
> repetition of a word or words already read
> incorrect phrasing or intonation

Whole language researchers (Goodman, Goodman, & Burke, 1977, 1987) view these as miscues rather than errors because they do not occur randomly, but rather as a result of the use and misues of available language cues during the process of reconstructing the author's message. Many miscues are meaning preserving and can only be logically produced because the child is processing the language in the text as in

> "Sarah looked everywhere for her dad"
> [Sarah looked everywhere for her *father*]

while others indicate that the child does not read at a level where the print and the language are well integrated as in

> "Sarah liked everywhere for her father"

Example Descriptive Reading Analysis

The following passage, written in a manner consistent with one from a reading inventory at the pre-primer level of difficulty was read orally by the 8½-year-old child with dyslexia profiled previously. He had read the accompanying word list with only two errors, both self-corrected. Thus, the ability to use orthographic information at this level to represent words was adequate. The child miscued, either by word substitution or omission, on many of the same words when they were embedded within the more complex discourse of the graded passage, indicating that he was not able to coordinate all of the necessary processes, or maintain a balance between them. The text presented to the child read:

> Bob went to the farm. He went for a walk. His cat
> went for a walk, too. They walked for a long time.
> Bob saw some apples. Some were red. Some were
> green. He did not take the apples. The cat saw some
> pretty birds. He did not go after them. They went
> home.

The child's reading, including miscues, reflected poor reconstruction of the message, as follows:

> Bob want to the farm. He went for a walk. He can't
> want for a walk, too. They walked for a long time.
> Bob say . . . saw some epple . . . apple. Some where red.
> Some where gree . . . green. He did not (skip) the
> apples. The cat saw some putting beerds . . . brids. He
> did not go after them. They want some.

When asked comprehension questions, the child responded correctly that Bob was at the farm, but did not indicate that he went for a walk when asked what Bob did at the farm. When asked why Bob did not take any apples, he correctly suggested that they were not his, but when asked why the cat did not go after the birds, he answered, "by walking away." Thus, for both word recognition and comprehension, the child's ability to deal with written discourse at a pre-primer reading level was frustrational, or at a level too difficult for independent learning to occur.

Analysis of Text Difficulty

Lists of isolated words require recognition of the orthographic or printed form of the word in a Decontextualized Situation, with no pictures or environmental objects present to suggest their meaning or reference. The Discourse context reflects unrelated, randomly chosen words, or Collections, and a Semantic context requiring only Labeling print, with no meaning necessarily attached. Thus, there is no context to either assist the child in word recognition through language cues or to interfere with word recognition due to the multilevel coordination required to process meaningful text.

The reading passage represents a more complex context, where relationships of meaning between the words have to be processed simultaneously with the orthographic structure of the printed words. The passage was Decontextualized, unaccompanied by a picture or other support, and it did not describe a directly experienced event, but rather required the child to take the perspective of an observer of the character's actions. The Situational context thus is at a level of Decontextualized-Egocentered, where all of the scenes, actions, objects, and reactions have to be re-created through the language itself. The story is a simple reporting of the events encountered on a walk in the order in which they occurred, or a Discourse context consisting of an Ordered Sequence along the Poetic dimension. The sentences used within the discourse were three to six words in length, and all were in a subject-verb-object order with no complex transformations. The Semantic context was primarily Descriptive, but relationships of causality or motive were necessary to the interpretation of two events (i.e., Bob didn't take the apples; the cat didn't chase the birds).

Text written at this level of Decontextualization was difficult for the child, even though the grammatical structure of the sentences, the descriptive level of the ideas, and the orthographic representation of the words were within his range of language ability. Evaluation of the miscue patterns produced revealed that the disruptions in processing that occurred were reciprocal, with miscues from both higher, or top-down, levels and lower, or bottom-up, levels contributing to the difficulties. For exaple, words like "went," "were," and "cat" that were recognized in isolation were miscued in context, indicating that the addition of context provided cues that the child attempted to use, but could not coordinate. After Bob had been established as the subject or agent of action in the first two sentences, the child did not have the flexibility to shift the perspective to that of possessor, so instead of "His cat," the child read "He can't," continuing to read as though the text referred to Bob. After determining that Bob cannot do something, the word "want" syntactically and semantically makes more sense than the word "went" in his sentence, and even though he correctly recognized the word "went" in the previous sentence, he miscued on it in this context.

Background knowledge was not easily activated, so that after identifying that the apples were seen, the child did not recognize the following two sentences to be descriptions of the apples, miscuing on the word "were." When the word "cat" appeared in another context, where it unambiguously functioned as the subject or agent to the child, the word was easily recognized. However, background knowledge was not activated to help the child predict what the cat might have seen. When asked for a logical reason why the boy did not take any apples, a perspective similar to that of the child's, he correctly responded; but when asked for a logical reason for the cat's actions, requiring an understanding of the cat's motives and behaviors, his reactions dropped to a level of describing *how* the cat left, a characteristic also seen in the oral language sample.

As the child groped for meaning during reading, top-down cues resulted in miscues at the phonetic level, such as substituting "some" for "home." It is not that the child visually confused these letters, or could not associate the appropriate sound with the letters, but rather that once he had semantically and syntactically reconstructed the message to be "They want ____," the word "some" is a better prediction than "home." Conversely, bottom-up cues also resulted in errors at the phonetic level, so that the word "apple" was originally read as "epple," where the pronunciation was consistent with the /ai/ and /ɛ/ cognate pairs. When that did not result in a meaningful word, he changed his pronunciation to that of a meaningful morpheme, reflecting a top-down function. Thus, this child is using many useful strategies, but he cannot coordinate them to reach a balance that will result in fluency or comprehension.

Example of Contextualized Reading

When greater support was provided by the Situational context, the child was able to coordinate the multiple levels of language needed for meaningful reading far more successfully. The following passage was written at the pre-primer level of difficulty, but the level of the situational context was Contextualized-Symbolic. Each page of the story consisted of an illustration and a single line of text that maintained an overlapping relationship, so that if the text read "Obadiah jumped in the fire," the illustration depicted the character jumping into flames. In the following excerpt from the book *Obadiah* (Melser & Cowley, 1990b), the child miscued only twice and self-corrected the miscues after examining the pictures for more information.

> Obadiah jumped in the fire. The fire was hot, so he jumped . . . in a pot. The pot was black, so he jumped in a sake/bag/sack. The sack was fall/full, so he jumped in a pool. The pool was wet, so he jumped in a net.

The change in the Situational context from Decontextualized to Contextualized revealed that this level of support was needed for the child to integrate all of the processes involved in reading at a level within the child's Zone of Proximal Development. The analysis suggests that intervention for this child should present meaningful, contextualized experiences with print, where the Situational, Discourse, and Semantic contexts are systematically controlled, beginning with simple Ordered Sequences in which most of the meaning is Descriptive, and gradually increased in difficulty to higher levels on all three dimensions.

Objective 7

Given a book in which the picture and text provide overlapping information, child will read text at a second grade level of difficulty, characterized by: 10–13 word sentences. Discourse structure at the Complete level of Poetic structure with 10 embedded episodes, each episode consisting of 5 to 10 actions, states, or events.

  Baseline: < Pre-primer level, 3–5 word sentences
  Discourse at Ordered Sequence level

Approximations Toward Objective   **Date Achieved**

Ordered Sequence of 4–8 word sentences
Reactive Sequences of 5–10 words
Reactive Sequences of 5–8 embedded
  episodes
Reactive Sequences of 10–13 word
  sentences, and 6–8 embedded episodes
Complete structures of 10–13 word
  sentences, and 8–10 embedded episodes

To determine what is developmentally appropriate for a child, text that is rated at a given grade level can be analyzed for the degree of complexity along the Situational-Discourse-Semantic continua. Grade-level ratings are done using Readability formulas, as well as descriptive analyses of the text (see *Readability: Its Past, Present, and Future,* Zakluk & Samuels, 1988). For example, several stories at a second-grade level can be examined to determine whether Situationally the pictures and text maintain a close or distanced relationship, the level of Discourse structure exhibited (including the number of embedded episodes and the number of actions, states, or ideas within each episode), and the percentage of the ideas that are Descriptive versus Inferential, and so forth. From this analysis, the interventionist can determine at what level of difficulty across all three dimensions the child will have to be able to understand and use language to successfully read and comprehend the passages.

◼️◻️ ASSESSMENT OF WRITING USING THE S-D-S MODEL

The S-D-S model can be used to elicit and analyze individual writing samples. Individual assessment allows for representative samples of written language to be obtained at different levels along the Situational-Discourse-Semantic continua, and for different functions. It enables the evaluator to determine if the child is able to write for different purposes and to take the needs of the reader into consideration. It also provides a basis for comparison between oral language obtained in a comparable context to determine if the written mode either inhibits or enhances expression and clarity.

◼️◻️ NATURE OF WRITING

Writing is much like speaking, in that the various levels of context must be organized and produced by the writer, rather than another speaker or author. Writing is an active process of constructing a message to communicate meaning for some purpose (Clay, 1991). When writing, the child is placed in a Situational context that falls somewhere along the Contextualized-Decontextualized dimension, from a level where environmental support for the writing process is present in the form of pictures, graphic organizers, maps, charts, or relevant objects, to a level where the entire context is created through language from sources such as written reference material, oral discussion, and background knowledge. Through writing, the child must create a Situational context, with the goal of producing a text at the appropriate level of decontextualization for the intended purposes of the composition (Calkins, 1986, 1991).

Similarly, the child must create a Discourse context that is appropriate to the meaning and purpose of the text. If the goal is to describe a procedure for completing a group project, then an *Ordered Sequence* along the Transactional function would be appropriate; if the goal is to consider the pros and cons of an environmental issue, then an *Interactive* structure of expository text might be required. Expressing ideas related to a topic such as "things that make you angry" can be organized as a *Descriptive List* of general and specific events along the Poetic function or can be organized as a story with one or more episodes. The writer also must select appropriate words and gramamtical structures to establish a Seman-

tic context that expresses the ideas at all of the necessary levels of interpretation for communication of the intended message (Halliday, 1985).

The young writer must coordinate all aspects of context and at the
same time apply conventions of letter formation, spelling, paragraph
structure, punctuation, and capitalization that are themselves only emerging. Fine motor control and eye-hand coordination also must be negotiated. It is not surprising that many children are reluctant writers whose
products reflect poor organization, lack of creativity, and poor use of
conventions. The child compensates for the inability to coordinate all of
the levels of processing required for writing by simplifying the task
along one or all of the dimensions involved.

Facility with Language Structure

Writing is a meaning-making process. The meaning that is constructed
by the writer depends on the writer's beliefs about the purposes of the
text, or the reason for writing it, and an understanding of how to communicate beliefs or information through words and other context. The
writer must choose language along all of the contextual dimensions to be
appropriate for an *implied reader*. The age, interests, and sophistication
with the topic and language abilities of the intended audience are just a
few of the judgments that the writer must make about the implied reader
(Bruce, 1981). From these presuppositions about the reader, the writer
must choose words and grammatical and discourse structures that are
neither too simple nor too abstract and complex for the audience (Calkins, 1986, 1991).

Beginning or poor writers have little sense of audience and write
primarily for themselves. The ideas expressed are often poorly developed and depend on context or shared information for interpretation.
The difficulty of maintaining a balance between all of the requirements
of writing results in the use of simple sentence structures that are repeated, with many fragments and run-ons. A metalinguistic awareness
of text is still emerging, and so spaces between words, conventions for
using punctuation and capitalization within sentences, and differential
use of punctuation marks are not clearly understood or consistently
used. An increasing interest in writing conventionally leads to greater
attention to form and sentence patterns among children in the second
grade, so that by third grade most children have sufficient skill in all
areas of writing to produce comprehensible and well structured sentences, with more variety in grammatical types (Calkins, 1986, 1991).

Children with less flexible language systems have all of the challenges related to learning how to balance the requirements of writing

and, in addition, have difficulty with vocabulary, morphological markers, complex grammatical structures, discourse structure, nonliteral reference, word retrieval, and metalinguistic awareness. They also have been shown to experience difficulty communicating a message in a register appropriate for the intended listener or reader. The writing process remains difficult and confusing long after peers have begun to master the complexities of the task. When a child is experiencing difficulty learning to write, it is important to help the child rehearse ideas and organize them into words at an oral level before they are asked to coordinate all of the additional aspects of the writing process. During intervention, it is important to help children put ideas into words and to provide feedback on the logic and form of the sentences.

Facility with Discourse Structure

All good writers, including children, write to make sense of experiences and to say something about what they have learned from life. The best writing does not come from writing about some unfamiliar topic, but rather from something that the child wants to say about personal experiences or personal interests. For most children, writing in the Expressive mode of discourse structure is easier than Transactional or Poetic and is often the first type of writing to emerge (Britton, 1982). Collections and Descriptive Lists, or a style of writing "all about" a topic, rather than an organized account of a topic or event, are commonly produced (Calkins, 1986).

For beginning or poor writers, the final product of a writing session often consists of only a few lines or sentences. Little or no elaboration of any one idea is seen. Much of the discourse occurs in the form of talking and drawing during the writing process, with little translated into written words. With increasing experience with writing, these oral and graphic symbols begin to be expressed in written words. Thus, talking and drawing are important and positive strategies for learning how to structure ideas into coherent wholes during writing. As the child is better able to coordinate all aspects of writing, the balance begins to shift so that less of the discourse is expressed through drawings and, finally, talking diminishes and thoughts are translated more directly into written words. By third grade, greater discourse structure is evident in the written product, with Ordered and Reactive Sequences or Complete episodes commonly produced. Cohesion between ideas is greater, with relationships of time and space linguistically marked between sentences using relational terms such as when, then, first, last, before, after, and a variety of prepositions (Calkins, 1986, 1991; Clay, 1991; McGee & Richgels, 1990).

Children with less flexible language systems are less able to make use of oral rehearsal strategies to structure written discourse. The discourse structures at the upper ends of the Transactional and Poetic dimensions are not exhibited in their oral language and, therefore, do not function to scaffold or rehearse well organized discourse before it is represented in writing. Therefore, the process of writing must be used to help them learn how to create more organized, coherent, and complex forms of discourse to facilitate the development of structures that have not emerged through oral language experiences. During intervention, it is important to use drawings and graphic organizers to enable the child to structure a complex discourse context, and to use these as scaffolds to produce oral discourse.

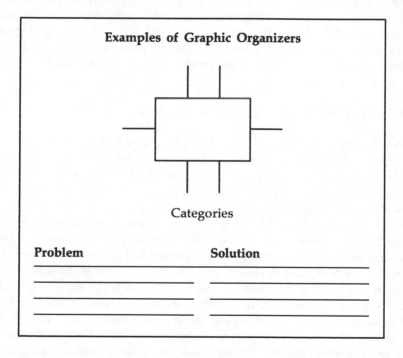

The process of actively constructing complex discourse enables the child to begin to internalize these structures and to use them more independently.

Activating Background Knowledge

Creativity and imagination in writing do not just occur, but rather have to be developed and nurtured. This ability evolves from possessing sufficient background knowledge about a topic to be able to maintain a focus on that theme and to reorder and recombine the information and events in new and interesting ways (Harste, Woodward, & Burke, 1984). The more that information is stored by a child within Experiential and Erudite Semantic networks of interconnected relationships, the easier this information can be accessed and actively used to create a setting and plot for a story, or to purposefully organize facts for exposition.

Information becomes networked through redundancy, or repeated exposure to the same information in a variety of contexts, and introduction of new information into a familiar context. Beginning or poor writers often fail to activate existing background knowledge as they attempt to write or do not seek or integrate new information when needed. They need experiences that will build a complex network of background knowledge to support a theme or topic, models of how to reorder and recombine this information in new ways, and active involvement in the creative process where the responsibility for generating and organizing the information is shared between the child and a facilitator.

Using the Orthographic System

Whole Language means that the entire language system, from the highest level of meaning to the lowest levels of speech perception, are integrated and function as one complex system. Each level within the system is simultaneously integrated with all of the others so that the perception of spoken or written words provides input into the system for it to refine, and it is itself refined by the higher order categories of meaning that govern which sounds or orthographic patterns are distinctive in a language. For example, in English, the aspirated and unaspirated /t/ are not distinctive categories in speech perception, not because the differences cannot be heard or produced, but rather because there are no meaningful words in English that are distinguishable from each other based on the presence or absence of aspiration. In certain dialects of Arabic, these are distinctive features, and their presence in a word differentially refers to two different concepts. Furthermore, the spelling system in English is highly integrated with the variations of meaning that are created by the addition of morphemes to root words, as discussed above (Hoffman, Schuckers, & Daniloff, 1989; Rumelhart & McClelland, 1986).

Reconstructing the orthographic system of writing at a level of refinement required for conventional spelling is a gradual process that emerges over years of meaningful use, much as the phonemic system of speech emerges over time during the preschool years. From exposure to conventional orthography during reading and experiences with spelling during writing, an increasing amount of structural knowledge is acquired that allows for further advances and refinements (Gentry, 1982, 1989; Hall, 1984; Read, 1986; Smith, 1983). These refinements must occur along the dual dimensions of phonetic structure and canonical, or syllablic structure. The manner in which these two aspects of orthographic knowledge emerge parallels the manner in which articulation development occurs and can be described in accord with the same phonological processes (Hoffman, 1990; Hoffman & Norris, 1989).

Phonemic Structure

The sounds, or phonemes, in words can be described in accord with the features that give them their distinctive characteristics. The /s/ phoneme, for example, is described according to the features +continuant, because the airstream is never blocked during its production, but rather flows in a continuous stream; +coronal, because the tongue tip is positioned high in the mouth and near the front; and −voice, because no vocal fold vibration occurs during its production. The /t/phoneme is nearly identical, except that instead of the airstream being produced in a continuous manner, the tongue tip actually touches the roof of the mouth allowing pressure to build up, followed by a quick release. Each sound of any language can be similarly described using a universal set of features. As children begin to mentally construct an orthographic system, an increasing awareness of these features can be seen (Read, 1971, 1986).

Awareness of writing begins with scribbling and drawing, followed by a distinction between the picture and the accompanying scribbles that the child perceives to be writing. The earliest actual spelling attempts, termed **prephonemic**, reflect emerging awareness of letter form, but no awareness of phoneme structure or syllable structure. Young children essentially babble with written letters, using lines, shapes, letter approximations, numbers, punctuation marks, and anything else they perceive to be writing to represent words. As they become aware of letter-sound correspondences, the phonetic principle begins to be applied to initial letters or stressed syllables, a pattern termed **early phonemic**. Often during this developmental period, the child confuses letter *names* with letter *sounds,* and uses the phonemes in the letter name to represent both consonants and vowels in words (i.e., S K P = *es ca pe*) (Gentry, 1982; Read, 1986).

Phonemic Simplifications

As more phonemes are represented in the middle and end positions of words and syllables, patterns that are **semiphonetic** are seen. In this pat-

tern, some, but not all, of the features of the phonemes may be represented in the spelling, in the same manner that younger children misarticu-
late because they are not able to coordinate all of the features of a sound
in their speech. In speech, these misarticulations can be described according to patterns, termed *phonological processes.* These processes have
been viewed as productive strategies and represent simplifications of the
adult production that the child does not have fully organized. These
identical phonological processes can be used to describe the phonetic
aspects of misspellings and probably occur for the same reason. One theoretical explanation for these simplifications is offered by Hoffman and
Norris (1989). The most common ones seen in children's misspellings include:

- **Stopping,** or the substitution or addition of a sound to a word
  that differs from the actual sound on the feature contrast stop
  versus continuant, as in /dit/ for "dress," /got/ for "go," or
  /ketten/ for "kitchen." Often these occur as the child is sounding out the word by silently producing it, and as the child holds
  the tongue position to think about the sound, the stop becomes
  the actual sound produced.
- **Deaffrication**, which occurs for the sounds represented with letters *ch* or *j*. These are complex sounds that begin by nearly stopping the airstream near the top of the mouth then end with a
  continuation of the airstream as the tongue drops. Children use
  letters that capture either stopping or continuation in their misspellings, as in /rehs/ for "reach," /wot/ for "watch," or /nasre/
  for "nature."
- **Affrication**, occurs for sounds that are represented by consonant blends in spelling, but in actual speech production are very
  close to affricates in the way they are formed. Examples in spelling are /jist/ or /jres/ for "dress," /shy/ for "say," or /chuck/
  for "truck."
- **Voicing/Devoicing,** or the substitution of one sound that is
  identical to the target sound except for the voicing feature, as in
  /tress/ for "dress"; /lidle/ for "little"; /reg/ (*g* with the same
  pronunciation as *j*) for "reach"; /sisiade/ for "society."
- **Assimilation**, which occurs when a sound in one position of a
  word is used in a consonant position in another position of the
  word, as in /kinnin/ for "kitchen"; /avive/ for "advice"; /sixsax/
  for "success."
- **Liquid Deficiency**, when a liquid sound /r/ or /l/ is omitted or
  some other sound, such as /w/, is substituted as in /buta/ for
  "butter," /bew/ for "bell."

Syllabic Simplification

Phoneme representation is just one aspect of word structure that has to be mastered in spelling. The order and appropriate number of phonemes within words also must be represented in the correct consonant and vowel sequences. Syllable structure begins to emerge in the early phonemic spellings of children, with longer words represented by more (often random) letters, and shorter words represented by only a few. As letters begin to approximate the actual consonant and vowel sequences of words, they are evident in the **semiphonetic** spellings. Just as not all features of phonemes are represented in these spellings, not all of the features of syllable structure may be present. Once again, these parallel the types of syllabic simplifications observed in younger children's misarticulations, and can be described in accord with phonological processes that relate to syllable structure (Hoffman & Norris, 1988). The most common ones seen in children's misspellings include:

- **Syllable Reduction**, when one or more of the syllables of a multisyllabic word (usually the unstressed syllable) is deleted, as in /et/ for "enter"; /spris/ for "surprise"; or /reble/ for "reasonable."
- **Cluster Reduction**, where one or more consonant members of a cluster is omitted. The reduction may retain one consonant from the cluster, or substitute a consonant with similar phonemic features, as in /mut/ for "must"; /jes/ for "dress"; or /ixlan/ for "explain."
- **Final Consonant Deletion**, or the omission of the final consonant from a syllable or word, as in /an/ for "and"; /avice/ for "advice"; /oder/ or /orde/ for "order."
- **Epenthesis**, or the insertion of a sound into a syllable or between syllables, generally resulting as the child slows or prolongs production of a syllable in an attempt to sound it out, as in /weyil/ for "will"; /deress/ for "dress"; or /orider/for "order."
- **Metathesis**, when the position of sounds or syllables is exchanged within words. This frequently occurs during the process of sounding out the spelling, as the child first writes the initial sound of the word, then the final sound, and then begins to think about sounds in the middle. The sequence in which the child thought about the sounds rather than the sequence of the actual spelling is the result, as in /muts/ for "must"; /dsres/ for "dress"; or /srpisur/ for "surprise."

Patterns of semiphonetic spelling are found in children's compositions well into high school, and even in the spellings of some adults.

Often a word will be simplified by more than one pattern so that two or more processes are applicable. Generally, the more process errors present, the less recognizable the word is to the reader, just as the word would become less intelligible to a listener in speech. Examples of spelling attempts for the word *hospital* with different numbers of process errors include /hospetl/ (no processes errors), /hopistel/ (one), /hospol/ (two), and /hoped/ (three). These patterns of spelling often comprise a high percentage of the misspellings produced by children with less flexible language systems who experience difficulty simultaneously coordinating the phonemic and syllabic aspects of orthography.

The spelling attempt /hospetl/ is not a semiphonetic spelling because all of the phonemic features of the sounds are correctly represented, and the entire syllable structure of the word is present. It is just not conventional, but rather **phonetic**. The word cannot be sounded out any further because it is complete in its representation. For greater refinement, the child has to become more aware of *conventional patterns* of spelling. The emergence of convention is seen in misspellings where the child uses an allowable orthographic pattern, but it is just not the correct one for that word. These types of spelling attempts are termed **transitional** and include misspellings such as /reech/ or /reche/ for "reach," or /natour/ or /naeture/ for "nature." Each of these spelling attempts represents refinements in the child's construction of the orthographc system, with greater awareness of conventions such as doubling vowels or using the final "e" (Gentry, 1982; Hall, 1984; Read, 1986).

Most children learn to spell a greater number of words with more complex syllabic structure and more irregular patterns of phonemic representation throughout the school years. But for many children, this refinement process is slow, and generalizations are minimal. It is important that intervention places a focus on the *child's* patterns of spelling rather than on conventional, adult spelling (Chomsky, 1979). Facilitating refinement from a child's current level enables the child to mentally construct the orthographic system as a gradual process rather than trying to rotely memorize complex orthographic patterns that do not make sense to the child and, therefore, will not be retained or used in actual composition.

■□ PATTERNS OF NONFLUID WRITING

Nonfluid or poor writing is characterized by overattention to only one aspect of writing, such as correct spelling, or an inability to coordinate all of the levels of language and motor skills that must be simultaneously produced. Like fluent reading, fluid writing involves multilevel processing of information that begins before actual writing is initiated, during the rehearsal phase, and continues throughout the final editing.

Many curricula teach writing in fragmented pieces with the assumption that children cannot be asked to compose until they have mastered prerequisite skills, such as handwriting, letter-sound correspondences, punctuation, left-to-right sentence formations, and the ability to spell an adequate vocabulary of words. This practice postpones the use of writing for meaningful composition by minimally a year, as the child rotely copies other people's words, fills in single words to complete sentences in worksheets, and punctuates sentences that are unrelated to any of the others on the page. Thus, when children do begin to write, they believe it to be an error-free process that is done in a linear, start-to-finish order. To accomplish this, they carefully choose simple sentence patterns and only use words that they can already spell, resulting in static and uncreative attempts at expression (Teale & Sulzby, 1986).

For fluid writers, writing is a process that occurs in recursive, overlapping stages that simultaneously create and evaluate. Much of the writing process is done before words are ever put on a page, during the rehearsal stage of composing. Oral discussion, drawing, examination of reference material, and idea formation and reorganization are strategies used during the *rehearsal phase* to assemble potentially relevant and useful information and to develop a focus or goal for the text. A *draft*, often in the form of an outline or flowchart, serves to select specific topics and information and leads to the selection of some level of **discourse context** in which to present the information. The *writing phase* involves the actual wording and structuring of the information into written discourse. Once the writing is a product, the *revision phase* can be used to objectively examine the text and to make decisions about points that need to be clarified, elaborated on, eliminated, or written from a different perspective. The *editing phase* refines the message to assure that the specific meaning and intention are communicated and corrects errors in form. These phases occur in cycles, rather than in linear order, as additions or refinements in one part of the text require changes in other sections (Calkins, 1986, 1991).

Writing, including composition and spelling, is developmental in the same way that language and speech are developmental. It is a meaning-making process from the creation of the idea to the selection of words to the representation in phonology in the same way that language and speech are meaning-making processes. Both reflect the active construction of a system that undergoes qualitative changes across time, rather than the rote learning of an already well-formed adult system. Both entail behaviors or patterns that would be considered "errors" if compared to the conventional adult system, but that actually represent the child's current level of organization of information across multiple levels of language. Because of the interaction across levels, one process, such as the capacity to use word order to organize ideas meaningfully, is reduced or simplified because of the amount of processing expended on another process occurring simultaneously, such as representing the words orthographically. Thus, writing must be assessed as a process, by evaluating what the child is doing as writing is attempted and by examining the interactions that occur across levels of language.

■□ ANALYSIS OF WRITING

The information included in a child's composition will be influenced by the type of contextual support provided for the writing process, including the familiarity of the topic, as well as the type of discourse structure used and the linguistic complexity of the ideas expressed. Consider the following writing samples produced by the 8½-year-old child with dyslexia profiled throughout this chapter:

THe BAs AND THe Bles ARe FuALiNg ouT THe END
(The bats and the balls are falling out   The end)

The first narrative was written in response to the same picture used to elicit the oral language sample described earlier so that a visual context was available for use in structuring the story. The story generated in writing was written in a more decontextualized style than the oral version. The referents (bats and balls) are specifically stated, as compared to the nonspecific language "all the stuff" used in the oral rendition. However, the story is even more limited in discourse structure than the oral story, consisting of only one sentence that described the main event or scene in the picture. Neither oral language nor written language was used to generate more than minimal discourse in response to this task, which did not represent a personal experience, motivating topic, or purposeful act of communication to the child.

PReA PAN is fTeiNg KAPTeMN Hook   THe END
(Peter Pan is fighting Captain Hook   The end)

In contrast, the second narrative was written in response to a request to write a story about the movie *Peter Pan*, a task that was Decontextualized-Decentered, providing no here-and-now context from which to structure the story, but which did represent a story structured for him by a movie, on a topic that was of high interest. The story that was generated was very similar to the baseball story, consisting of one sentence that described a main event or scene and containing specific referents for the actors and actions. However, he created considerable context using both oral language and an accompanying illustration, both of which he used in preparation for writing. When asked to write the story, he began by rehearsing an oral story.

> "Well, the croca um, the Peter Pan and Captain Hook were fightin' and Peter Pan was right up by the crocodile thing and it moved. And Captain Hook's hook went right in the way of the thing that was holdin' the crocodile up, and he went, 'No, get it out of here!' And he pulled it out. And the rope started breakin' and stuff, and he went, 'No, no, no!' And he ran and he ran away and the crocodile went 'vuuut,' like that."

His accompanying illustration showed Captain Hook and Peter Pan fighting with a sword, each wearing representative clothing for the characters. Thus, although the written product was minimal in discourse structure, sentence structure, and linguistic context, each dimension was more elaborated on at the prewriting stages of the writing cycle.

While interest in the topic was an important factor regarding the amount of oral and illustrated context generated by the child in response to the writing task, the amount of background knowledge and the degree to which the story was structured by others also were influential. In the third written sample, below, the child drew an elaborated picture of a bat with more detail than shown in the Peter Pan scene, but the picture showed no action and none was provided by the accompanying oral language. His written text merely labeled the drawing.

> My PikcHr LookT Leike a Biet
> (My picture looked like a bat)

When the Discourse context was simplified, consisting of a personal experience

> I HA LiTTLe RABBit. I'm LeTTiNg yuo go
> (I had little rabbit. I'm letting you go)

and an Expressive comment

> I WiNT To see Faivl Go's WasT! AND I LoVeD It.
> (I went to see Fivel Goes West! And I loved it.)

the text was more elaborated, consisting of two sentences each. Both are written in the first person. Punctuation is seen for the first time, perhaps because the two sentences created a perceived need that was not present for single sentences, or because the simpler discourse levels enabled the child to coordinate the use of punctuation. More complexity in the grammar and maintenance of noun-verb agreement was seen in the Expressive comment, which is the easiest Discourse context.

When multiple sentences were produced but the Situational and Discourse contexts were Decontextualized and Poetic, punctuation no longer appeared. Instead, run-on sentences were used, connected by "and" as in

> INDeANieA JONS iS rANiNG to HiD FoRM THe BAD Gis
> (Indiana Jones is running to hide from the bad guys
>
> AND He JOPT iN tHe YoDR   THe END
> and he jumped in the water   The end)

This story had been rehearsed in an oral discussion between the child and an adult and had been symbolized in illustration before writing was begun. It was produced as an Abbreviated Episode designating causality in the character's action. When activities immediately preceding the writing established extensive background for the topic of the space shuttle using pictures, oral discussion, Transactional text read in a group, and diagrams drawn of the shuttle, the most elaborated written story was produced, accompanied by only a minimal drawing. The child used written language to create an imagined experience and organized the events into an Ordered Sequence. All of the information consisted of simple Descriptions of actions or the sound of the shuttle.

I PaUT ON My SPSoeT AND WHT TO THe SPass ShDOL
(I put on my spacesuit and went to the space shuttle

AND WHT To SPass AND tHis is tHe SaOD
and went to space and this is the sound

iN THe SPaS SHDOL   TH TH TH !!!
in the space shuttle Th-Th-Th !!!)

The writing samples demonstrate that many aspects of composition are emerging for this child, but they cannot yet be coordinated (Ferreiro, 1986). When difficulty increased along one contextual dimension, then productions simplified along another. When time is spent establishing background information and organizing the ideas prior to writing, the writing is more elaborated in Discourse structure, grammatical structure, and Semantic complexity. The externalization of the process through oral discussion, drawing, and examination of reference materials was effective in helping the child to internalize the information needed for translation into written words.

Compare this to the story composed by the child with no language or learning disorder, written at a level of Decontextualized-Symbolic and maintaining a Poetic-Complex level of discourse. The context was familiar to the child, whose own family experienced the addition of a baby *brother* within the past year.

Once upon a time there was a family But, not an orrdinary faimily — a mushroom family. Tonight is a very speshul night because mama is going to have a baby. It is midnight. Mom woke up dad and dad woke up the rest of us. My dad told my brother who is a pig eating chips, to go and get the car. Dad told me to pick mom's clothes. All of a suden we were at the hospital waiting for the news. At 1:05 am I finally had the cutest baby sister I could ever see. Now my sister is home and were a very happy mushroom family. Exept sleeping is hard. The End.

■□ ANALYSIS OF SPELLING

Analysis of the spelling patterns produced in the seven stories written by the dyslexic child revealed that most of the words attempted were single syllable words (82%) or a single syllable root word with the present progressive /–ing/ morpheme attached (5%), resulting in only 13% of all words attempted having complex syllable structure. The seven words "the," "end," "and," "a," "is," "I," and "to" occurred with high frequency, comprising 40% of the words used in the stories, and they were always spelled conventionally. Of the remaining words, 35% were spelled conventionally, 12% transitionally, 31% phonetically, and 22% semiphonetically. These patterns demonstrate that the child has developed principles of phonetic representation and is beginning to organize patterns of orthography for vowel rules and consonant blends and digraphs.

Of the 11 words spelled semiphonetically, 2 were characterized by the process of metathesis, both occurring as a result of adding midsyllabic sounds after the final sounds had been written ("Peter," first produced PR, then the vowel added = PRea; "sound," first produced sod, then the *n* was squeezed into the middle = SNOD). Final consonant deletion occurred three times (bats = BAs, have = HA); gliding occurred once (/y/ substituted for /w/ in water = yoDR). Epenthesis, or the addition of a vowel occurred twice, as the child prolonged the syllable while sounding out the word (bles = balls, form = from). Five words failed to represent the vowels with letters.

The phonetic misspellings were highly influenced by phonetic and acoustic cues so that the element of stopping present in the /ch/ sound was captured in the spelling PikcHr, the unvoiced production of the past tense marker was represented in LookT and JOPT, and the relationship of long to short vowels was shown in the spellings of "went" as "wint," and "west" as "wast." The features of the /m/ sound were captured by the /p/ (unvoiced bilabial continuant) rendering the letter *m* phonetically unnecessary in the representation of the word "jumped" as "JOPT." The transitional spellings, such as FUALiNg or Leike, represented emerging awareness of conventional patterns such as double vowels or final "e"s to represent vowels.

Thus, while this child's spelling at first examination appears poor, on analysis it is evident that the misspellings are developmental and entirely consistent with principles of phonetic representation of sounds with letters (Ferreiro, 1986; Gentry, 1982). Although few multisyllabic words are attempted in his compositions, those words that are produced contain few syllabic simplifications. Thus, both aspects of phonological knowledge are emerging within simple words. The spelling patterns displayed by this child are immature for his age, but commensurate with the overall delay exhibited in all aspects of his writing. His enthusiasm for writing that is exhibited whenever environmental support and organization is provided suggests that much of the delay is related to a severe lack of experience with writing that would lead to further refinement.

Objective 8

Given a short topic of the child's choice that is contextualized by either a drawing or a graphic organizer, the child will write a story or text at the level of a Reactive Sequence (temporal order, cause-effect relationships) consisting of seven 4- to 6-word sentences.

Approximatoin Toward Objective	**Date Achieved**
Six sentence Ordered Sequence (4–6 words)	
Five sentence Reactive Sequence (3–5 words)	
Seven sentence Reactive Sequence (4–6 words)	

Objective 9

Given a passage written by the child as described above, the unedited text will be spelled with 80% conventional spelling, and 20% phonetic or transitional.

Approximation Toward Goal	**Date Achieved**
60% conventional, 40% phonetic or transitional	
70% conventional, 30% phonetic or transitional	
80% conventional, 20% phonetic or transitional	

■ SUMMARY

As this chapter has demonstrated, many variables affect a child's ability to successfully use language in a complex environment such as school. Assessment not only is conducted to determine the types of behaviors that the child is unable to perform, but also the contexts and variables that result in successful independent performance, the qualitative or developmental patterns that the child is exhibiting, and the contexts and strategies used by others that facilitate learning and refinement for the child. This holistic view of assessment results in conclusions about the child as a dynamic, complex learner and leads to implications for providing intervention in integrated and holistic contexts, where language can both be learned and successfully used as a tool for learning.

The holistic assessment also reveals the problems inherent in giving a diagnostic label to a child, such as "dyslexia," without considering how the child actually uses language to organize and express information in real communicative situations. Standardized testing revealed average or above performance in all language areas, while the contextualized assessment revealed characteristics of a severely inflexible language system in both oral and written modes. If the intervention plan for this "dyslexic" child focused only on the orthographic processing problems, then the range of language needs that are all contributing to poor language development and use would not be addressed. This focus on one level also isolates one cuing system from all of the others needed for fluent reading and comprehension and removes all of the cues that the child was shown to benefit from when the situational-discourse-semantic context was varied during assessment. Thus, the nature of and the implications that result from a Whole Language assessment are qualitatively different from those of skill-based assessments and represent different ways of viewing children and their learning.

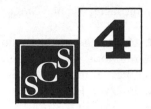

Developing Explicit Understanding of Language: Intervention for the Lower Academic Level Child

Whole language philosophy as it is implemented in the classroom encourages children to explore topics within self-directed groups. Children use oral and written language as tools for acquiring new knowledge and, in turn, acquire new vocabulary and language skills. Children with less integrated and flexible language systems, including those with learning disabilities, mental retardation, specific language disorders, hearing impairments, low achievement levels, or other developmental delays will learn in a manner consistent with Whole Language principles. However, these children must learn many of the complexities of oral and written language that their peers have easily mastered and at the same time use their current level of language to acquire and direct new learning. This chapter provides specific activities and strategies that can be used to assist these children to simultaneously acquire oral language complexities, written language abilities, and to engage in content area learning using Whole Language principles. This chapter explores

- How children learn how to learn
- Methods for establishing an effective learning environment
- Intervention strategies in oral language contexts
- Intervention strategies in the context of reading
- Intervention strategies in the context of writing

Many methods used to teach children, including methods of language intervention, focus on the identification of important skills or behaviors. Once identified, these skills are individually and sequentially taught, selected in accord with a developmental sequence or to meet an identified need. This method of teaching by definition reduces language, which is a complex and integrated system (i.e., a *whole*) into a discrete and disintegrated collection of *parts*. This makes the procedure for teaching language behaviors easy and systematic. The problem is that once language is disintegrated into parts, it is no longer language. It no longer functions as language to accomplish purposes and goals, it no longer creates shared meaning between participants, it no longer organizes a message within a coherent discourse context, and it no longer provides the user with meaningful consequences that are consistent with the language used.

For example, targeting the auxiliary verb form "is + verb + ing" and then providing 10 trials to produce the form in response to picture cards teaches the child to attend to a stimulus only long enough to say one thing about it, to shift the topic with each sentence produced, to say sentences for purposes of pleasing an adult, and to expect the words to be meaningless. If the child correctly says "The cat is sleeping," the teacher would reply "Good job," thus communicating to the child that the meaning of *what* was said was irrelevant and unimportant, as long as *how* it was said conformed to the teacher's rule. There is no comparable experience in the real world of language use, where saying "The cat is sleeping" would result in another person saying "Good job," unless they had been trying to settle down a nervous cat. In that case, saying "The cat is sleeping" would serve the meaningful function of informing the listener on the current status of the cat, and the reply would function as a grateful acknowledgment of the person's efforts to calm the animal. The difference in the two situations is the difference between Whole Language and something that is less than whole.

Teaching language in a manner consistent with Whole Language does not mean that the parts are never examined or focused on. Nor does it mean that aspects of language that teachers typically identify with the form of language are ignored, such as the structure of sentences, organization of discourse, or patterns of sounds and syllables within words. These things are part of language, and thus they are part of Whole Language. The difference is the manner in which they are examined or focused on. Some of these differences include that in Whole Language

- Parts of language are examined as they are encountered within a context, and not in isolation.
- Parts of language are examined because the examination would be useful to the child in that particular context and at that particular time.
- Learning the "part" is neither a goal nor an objective, but rather an outcome of learning about something that is meaningful and purposeful.
- Parts are not targeted for learning and, therefore, activities to teach them or situations designed to elicit them do not need to be planned.
- Language forms are viewed as organizational strategies used to effectively communicate meaning and accomplish purposes.
- Models are not provided to assist the child to produce the parts correctly, but rather to help the child discover some properties or features that will enable the child to make a change or refinement in existing knowledge.

This chapter provides specific examples of strategies that can be used to facilitate language learning in the context of exploring topics consistent with the school curriculum, such as literature, science, and history. The strategies use both auditory input, or oral language experiences, and visual input, or written language experiences, to assist the child to make simultaneous discoveries about the content, form, and use of language. In the process, the child not only acquires better language skills, but also increases reading and writing abilities, learns about the physical and social sciences, and acquires skills necessary for continued independent learning. The strategies presented in this chapter are not "Whole Language," but rather are consistent with the Whole Language philosophy. Many other techniques and strategies beyond those presented in this volume also are consistent with Whole Language. Each strategy presented in this chapter will be discussed relative to its level of complexity along the continua of the Situational, Discourse, and Semantic Contexts as discussed in the model developed in Chapter 2. The intent is not to apply these strategies rigidly, but rather to present a wide range of intervention methods that can be adapted using the model to fit the needs, purposes, and developmental levels of the participants.

The following topics related to language learning and intervention will be developed in this chapter. Beginning with a discussion of learning as it is viewed from a Whole Language perspective and ending with specific methods for facilitating language development and learning, the chapter will explore:

■ Learning how to learn
■ Creating effective learning environments
■ Providing intervention in oral contexts
■ Providing intervention in the context of reading
■ Providing intervention in the context of writing

Although the examples provided are designed for children at lower levels of academic achievement, including those at early grade levels or older students with poor oral and/or written language skills, the same strategies can be adapted upward and used with older, higher achieving children. The strategies may be implemented within a classroom or in a therapy situation, and may be adapted to large groups, small groups, or individuals.

■□ LEARNING HOW TO LEARN

Learning involves attending to the most important and relevant features of an event within a Situational Context, recognizing and organizing the information at an appropriate level of complexity within the Discourse Context, and assigning an appropriate level of meaning to information in the Semantic Context. These three dimensions of meaningful context interact within any event and determine how successfully learning will occur. These contexts refer to the amount of support for learning provided by the environment in the form of objects or other cues, the familiarity of a topic, the amount of assistance provided by adults, peers, or others in learning about that topic, the type of discourse context in which the information is embedded, and the level of abstraction at which the information is presented. Each of these factors interact to create a range of complexity at which learning can occur (Hudson & Shapiro, 1991; Purves, 1991; Sulzby & Zecker, 1991). Intervention is based on understanding the range of complexity that can be created by varying the levels at which an activity is conducted along the Situational-Discourse-Semantic continua.

For example, observation might reveal that a child is not attending to a classroom discussion, but instead sitting passively and looking out the window. When asked questions, the child asks for a repetition. This observation would suggest that the instruction is occurring at a level that is too difficult for the child to learn from, and thus attention is poor. The teacher can change the interaction in any one of (or combination of) three ways to better meet the needs of the child. The teacher may

1. reduce the level of the Situational Context by adding visual support for the language (i.e., pictures, diagrams, representative objects)
2. reduce the level of the Discourse Context by simplifying the discussion to an Ordered Sequence or other more appropriate level
3. reduce the level of the Semantic Context by providing more descriptions, pointing to things within the picture or diagram that correspond to the information talked about, and engaging the child in active participation by asking questions that require only labeling or describing, or by allowing the child to contribute comments that can then be elaborated on.

Vygotsky (1978) referred to the range at which learning can occur for any individual child in any given situation as the Zone of Proximal Development (ZPD). The ZPD represents the range of the child's mental functions, or the capability to learn when provided guided assistance. It thus represents the child's *potential* for learning and development. Vygotsky believed that this potential could either be facilitated or suppressed, depending on the types of experiences and social interactions provided by the environment.

The lower end of the ZPD refers to the actual, or completed, part of a child's development and represents the behaviors that the child can perform independently or that can be applied in a generalized manner to new situations or contexts. The grade equivalency at which reading is independent as measured by a reading inventory would be an example of this level. The upper end of the continuum refers to the maximum level at which learning can occur when there is sufficient environmental support for that learning. This support could take the form of modeling and demonstrations, instructions given in small steps, sensorimotor experiences with manipulable objects, a reduced level of language input, assistance in formulating an idea or expressing it in language, or other strategies that either reduce the complexity of the activity along the Situational, Discourse, and Semantic dimensions, or that increase the child's ability to understand and talk about information at higher levels within these continua.

■□ LEARNING WITHIN
THE ZONE OF
PROXIMAL DEVELOPMENT

Vygotsky (1978) believed that it is important to immerse children in learning experiences that are near the upper limits of their zone. When learning is directed at the lower end, or one step more advanced than child's current developmental level, then overall development is not stimulated. This level of instruction occurs when oral or written language skills are taught in accord with a developmental sequence, as, for example, when a child who is using forms or constructions at Brown's Stage IV of language development is taught those that typically emerge during Stage V (Brown, 1973), or when written word identification skills are taught in a predetermined progression. This practice serves to limit the type and level of information provided to the child, systematically eliminating opportunities for exposure to more abstract or complex aspects of knowledge and language. Any emerging tendencies toward abstraction and complexity will be suppressed because they are not reinforced or elaborated on, and they are often ignored when they do occur because they are not on the list of targeted goals and objectives.

To facilitate more abstract processing, the child requires exposure to higher level information or behaviors. Exposure to information in advance of expected emergence serves to establish a foundation for and experiences with this knowledge. By immersing children in activities that are near the upper limits of their ZPD and supported by mediation from others, as shown in the diagram below, children experience a qualitatively different way of thinking and using language. They participate in and learn something that is more advanced than their own current level of development could support. To assimilate this information into existing mental structures, the mental representations of knowledge must be reorganized in new ways that are more complex and abstract, a process called accommodation (Piaget, 1970). These new mental organizations enable a child to think about both old and new information in qualitatively different, more advanced ways, as shown by the changing relationships between the lower and upper levels of the ZPD in the diagram. Learning thus *leads* or guides the developmental process in a whole-to-part manner, as a general understanding of a more complex behavior or activity allows for a more specific and detailed level of knowledge to emerge over time.

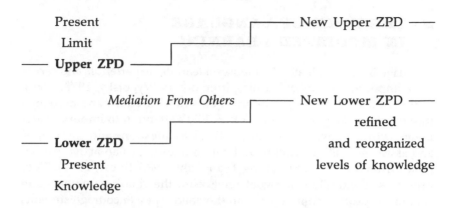

Present Limit
—— Upper ZPD ——
⌐—————— New Upper ZPD ——

Mediation From Others ⌐—————— New Lower ZPD ——
refined
—— Lower ZPD —— and reorganized
Present levels of knowledge
Knowledge

Learning that is designed to range within a child's ZPD creates a dynamic state of organization and reorganization of knowledge. This type of learning requires guidance and social interaction with others because the advanced developmental processes required for functioning at this potential level are able to operate only when the child is helped to use them through the assistance of others. Adults or more mature peers function to mediate learning for the child by providing interpretations and adding meaning to unfamiliar or confusing events. As a child attempts to solve a difficult problem, others mediate this process by asking the child leading questions, providing a model of how to do the task, or engaging in collaborative problem solving (Vygotsky, 1978). The child actively behaves at a level beyond his developmental age, so that learning actually is in advance of development.

The active participation at a level where the child can achieve success, the assistance to collaboratively engage in behaviors that the child could never experience independently, and the interpretations, elaborations, and feedback given through the mediation provided by others with greater skill all serve to enable the child to make assimilations and accommodations in existing mental structures. These higher level patterns of language and thought eventually become internalized, or reconstructed, through this process of mental reorganization. Once internalized, they become part of the child's independent developmental achievements or abilities (Vygotsky, 1978, 1986). This is seen as a qualitatively different way of approaching a task or thinking about a problem and of using language to accomplish goals and to create new concepts. This qualitative change enables the child to independently perform at higher levels along the continua of **Situational, Discourse**, and **Semantic** contexts.

■⊐ THE ROLE OF LANGUAGE
IN MEDIATED LEARNING

Language is both facilitated by mediated learning experiences and serves as an important means of learning from others (Vygotsky, 1978, 1986). In the context of formal and informal experiences, adults and more mature peers use language to direct the child's attention to important elements within an event, provide feedback to questions and comments, and assist the child in talking and communicating as an active participant within the context (Collins, 1986; Lehr, 1985; Snow, 1972). They provide semantically contingent remarks to the child's comments and wait for or prompt comments from the child. They encourage students within a classroom to generate questions for each other and to facilitate cooperation in answering the questions or seeking additional information (Hillocks, 1986). They help the child become aware of misconceptions by focusing on what is known and not known. They help to refine existing information and expand oral language abilities. They ask questions to focus the child's attention on relevant information or to ensure that the child comprehends important facts (Cazden, 1983; Martinez, 1983), and they provide elaborations and expansions on both the implicit and explicit meaning surrounding actions or events (Raphael, 1986).

The communicative assistance provided by facilitative adults and peers has been referred to as **scaffolding**, initially by Bruner (1978) in the context of learning in young children and later applied by Lehr (1985) to the context of instructional scaffolding that can be used within classroom discussions. Scaffolding allows the child to use language at a higher level of decontextualization, discourse structure, and semantic complexity than could be independently accomplished. Through scaffolding, adults or peers initially provide a relatively high degree of verbal structure that supports attempts made by the child to communicate an idea or to structure some level of discourse. As the child becomes increasingly capable of communicating and organizing information more independently, the adult provides progressively less assistance, until finally the child has internalized the structures that allow for complete independence.

> **Scaffolding Strategies Used To Mediate Learning**
> ■ Direct attention to important elements
> ■ Provide feedback to questions and comments
> ■ Assist child to talk and communicate
> ■ Provide semantically contingent remarks

> - provide child with time and prompts
> - Encourage peer teaching and cooperative learning
> - Assist child to formulate questions
> - Engage child in active problem solving
> - Provide elaborations and expansions
> - Model both implicit and explicit meaning
> - Provide progressively less assistance

Scaffolding serves as a mechanism to facilitate changes in both language and thought. Through the actual use of the language, and the active process of reorganization that occurs as the child is helped to make sense of the complex ideas, the language itself is learned (Bruner, 1978; Lehr, 1985; Nelson, 1985, 1991). At the same time, the language used in the context of the activity or discussion helps the child to attend to important elements and to organize the content of the discourse in ways that draw comparisons, highlight contradictions, or refer to order and causality. The language thus serves as an instrument for reorganizing thought in a manner that is qualitatively more abstract and critical (Vygotsky, 1978, 1986). As new schemes and strategies emerge, the child can approach difficult tasks using language to search for a new plan and to independently direct activities without relying on the mediation provided by others (Nelson, 1992).

▪️⌐ ESTABLISHING AN EFFECTIVE LEARNING ENVIRONMENT

The goal of language facilitators is to help children learn about the world through the use of language and to use language to control or influence their world. It is simultaneously a social and cognitive process. To be effective facilitators, we must establish a learning environment and a curriculum for children that assists them in the meaning-making process and provides social opportunities to learn from and to influence others. Ken Goodman (1986) writes that language is easy to learn when it is real and natural, when it is not fragmented into parts such as a lesson on verbs or the /s/ sound, when it makes sense to the learner, is interesting and relevant, has social utility and purpose, and the learner has both the choice and power to use it. This means that the adult cannot choose for the child what language to learn or use on any worksheet or language picture card or within any activity or story. The adult can only make language accessible to the child so that the child can experiment with the words or ideas that make sense, and refer to events or ideas that are interesting and motivating.

This type of learning environment is the goal of Whole Language. Whole Language represents a philosophy of learning, and not a method or curriculum. There is no one "right way" to establish an effective learning environment that is equivalent to Whole Language. Rather, the methods, activities, strategies, or curricula are interpretations of the underlying philosophy. The specific methods and curricula that are implemented will depend on a myriad of factors, such as whether intervention takes place in the regular classroom or in a small group, whether the classroom operates under principles of Whole Language or a more traditional model, the resources that can be committed to a child's program, including time, personnel, and materials, and the opportunities for collaboration between professionals and between the child and his peers. However, general principles will be apparent in a Whole Language learning environment, whether that situation is a regular classroom or a small group of children specifically seen for intervention.

Characteristics of a Whole Language Environment

Learning is a process of actively constructing knowledge about the world, including information about the physical and social environment, and the logical systems such as language or math that allow for order to be imposed on experience. This process of assimilating new information into existing knowledge and making accommodations in mental structures to account for differences takes time and frequent exposure to similar information. This is true for all learners, but it is particularly true for children with less flexible language systems who have difficulty learning the logical operations of language and using language to interpret the world once it is acquired. When providing children with an effective learning environment, it is important to remember that *less quantity* often results in *more learning* with greater quality. There are many factors that fall within the domain of "less" quantity. These include:

◼️ *Fewer topics to simultaneously explore*. In a traditional curriculum, each content area has its own agenda and disparate topics, while in Whole Language the curriculum is integrated, so that if a question about the politics of South America is explored, then the current and previous history of the area is examined in social studies, the ecological issues involving the plants and animals of South America are studied in science, the culture is examined by reading South American literature in English, and South American painting is emulated in art. Even these subject area boundaries are eliminated in classrooms where one person teaches across the curriculum.

■ *Fewer writing assignments are made.* Instead, children are given the time to rehearse, compose, and edit a single, refined composition designed to reflect on or report on what was learned, rather than a series of hurriedly completed papers.

■ *Fewer pages are covered in a reading assignment.* Reducing the amount that is read provides time for oral discussion and critical evaluation to occur, with the goal of learning from the literature, rather than "getting through it" in order to move on to the next assignment.

■ *Instruction is directed at fewer skills or patterns of language.* Instead of addressing all skills in accord with some textbook designed scope and sequence, specific patterns are addressed when there is a need for them in a meaningful context of language use. If a specific skill is not problematic to a child, then errors involving that pattern, such as reading miscues or spelling errors, will not occur frequently and so time is not spent addressing it. If a skill or language pattern is a problem, then difficulties will occur with high frequency in the context of speaking, reading, and writing, and there will be many naturally occurring opportunities to focus attention on that pattern.

■ *Less complexity along one or more dimensions* of Situational, Discourse, or Semantic context is presented to facilitate understanding of some higher level skills along another dimension.

In other words, the goal is to teach children, rather than curricula. By addressing fewer topics over a longer period of time, children have the opportunity to reconstruct and reorganize the same information at higher levels of abstraction and complexity. All of the skills that are considered important to school achievement are acquired, but with greater depth of understanding and flexibility of use. This is true for all learners, but it is particularly true for children with less flexible language systems who require time and socially mediated experiences to interconnect information within and across all of the many levels of context.

Creating Networks of Concepts and Language

Learning that is useful in accomplishing purposes and generalizing to new situations is not organized as isolated bits of information, but rather in interconnected networks. For example, you could learn that

Asia is a continent
China is a country
Rice is grown in China
Old rulers were called Mandarins
China has the largest population
South China contains the Red Basin
The writing system is pictographic
Many languages are spoken
Many families are poor

This information is random, and to remember it, each fact would need to be memorized and is likely to be quickly forgotten. But when relationships of meaning, or interconnected networks are established between the facts, the information becomes meaningful, as in:

China is a country in the Asian continent that has the largest population of any country. Because of the large population, many families are poor and eat a diet of rice which is grown where the climate is hot enough in the Red Basin of southern China. Each area of China speaks its own language, and so to communicate with each other they have developed a pictographic writing system that does not depend on any one language.

When the networks with all of the interconnected relationships of meaning are established, the information is usable and generalizable. Other countries can be compared for location, population, economy, language, and writing systems. These types of meaningful comparisons help a child to develop a scheme for the kind of information that is important and how it might be organized. Once developed, the scheme can be used to interpret other, related information. The scheme also can be used to recall the content information about China, since these facts are not merely stored randomly in memory, but rather are part of the logical network that they helped to form. Thus, two types of information are learned and networked, that is, the specific content or world knowledge about China and the more generalizable logical structure or scheme for interpreting and organizing geographic information meaningfully.

Language exists and develops within the same types of interconnected networks. It does not emerge by learning the names for isolated objects, one at a time until sufficient vocabulary exists for word combinations to appear. Rather, language emerges from within complex interconnected events, such as daily routines (Nelson, 1991). Words initially refer to the entire meaning of the event, including the actions and intentions related to the object, and only gradually begin to acquire more specific, adult meanings (Carey, 1982). Adults facilitate this learning by focusing the child's attention on specific objects or actions when they are relevant within the routine and talking about them. Thus, from the whole event, the specific objects and the words used to talk about them and their related actions begin to *parse* out from the whole.

This can be visualized as a tree growing from a seed, to steal an analogy from Yetta Goodman (1980). What is seen is the tree (i.e., a new word), but what is not as apparent is the complex root system or network that supports the tree (word) and allows it to emerge. As a concept is parsed from the whole event and is represented in language, it maintains its interconnection to all of the other concepts related to the event. However, most concepts are not specific to just one event, but rather overlap across many. Thus, they have a root system, or network, that crosses boundaries between experiences or events. Thus, the concept parses away from the direct experience as something that is part of each of the events from which it formed, but also separate from and more abstract than any one event. The network supporting the concept becomes more complex, interrelated across many situations and many events.

Creating Semantic Concepts

As concepts become more abstract, they are increasingly created from the linguistic representations themselves. Concepts that do have an experiential base, such as "toys," "turns," and "grabbing" are recombined in a new way to form the more abstract concept of "sharing." Sharing is recombined with "good" and "equal" to form "fair"; fair is recombined with "reasonable" and "justice" to form "equitable"; equitable is recombined with "absence of bias" to form "impartial," and so forth. Each shares with the others links within the network that created them, and allow them to be used in a flexible manner within a variety of contexts where they may never have been experienced or heard.

toys + turns =

sharing + equal =

fair + reasonable =

equitable + ? =

Thus, the interrelated network enables the word to be used to represent concepts in a flexible and variable manner. The network acts as an enormous interconnected web of information that itself is inseparably interconnected to the linguistic representations that can be used to refer to these concepts. The more links between elements of the network, the easier a word is to retrieve for use in a wider variety of contexts. When the interrelated network is weakly linked, then there is limited flexibility and variability in the possible connections between concepts and their linguistic representations. The child struggles to find words to represent the meaning in context, as seen by the production of fillers, nonspecific vocabulary, false starts, and other linguistic nonfluencies, as exhibited by the child with dyslexia profiled in Chapter 3.

The goal of intervention is to build interconnected networks of concepts and their linguistic representations, rather than to teach discrete skills, facts, or linguistic behaviors. From these networks, refinement and complexity occur as a process and can be seen in the outcomes or products, including more vocabulary with greater abstraction, longer utterances with more strategies for combining ideas in grammatically complex ways, longer monologues with greater organization and complexity in discourse structure, more organizational schemes for functioning within a wider variety of contexts, and more world and social knowledge that can serve as a background for interpreting new information in more elaborated and generalizable ways.

■□ CREATING AN EFFECTIVE LEARNING ENVIRONMENT

Effective learning environments are designed to help the child develop interconnected networks of concepts and language. The learning environments themselves must be interconnected and meaningful, with numerous opportunities for language use and development. Whether the physical environment is a classroom or a small group of children in a therapy room, the learning environment should maximize opportunities to refine knowledge by establishing variable and flexible relationships of meaning between concepts and their linguistic representations. To accomplish this, several characteristics should be present within the organization of learning, including thematic organization, redundant organization, whole-to-part refinement, and social collaborative organization.

■□ THEMATIC ORGANIZATION OF LEARNING

Thematic organization involves the use of language to explore a topic from many different perspectives. The topic maintains continuity within and across days, so that new information and language are continuously integrated into overlapping networks of prior knowledge about the topic. It provides a context for exploring content knowledge and developing oral and written language skills in a manner that continuously focuses on refining meaning. Content knowledge is integrated so that science, math, natural, physical, and social sciences, reading, and writing often occur simultaneously within the same activity, and exploration in one area is done to inform or elaborate on another area. Integrated, interactive experiences with a topic are explored to help children achieve integrated ways of thinking about the world and interactive levels of Poetic, Expressive, and Transactional discourse structures for talking about and organizing experience.

Thematic organization exists along a continuum from adult-designed theme units to child-directed theme cycles (Edelsky, Altwerger, & Flores, 1991). At one end of the continuum, the teacher chooses the topics and uses them to teach information in each of the content areas, so that spelling words, art projects, literature selections, and writing assignments all are integrated into the curriculum and used to teach subjects or skills. For example, each content area focuses on the topic of the Amazon forest and studies elements of the culture and geography of that area. Activities are chosen because they teach targeted goals and are consistent with a topic, with the focus on learning content knowledge and skills.

At the other end of the continuum, theme cycles begin by involving the children in generating a question or questions about a topic, starting with information that they already know. For example, the question might be "Why is the Amazon forest being cleared, and what are the positive and negative effects?" The subsequent explorations of the topic are then conducted to answer that question. Generally, in the process of trying to answer one question, other issues or questions arise that require exploration to fully understand the problem. This results in the exploration of a chain of subtopics that unfold in cycles of questions and answers, driven by the need for more information to understand the original issue. The focus is on learning how to learn, and the skills and content knowledge are viewed as *outcomes* of the learning, but not the goal or process of learning itself.

The level along the continuum at which themes are used by a speech-language pathologist or other special service provider will depend on many factors, including whether intervention is classroom based or pull-out, the degree of independence exhibited by the child, the amount of time available for explorations of a topic, and the needs of the child (see Table 4–1). However, thematic learning is critical to the child with a less flexible language system who is less capable of networking information and generalizing information than peers. If information is not organized as an integrated part of a larger, meaningful network, then any learning that occurs is likely to remain disconnected, therefore reinforcing the inflexibility already exhibited by the child. More information may be acquired because it was taught, but the child is not helped to learn how to learn and does not have a more elaborated network in which to embed and compare new experiences.

Topic-Centered Theme Cycles

There are many options for selecting the type of service delivery that will be provided for children with less flexible language systems and the themes used in intervention. Table 4–1 profiles many of these options.

TABLE 4-1
Choices that govern the type of intervention provided.

1. Determine the most appropriate **model** for service delivery

| •Regular classroom | •Self-contained classroom | •Pull-out of classroom |

2. Determine the most appropriate **role** in service delivery

| •Consultation with teacher | •Team teaching with regular or Special Education Teacher(s) | •Direct service provision |

3. Determine the most appropriate **grouping** of children

| •Individualized assistance within classroom | •Small group within classroom | •Small group outside of classroom |

4. Determine the most feasible **time** schedule

| •Intensive short-term blocks | •Short Periods several times weekly | •Variable time scheduling |

5. Determine the most appropriate **Theme Unit or Cycle**

| •Topic-centered | •Narrative-centered |
| •Classroom curriculum content | •Developmentally appropriate content |

6. Determine the appropriate **level of material or activity** along the Situational-Discourse-Semantic continua

| •Language level | •Reading level | •Interest level |

Any combination from this table is possible, so that after the first decision is made to provide intervention in the regular classroom, for example, the second decision could be to provide these services by consulting with the classroom teacher, or by going into the classroom on a regular basis and providing direct services there. Many of the decisions in Table 4-1 will be governed as much by circumstance as by best practices (i.e., caseload size, classroom curriculum, other service delivery team members), so flexibility and collaboration with others to develop the best program possible is important. Models for helping to make these service delivery decisions can be found in Secord (1990) and Secord and Wiig (1991).

Current practices suggest that one of the best contexts for providing language intervention is the child's regular classroom (Nelson, 1989; Secord, 1990; Simon, 1987). If the child's regular environment is a Whole Language classroom, then scaffolded interactions, **including any of the strategies discussed in this book** can be used within the classroom setting to develop oral and written language abilities. The interventionist can work with individuals or small groups of children to develop language using materials from any content area, such as literature, social sciences, or physical sciences. Intervention can be provided by working collaboratively with a child to address a topical question, issue, or problem selected by the child, the teacher, or a group of peers. Intervention can be implemented in the form of direct services provided within the classroom, or indirect services provided through modeling and consultation with the teacher, an aide, and/or peers working on the same problem. The greater the number of individuals who understand how to facilitate language learning in context, the greater the benefits will be to the child, so obviously collaboration and team efforts are encouraged.

Unfortunately, not all classrooms are receptive to or conducive to classroom-based intervention. Scheduling complications also may preclude implementation of this type of service delivery. Thus, a second option is to ascertain what topics will be covered in the classroom during the semester and to select and develop a theme to pursue with the children from these topics. While not ideal, the advantages are that the children will have considerable background knowledge for understanding that topic when it is encountered in the classroom and will, therefore, perform better in the class for that specific content. More importantly, the real goals of theme-based intervention are to enable children to learn *how* to learn, and these strategies and skills are generalizable to all classroom content. The goals of improved problem-solving strategies and higher level oral and written language abilities will facilitate more independent learning across all content areas and topics. Furthermore, many teachers are willing to contract with a child for individualized learning projects and will substitute this work for other classroom requirements, thus lessening the child's burden of attempting to keep up with the classroom assignments as well as those specific to intervention.

Many special service providers, such as speech-language pathologists or special education resource teachers, serve large caseloads of children distributed across many schools, grade or age levels, classrooms, and ability levels. Classroom service delivery, or even classroom content-based themes may not be realistic options because of the heterogeneous population of children that must be served in any one setting. Thus, a third option is heterogeneous grouping across grade levels, where the same theme is simultaneously developed at more than one level, but within the Zone of Proximal Development (ZPD) for all group members.

All grade levels teach much of the same curriculum, but at more sophisticated and detailed levels of information with increasing grades. For example, dinosaurs, the weather, life cycles of plants and animals, the solar system, United States and world geography, and political systems are all topics that are covered in almost every grade from kindergarten through high school. The same topic or problem can be addressed in a group of children at heterogeneous grade and ability levels through oral discussions and use of materials where the interactions are focused at lower Situational, Discourse, and Semantic levels for the less mature learners and at higher levels for others. The more mature learners in effect provide the less mature with exposure to the more abstract elements of the problem, or the upper limits of their ZPD, while at the same time much of the learning in the group specifically focuses on the needs of the less advanced child.

A fourth option may be chosen if the content or level of the material presented in the regular classroom is developmentally inappropriate to the learning needs of the children served. Many children with less flexible language systems exhibit a wide range of language and learning problems by the middle elementary grades. Their reading level may be two or more grade levels below the materials presented in their textbooks, their poor oral and written language skills may have resulted in limited acquisition of world, scientific, or cultural knowledge needed to interpret grade-level text, and their language abilities may be significantly delayed compared to the language encountered in the curriculum. In this case, the classroom curriculum would be above the child's ZPD and, therefore, too difficult to learn or benefit from.

Any topic that is interesting and motivating to these group members could serve to provide the basis for a theme. The theme may or may not be directly related to classroom content for any group member. Since the goal of Whole Language intervention is to *learn how to learn*, and not to acquire discrete skills or facts, the content presented is largely arbitrary, with no one topic being inherently better than another. The goal of intervention is to increase the child's ability to use language with greater sophistication and refinement. The objectives are to increase oral or written language abilities to be closer to the upper limits of the child's ZPD. Learning specific skills or facts would be included among the many *outcomes* of intervention.

The goals and objectives of Whole Language intervention should not be confused with outcomes. When the outcomes, or *products* are placed before learning how to learn, or the *process*, then discrete skill targeting and teaching becomes the focus. It is sometimes tempting to adopt a tutoring role, teaching the skills or information that a classroom teacher expects the child to respond to on a test. However, since this form of tutoring does not facilitate change in the child's language system and does not help to form the networks of information needed to support the use of language for problem solving and other critical and creative functions, it results only in short-term learning. The child becomes a passive learner who is increasingly dependent on others for tutoring — an undesirable pattern of learned helplessness.

Instead, strategies for learning how to learn, such as note taking, using reference materials, searching for needed information in a text, developing a topic with supporting facts or events, establishing goals and plans, and organizing information into logical categories and structures (i.e., language at the higher levels of the Situational-Discourse-Semantic continua) can be acquired in the context of any theme that focuses on meaningful and motivating content. As these strategies are learned, the child can be helped to apply them to the content of the classroom curriculum. Thus, it is critical that these long-term language learning goals and objectives remain the focus of intervention, rather than learning discrete skills or facts to temporarily enhance performance on worksheets or tests. The needs of the child should dictate the curriculum, including the type and level of materials used, rather than some arbitrary scope and sequence dictated by a textbook or teacher's guide.

Narrative-Centered Theme Cycles

All of the thematic approaches described above have represented **topic-centered** theme cycles, where discourse along the Transactional dimension was used to focus the theme. A fifth option is to use **narrative-centered theme** cycles (Norris, 1992a; Norris & Damico, 1990; Norris & Hoffman, 1992a). Narrative-centered themes are constructed around a single book or story, with episodes or concepts important to the understanding of the story used to develop the theme. For example, on the first day of a theme unit using the book *The Hungry Giant* (Cowley, 1990f), the cover page can be used as the focus, with all topics explored on that day designed to enhance understanding of the concepts related to that page. In this book, a picture of the giant on the cover page can be examined and discussed, including concepts of size, shape, color, number, comparison, action, interpretations of facial expressions or states, predictions, evaluations, and so forth. Throughout that day, all other experiences would be related to the concept of giants, including reading *Jack and the Beanstalk* (Moon, 1988b), experiencing gianthood by using miniature dishes and equipment for real purposes, reading *Bogle's Feet* (Cowley, 1989a) about a giant's huge feet, followed by designing large feet in art and practicing walking in them using giant steps, and studying facts about growing using the book *It Takes Time To Grow* (Cutting & Cutting, 1988d), followed by recording each child's length at birth compared to their current height.

Thus, in narrative-centered themes, Poetic Discourse serves to coordinate the learning within the theme, and Transactional Discourse is used to develop the background of scientific, historical, and cultural knowledge needed to understand the story at increasing levels of complexity. Expressive Discourse is used to relate the experiences of the characters to personal experience and response. The activities described above would provide many experiences along the Contextualized end of the Situational Context, including reading and discussing several factual and fictional books written with a wide variety of Poetic and Transactional Discourse structures. Many outcomes from numerous content area domains would result from these interactions, such as measurement skills, addition and subtraction facts, the ability to read charts and graphs, knowledge of the life cycle and the factors that contribute to growth and change, knowledge of spatial orientation, fine and gross motor skills such as drawing, cutting, and balance, following directions, critical listening, active problem solving, critical observation, knowledge of discourse structure, print awareness including word and letter recognition and the language used to refer to the content, the pragmatic interactions between participants, and all of the many concepts and subskills inherent in each of these activities.

On the second day of the unit, the information examined on the first day is reviewed, and a new page(s) representing the beginning of the story is introduced. In this story, the giant makes demands and threatens the townspeople, yelling

> "I want some bread!" roared the giant. "Get me some bread, or I'll hit you with my bammy-knocker."

On this day, the concept of a bully could be explored, including the children's personal experiences with one and things that can be done if you encounter a bully. Role play modeling how a bully would act versus constructive ways to deal with problems or conflict can be enacted and written about. These activities provide experiences at the Decontextualized end of the Situational Context, with discussion serving to assist children to Semantically make inferences and generate evaluations. Many outcomes related to writing, personal expression, problem solving, pragmatic uses of language to influence the behaviors of others in problematic social situations and so forth would result.

On the third day, the giant demands butter from the townspeople, and the efforts that they expend to make him enough can be examined. The process of making butter, from initially milking the cow to the importance of refrigeration, can be explored in a variety of activities. Butter can be made by the group, flavoring part of the batch with honey versus apples for taste comparison. Once again, information from many content areas (e.g., science, nutrition, psychology, geography), as well as many levels of oral and written language learning along the Situational-Discourse-Semantic dimensions would result. On the fourth day, the giant demands honey, and so bees are studied extensively, including their ability to make honey. Their community structure, communication system, and respective jobs within the community are studied and compared to the classroom community.

On the fifth day, the townspeople "looked everywhere for honey" but were unable to find it. On this day, the home, or the hive of the bee is studied, and children try to construct a honey comb either emulating the geometric pattern of the bees or experimenting with shapes of their own. Additionally, places where the townspeople might look are explored by looking at different animal and insect homes, using books such as *Who Lives in this Hole?* (Williams, 1990b), *Underground* (Williams, 1990a), and *The Tree* (Cutting & Cutting, 1988h). The theme unit continues until the book is completed, or longer if the group members choose to continue to explore related topics. In the process, learning from all content areas and all language domains occurs.

Narrative-centered themes provide a means of exploring a variety of different topics in a manner that integrates them within a whole. They are designed in particular to facilitate language and literacy development, following principles found to enhance learning in normal development such as repeated readings of the same book. Repeated readings across long periods of time, often extending across several weeks, enable the children to internalize more about the concepts and the Situational-Discourse-Semantic dimensions of the language of the book with each examination. With each reexamination, the children bring a more extensive network of concepts and language that can be independently used to interpret the picture and text. This foundation allows for more abstract levels of the Semantic context to be verbalized, such as evaluating whether a person who is bigger and stronger than others should take advantage of his size. It also allows for more attention to be directed at Metalinguistic levels of language, such as analysis of the print for letter-sound correspondences, syllable structure, or conventions of capitalization and punctuation. Specific strategies for developing Metalinguistic awareness of written language in the context of repeated readings will be provided later in this chapter.

Advantages of Narrative-Centered Themes

The gradual reconstruction of the story across time enables children to begin to internalize the narrative structure of the story (i.e., Discourse Context), and through retelling, to learn how to express more organized and detailed information with greater displacement and independence from pictures (i.e., Situational Context) (Norris, 1992a). It provides a naturally occurring context for learning to use world and scientific knowledge to interpret and expand on experience (i.e., Semantic Context). It enables even the poorest readers to experience fluent reading, and it provides a sufficient scaffold for them to begin to discover how print functions to communicate meaning and internalize the patterns and form of print. It thus serves as a strategy for addressing multiple levels of language needs for children with less flexible language systems simultaneously, and it provides a mechanism for maintaining continuity across intervention sessions. It provides a naturally occurring context for learning how to reorganize the same information at different levels of summarization and how to link ideas or events across transformations of time and location, as the old information related to the story is reestablished before a new episode or event is introduced. All of these abilities are critical to successful performance in any academic content area.

The narrative-centered themes can themselves be embedded within larger themes (see Table 4–2). For example, *The Hungry Giant* (Cowley, 1990f) was one of five narrative-based units within the larger theme of "Self and Home" that was implemented over a 3-month period in an at-risk kindergarten program (Norris & Hoffman, 1991). Within this large theme unit, the first book, *Grumpy Elephant* (Cowley, 1990b), was used to introduce the general concept of moods, feelings, and self-expression; *The Hungry Giant* (Cowley, 1990f) explored the concepts of empowerment and control, as well as community structure and function; *Little Pig* (Melser, 1981) provided experiences with self-identity within the community, including developing independence, role within the family and

TABLE 4–2
Theme units in kindergarten curriculum.

Community and World

[August	September	September	October]
STOP!	WHO WILL BE MY MOTHER?	BOO HOO	HAIRY BEAR
Farm	Farm	Animals	Crime
Farm Animals	Family Roles	Problem	Police
Farm Vehicles	and Structure	Solving	Safety
Community	Other Cultures	Cause-Effect	Fear
Helpers	and Societies	Buy-Trade	Problem
City Vehicles	Animal Care	Happy/Sad	Solving
Community	and Habitats		
Problems			

Holidays and Customs

[October	November	November	December]
MONSTERS PARTY	MEANIES	JIGAREE	ONE COLD NIGHT
Halloween	Friends	Thanksgiving	Seasons
Fear	Other Countries	Other People	Weather
Celebration	Other Customs	and Customs	Clothing
Talents	Animals from	Solar System	Shelter
Customs	Other Countries	Friends	Animal
			Adaptation

Self and Home

[January	January	February	February	March]
GRUMPY ELEPHANT	HUNGRY GIANT	LITTLE PIG	TO TOWN	OBADIAH
Moods and	Empowerment	Home	Home	Senses
Feelings	and Control	Safety	Town	Vision
Self-Concept	Communities	Defiance	Travel	Movement
Self-Expression	People	Independence	Vehicles	Taste
	Animals	Communication	Maps	Touch
Responsibility	Cooperation	Role within	Geography	Sound
Civil Rights	Learning a	Community	Mardi Gras	Smell
	Lesson			

(continued)

TABLE 4-2 *(continued)*

Weather and Environment			
[March	**April**	**April**	**May]**
MRS. WISHY WASHY	*TOO BIG FOR ME*	*RED ROSE*	*IF YOU MEET A DRAGON*
Seasons and Weather	Life Cycles Insects	Life Cycles Plants	Dinosaurs Reptiles
Rain and Mud	Spiders	Prey and	Jungle
Cleaning	Defenses	Predators	Swamp
Bathing and Hygiene	Size Easter	Colors Chain	Ecology
Health		Reactions	

community, and communications: the book *To Town* (Cowley, 1983a) explored travel and transportation near to and far from home; and the unit ended with *Obadiah* (Melser & Cowley, 1990b), which provided a narrative theme from which to explore the senses and how they are used to learn from and function within the environment.

Narrative-centered themes can be used with any age or ability level, following the same principles. For example, the story *Old Nelson Godon* (Jones, 1986), written at a fourth-grade level of difficulty, begins with the introduction of one of the famous Maracas bulls of Trinidad named Old Nelson Godon. This setting could be explored on the first day of the unit by studying Trinidad, locating the mountain range and rivers that identify the Maracas Valley, and exploring the geography, culture, and bulls of the region, thus establishing the setting for the story. Pictures, maps, globes, and models could be used to provide Situationally Contextualized examples of the highly Decontextualized-Symbolic information (i.e., another country, another part of the world, another culture) presented in the story. The elaborated discussion and Contextualized experiences would enable the children to include Erudite meanings in their interpretations of the sentences as they are read and discussed. Reading with children in this manner teaches children to *expect* and desire this level of meaning and background when they read and immerse themselves in the use of strategies to acquire the necessary knowledge. Through this immersion, the strategies become internalized, and the children become increasingly more able to apply them independently.

On the second day, the initiating event is introduced, that is, Old Nelson (who "thought a lot of himself") declares himself to be king of the other animals. On this day, issues such as empowerment, prejudice, and control can be examined, including how the children experience these in their own lives and how they are manifested in the national and world cultures, thus expanding the Semantic interpretations to include more implicit and Erudite levels of meaning. The combination of the Poetic Discourse of the book, the Transactional Discourse used to discuss topics such as empowerment and prejudice, and the Expressive Discourse used as the children make generalizations to their own lives enables the participants to integrate these different ways of thinking and talking into a coherent whole perspective on a topic.

On the third day, the Spider Monkey, Tigercat, and Boa Constrictor each reject Old Nelson as ruler and specify what actions they will take to avoid his control. Concepts such as civil disobedience and protest over political suppression can be discussed relative to strategies, historical movements, and current events (i.e., Erudite meaning). On the fourth day, Old Nelson seized power over the weaker, less aggressive animals of the plains, and used his power to keep all of the best grass, shade trees, and ponds for himself. The difference between carnivorous and herbivorous animals could be studied and compared with flowcharts or other graphic organizers (thus reducing the level of the discussion from Decontextualized to Contextualized-Logical) to understand why Old Nelson was able to gain control over the herbivores but not the carnivores. Parallels to the struggle over environmental resources conducted by humans can be drawn (Poetic to Transactional comparisons). Once again, this narrative-centered theme could continue until the book is completed, providing the older child with all of the advantages of repeated readings and story-focused topic integration for language learning across Situational, Discourse, and Semantic contexts.

Language and Theme-Centered Learning

Thematic organization is a property of the language system itself. Language is structured within sentences that establish relationships of temporal and spatial sequence, causality, conditionality, exclusion, inclusion, negation, or contradiction between semantic elements; discourse establishes the same types of relational ties across and between sentences to create unified text; discourse is structured within a situation that itself maintains continuity of topic. If our goal is to facilitate well structured and coherent language development and use in children, then the information that we present to them for learning should have these properties.

The practice of systematically teaching discrete language or academic skills lacks each of the above properties. It disintegrates the whole into parts, without providing the child with a context in which to embed them, or a scaffold to understand how the aspects of the whole fit within the unified whole. Thus, although it is tempting to teach short-term, discrete skills to achieve some superficial outcome, especially if the time available for providing intervention is short, the benefits are limited and contradictory to the manner in which language is intrinsically structured and used.

Themes can be used no matter how limited the time for intervention. In fact, the less frequently sessions occur, or the less amount of time that is spent in intervention, the more important the continuity within and between sessions. Themes provide this continuity by exploring the same topic, integrating new ideas and concepts with those previously established, using many of the same and additional materials in both familiar and novel ways. Themes allow for a foundation to be established that is then elaborated on and refined across increasingly more complex dimensions of Situational, Discourse, and Semantic contexts. Themes provide for the same language to be used to accomplish multiple goals at different levels of meaning across time. Even if the intervention time with a child is minimal, the learning that occurs can be maximized through the use of themes.

■□ REDUNDANT ORGANIZATION OF LEARNING

A second characteristic of an effective learning environment is the principle of redundant organization. Redundancy is very different from repetition, or the presentation of the same information in the same way until it is overlearned sufficiently as to not be forgotten. Redundancy means that the same information is encountered numerous times, but in slightly different ways or in slightly different contexts each time. In each encounter there will be an overlap of information and skill, but many differences in application, content, knowledge, and levels at which the information is considered. From this myriad of experiences that are simultaneously familiar and unique, the learner develops highly generalized concepts that are networked to an almost infinite array of different concepts and behaviors. The language related to the topic and the potential pragmatic uses of this language for the learner is highly refined and flexible in utility. It can be used Semantically to label, describe, attribute characteristics, draw inferences, create metaphors, or analyze a situation. In Discourse, the language can be used to organize the information to express Transactional, Expressive, or Poetic functions. Situationally, the language can be used to refer to ongoing Contextualized events, or to create hypothetical Decontextualized situations.

Redundancy Within a Theme

For example, when attempting to address the issue of clearing the forests of the Amazon, the book *Forests Forever* (Walker, 1992b) can be used to help the children to become aware of the many perspectives on this issue. First, the changes that occur within the environment when forests are cleared, including erosion, can be explored. The different types of trees, including deciduous and conifers, can be studied to determine how they help to prevent erosion. The effects of erosion, including floods and poor soil, can be considered in relationship to the types of plants that can no longer grow. The importance of these plants and trees for food, medicine, and shelter can be studied, balanced against how the consumption of these plants and trees for these purposes contributes to the clearing of the forests. Through the exploration of overlapping topics from different perspectives, the same concepts, information, and language will be repeatedly encountered in a manner that is redundant rather than repetitious.

Similarly, the same information can be explored using different symbolic systems and means. The differences between deciduous and coniferous trees can be explored by reading Transactional text, creating a mural for purposes of organizing and exemplifying the differences discovered by the child's research, writing about some aspect of the topic as a method for sharing, integrating and internalizing the information, drawing to scale differences in tree leaves and needles, and reading narratives that reflect individual and cultural attitudes toward and uses of trees. Thus, the same information about a topic will be explored and expressed through oral and written language, Transactional text, Poetic expression, art, graphic representation, and writing. The redundancy across these different means of expressing the same information provides the child with the experiences needed to enable the concepts to parse out as something that is a generalized concept, more abstract than any of the individual contexts from which it evolved, while remaining attached to each of them. In other words, displacement and complexity are developed within the network.

Redundancy Within Language

Redundancy is important to the development of a flexible language system and is, in fact, a property of language (Brown, 1973). The language contains expressions of this redundancy, including syntactic structures and vocabulary that serve as cohesive ties. A text, whether it be Transactional, Expressive, or Poetic Discourse, by definition is any unit of language that has *unity,* or continuity between the ideas expressed so that the text hangs together around some recognizable topic. The text maintains *coherence* through linguistic strategies that enable reference to be made to repeated or redundant information.

The eight levels of complexity along the Discourse Continuum in the Situational-Discourse-Semantic (S-D-S) model reflect increases in linguistic strategies for capturing and expressing redundancy. Children with less flexible language systems often do not have well internalized knowledge of these structures, or the cohesive ties used within these structures, to refer to redundant information. Without this internalized knowledge, children misinterpret information heard or read when they encounter these forms and fail to use them to organize their own discourse when they speak to others. The four categories of cohesive devices or ties that serve to capture redundancy in language are:

- **Reference**, or the use of grammatical strategies to refer to already stated, or old, information. The first time a referent is mentioned, it is introduced with the indefinite article a/an and is specifically named. After that point, the definite article "the" is used to refer to it, indicating that it is a redundant rather than new referent. Pronouns are another means of establishing reference to old information, including words such as this, that, one, or various forms of subjective, possessive, objective, and reflexive pronouns. Children with inflexible language systems typically experience difficulty acquiring these forms as preschoolers and at school-age have difficulty understanding how they function to coordinate ideas across boundaries of sentences and paragraphs.
- **Ellipsis** refers to the omission of elements of grammar or vocabulary from the text if the information they express is redundant. Many complex grammatical strategies, or transformations, serve this function, as in the two sentences "The Chinese families eat rice," "Many Chinese families are poor" that can be restated "Many poor Chinese families eat rice." The redundant information is combined through ellipsis, or elimination of the words that are common to both ideas. Another example is found in the sentence "The rice that I like is whole grained," which, with ellipsis, can be restated "The rice (that) I like is whole grained." Ellipsis removes the redundancy from the surface of the sentence and actually adds complexity to the sentence. Many children with inflexible language systems have difficulty with sentences that have been altered in this way.

■ **Conjunction** is a third grammatical strategy for combining ideas that share redundant information, as in "The Red Basin grows rice," "The Red Basin has a hot climate" that can be restated as "The Red Basin grows rice because its climate is hot." Many children with inflexible language systems understand and use the strategy of conjunction to establish links between ideas, but may not use it to reduce redundancy. The conjunction is used to list, rather than to coordinate ideas, as in "The Red Basin grows rice and the Red Basin has a hot climate." The primary conjunctions used are additive, as in "and" or "and then," with limited use of more complex forms such as "unless," "therefore," "until," "while," "even though," "if-then," "rather than," and so forth.

■ **Lexical** cohesion uses synonyms and repetitions of the same word to refer to old or closely related information to signal that the same topic remains in focus. Sentences such as "The Chinese grow **rice** in the *Red Basin*. This area has a hot climate that is ideal for this **crop**" use words that maintain a level of synonymy to eliminate redundancy from the surface of the sentence, while maintaining the redundancy of the underlying meaning. Children who know the meanings of words but who lack the integrated networks between them will fail to understand how the sentences interrelate, even though they can define every word.

Redundancy as it is expressed in oral and written discourse can only be understood and used by children if they have information organized into networks of redundant and overlapping relationships. Transactional, Expressive, and Poetic Discourse lack unity and coherence without redundancy, resulting in discourse structures characterized as Collections or Descriptive Lists, and expressed through nonspecific language and unclear reference. Lack of redundancy also is manifested in inefficiency of expression, as the child states and restates the same information without eliminating reference to old or already established elements of meaning. These children seem to talk a lot but express very little information.

Redundancy allows for greater amounts of information to be organized into one unified text, while at the same time allowing this information to be expressed with fewer words and sentences. Greater redundancy also allows for the same ideas and concepts to be used in many contexts and at many levels of abstraction. Thus, establishing an understanding of and developing linguistic strategies for expressing redundancy are important goals of intervention. To facilitate this development,

children need to be provided many opportunities for the same information to be encountered and talked about in many contexts of overlapping relationships.

■□ WHOLE-TO-PART ORGANIZATION OF LEARNING

A third characteristic of an effective learning environment is that smaller
topics and/or elements of language are parsed from the larger theme or
context to place them in focus for examination and elaboration. This is a
whole-to-part process, or essentially the opposite approach of that presented by many traditional curricula. For example, a traditional program
might view vocabulary acquisition as a goal or objective instead of an
outcome and thus teach vocabulary units (i.e., names of foods, names for
emotions, labels for body parts, categories of occupations). Whole Language instead views vocabulary acquisition as a natural and logical outcome of exploring new and interesting topics for purposes of understanding the events within a story, or deriving solutions to a problem.
The teaching or examination of vocabulary would occur whenever an
unfamiliar word is encountered in a context of use (Baumann & Kameenui, 1991). For example, while reading, an unfamiliar word may be pointed to and discussed in a manner that elaborates on its meaning and
function in relationship to understanding the message and what the
word means in that context. Other words that serve a similar function
might be generated and compared. Thus, the focus on this smaller "part"
of language occurs as a result of a need for refinement of the whole idea
expressed by the sentence or text, and it is defined in its relationship to
the whole.

Thematic organization similarly facilitates whole-to-part processing. The learner explores small topics with the big picture in mind, rather
than learning about a series of small topics and only eventually synthe-
sizing them into a whole. The parts and the whole continuously reshape
and modify each other, as new information on a subtopic motivates a reinterpretation of previously learned information or a redefinition of the
overall topic or problem. This is an active reconstruction process. When
new information contradicts current beliefs or concepts, a state of imbalance or discontinuity results. To reduce discontinuity and regain balance,
new assimilations and accommodations to existing cognitive schemata
must occur, which requires more information on relevant topics and/or
a change in perspective that will result in the reorganization of existing information.

The degree to which smaller topics are parsed from the whole depends on the needs of the learner. When specific information is needed or is relevant to a decision or situation, each of the smaller topics is focused on until enough information is understood to make a decision or complete the necessary task. The more specific concepts and the language that represents this refined knowledge emerge in parallel, as the language serves as an instrument to create the concept and then to refer to it once it is established. Thus, as we have seen earlier, language itself is a whole-to-part learning process. To facilitate language refinement, a focus on smaller topics in a manner that elaborates on them in relationship to the whole from which they are parsed is an important characteristic that must be maintained in intervention.

▪□ SOCIAL ORGANIZATION OF LEARNING

A fourth characteristic of an effective learning environment is the principle of social collaboration. Learning is *social* when it occurs as a result of interaction between participants who share a joint focus on a topic. Learning is *collaborative* when the participants must work together to achieve a common objective. Both concepts evolve from Vygotsky's (1962) view that social interaction serves as a catalyst for intellectual growth and language development. In a social or collaborative situation, one participant may have more information or skill related to a topic and, therefore, serve to mediate learning for the less competent or knowledgeable individual, or peers with equal ability or knowledge may provide mutual support that enables problems to be solved that neither participant could solve independently (Lehr, 1985). In either case, the interaction and mutual support provide the structure and the knowledge that makes learning possible.

In a traditional intervention model, there are limited opportunities for children to use and refine language. Talking is restricted to an interactional pattern consisting of a question initiated by the interventionist, a response to the question elicited from the child, and an evaluation of the correctness of the response provided by the adult (Cazden, 1988). When children do attempt to engage in meaningful communication, it is viewed as an off-task behavior and thus discouraged. Opportunities for the children with the least flexible language systems are further limited by classroom practices such as ability grouping when these groups focus on skill learning. The lowest ability groups maintain a low level of performance, with characteristics including less discussion, few opportunities for critical thinking, more structured paper and pencil activities, fewer opportunities to demonstrate competence, less self-directed learning, lower expectations, more frequent interruptions, and few opportunities for meaningful learning (Good & Stipek, 1983; Sorensen & Hallinan, 1986).

In contrast, social collaboration models treat children as far more capable than their independent abilities can support. In normal development, young language learners are assisted to explain or recount an event to an unfamiliar listener by adults who suggest ideas that they should include, provide words that would express the intended meaning, finish a sentence for them, or interpret an unclear or unintelligible utterance. As children are able to use language to tell about the event independently, they are helped to embellish with adjectives, adverbs, metaphors and other refinements through suggestions that they express how someone felt, what something looked like, what caused an event to occur, or what they learned from the experience. The adult functions as a facilitator and scaffolds the interactions, adjusting to the child's changing developmental abilities, thus providing the means and the need for new language structures to emerge (Snow, 1972).

Learning from this perspective is not viewed as linear and error free, but rather as an interactive process that involves a variety of false starts and tentative explorations. Talking is encouraged in a wide variety of contexts, including group discussions, peer tutoring, and cooperative learning groups as a method of refining knowledge and language. The same information is explored and talked about repeatedly as group members discover new information related to a topic and attempt to integrate it with old information, or as they edit and revise stories or reports related to their topic. Information is reread, retold, and rewritten as children use the data to draw conclusions or address a problem. In these groups, the members have control over the activities, topics, and outcomes of the learning, and the group as a whole takes responsibility and credit for the learning, so that cooperation rather than competition is encouraged (Indrisano & Paratore, 1991). The redundant exploration and reorganization of this socially embedded and transmitted knowledge gradually becomes part of the child's internal schemata, leading to generalization to new contexts and thus facilitating more rapid learning.

The adult's role is that of a collaborator or facilitator, rather than a disseminator and evaluator of information. The adult provides guidance, helping the child to think about and organize information at higher levels of Situational, Discourse, and Semantic context, and providing feedback for purposes of elaboration and clarification, rather than evaluation. Evaluation of the correctness of information or skill only serves to discourage risk taking and exploration and treats unrefined approximations as errors to be corrected rather than as reflections of the child's current level of organization (Applebee, 1991; Lehr, 1985). Peers serve many of the same facilitative functions for other group members, a process of cooperation that is viewed as natural, consistent with what occurs in adult work places or home environments and, therefore, positive and appropriate. This is in contrast to the traditional classroom expectations, where collaborative and assistive efforts are viewed as cheating (Slavin, 1986).

If development and refinement of language are the goals, then a facilitative social context must be provided for its exploration and use without risk of failure. Adults and peers must be available for providing a scaffold to mediate learning and to enable a child to engage in language learning and use that would be too difficult if approached as an individual effort. The social group not only provides facilitation for learning, but also provides meaningful opportunities to communicate information to others and to receive feedback on the success of these communicative attempts. Through these interactive attempts, the child gains increasing competence in organizing information with sufficient structure to clearly inform others, adjusting style of speech for the intended audience and purposes, recognizing differing points of view and perspectives, analyzing information in relationship to a problem, and considering the differences in background and information held by different listeners (Strickland, Dillon, Funkhouser, Glick, & Rogers, 1989). Each of these competencies contributes to greater flexibility in language functioning.

■❏ PROVIDING INTERVENTION IN ORAL LANGUAGE CONTEXTS

The Situational-Discourse-Semantic model can be used to plan, organize, and evaluate oral language intervention. The activities and strategies used will depend on the goals or purposes of the intervention. For example, if the goal is to increase the level of complexity and organization in the Discourse used, then materials that provide a high degree of Contextualized support might be chosen along the Situational dimension, such as toys or pictures (i.e., Contextualized-Symbolic). The objects or pictures provide a means of "keeping in mind" the persons, places, or things talked about (i.e., the Semantic dimension) and for using spatial location of the objects or elements in the picture as a means for organizing them so they can be talked about in temporal, causal, conditional, or other order at a level of Discourse structure.

If, on the other hand, the goal is to increase the level of Decontextualization at which the child can clearly communicate and specify all needed information for the listener (a Decontextualized Situational context), then a lower level of Discourse structure might initially be used, such as a Descriptive List or Ordered Sequence. A lower Discourse level reduces the linguistic burden of remembering and clearly communicating all of the information *and* at the same time using language to establish complex relationships between all of the elements. Failing to change one dimension requires a coordination of both a high level of Situational and Discourse contexts that may well be beyond the child's Zone of Proximal Development (ZPD).

The degree to which the topic under consideration is familiar and the amount of background information possessed by the child related to that topic will affect the level of Decontextualization that can be presented. To facilitate talk at higher levels of Decontextualization, familiar topics should be presented. Familiarity also will affect the ease with which a child will be able to internalize more complex Discourse structures and more abstract or implicit meanings related to the situation. If the goal is to develop an understanding of new and unfamiliar content information, then learning may be enhanced by increasing the amount of Contextual support by presenting more pictures and/or hands-on experiences and presenting the information at a relatively linear and uncomplicated level of Discourse structure. In contrast, information that is already familiar may be used to immerse the child in the production of more complex and logically ordered levels of Discourse and to talk about this content with minimal support from pictures and objects.

In addition to manipulating the difficulty of the information presented, the amount and type of social mediation provided to the child will impact learning. Social interaction is the interventionist's means of helping the child to focus on important information and to begin to mentally represent these ideas. Through verbal scaffolding, the interventionist can provide greater or lesser degrees of assistance and support for communication and provide the amount and type of support required to either introduce the concepts or to guide refinements. This can range from direct models of things that can be talked about and words that can be used to refer to these ideas through open-ended questions or comments that merely guide thinking.

◼️ CONTEXTUALIZED INTERVENTION ACTIVITIES

Intervention activities that are Contextualized are characterized by the use of objects, illustrations, or situations that support the language used within that context. This support is one factor that enables children to communicate at the upper level of their ZPD. The importance of Contextualization has been extensively documented by Piaget (1954, 1960), who has demonstrated that young children are limited in their reasoning strategies first to objects that are actually physically present and manipulable (Preoperations), then to problems that can be thought of in terms of real objects (Concrete Operations), and finally to hypothetical problems (Formal Operations). Providing a picture or objects, for example, enables a child with more concrete strategies to reason about changes in time, location, and state and the factors that might cause them, and to include that information in a story or discussion of a topic. Similarly, Blank, Rose, and Berlin (1978) demonstrate that the presence of objects or pictures enables the child to attend to more abstract characteristics. For example, a picture showing a broken chair may enable the child to make the Interpretation that Goldilocks was too big for it, an idea that the child might not otherwise have been able to deduce.

The following are examples of the types of Contextualized activities that can be used to facilitate language development and use.

Contextualized-Relational Activity

The Contextualized-Relational level of the Situational context involves real objects used in relational actions, such as cooking. For example, in the story *Boo Hoo* (Melser & Cowley, 1990a), the main character bought and sold in succession a cow, horse, pig, sheep, goat, and cat. A follow-up intervention activity might set up a store for the children to experience buying and selling, including learning to count and exchange money, conduct negotiations between buyer and seller, and to set up categories of things that might be purchased in the store. One type of merchandise could be animal cookies that the children make before opening the store to buy and sell. The actual cooking utensils and ingredients must be used in relational combinations of unpackaging and measuring, measuring and pouring, pouring and stirring, rolling and employing animal cookie cutters, greasing and arranging, and heating and baking (i.e., an Ordered Sequence of relational events).

Rather than reading the recipe to the children, scaffolded interactions can be used to involve the children in planning and organizing the sequence of events. Scaffolded interactions involve the use of cues, prompts, and visual supports such as a recipe written in words and picture symbols on a board. These interactions put the thinking process into words as the actions are performed. The scaffolding helps the child to link a continuous sequence of ideas rather than answering a series of discrete questions. The interaction might proceed as follows:

> A **preparatory set** is used (i.e., examining the recipe) to establish information that is important to consider in the activity.

Adult: Tom, we need some information about making cookies (pointing to the recipe). How should we start?

> A child is given a **communicative opportunity** to organize the action and to put the thoughts into words, or the process of *internalization*.

Tom: We need butter.

> The child provided only one part of a Semantically Descriptive idea. The adult acknowledges the child's information and then uses **cloze** (i.e., shared completion of ideas) and **pointing** to relevant objects to help the child link a series of actions into a unified event.

Adult: Right, we need to measure _____
Tom: the butter
Adult: using _____ (handing him the measuring cup)
Tom: the measuring cup
Adult: to make sure we have (pointing to the recipe)
Tom: a half a cup, and then put it in the bowl

> The adult uses **relational terms** that cue meaningful relationships between ideas such as "because" (causality) or "next" (temporal), or "if" (conditionality).

Adult: because next _____
Sarah: we have to add sugar
Tom: Yeah, we have to add sugar and mix it up

> When children do not appear to have information or cannot spontaneously recall words, the adult may provide a **binary** choice.

Adult: with _____ (no response) mixer or a spoon?
Tom, Sarah, and Jeremy: a mixer!

> In confirming the children's ideas, the adult frequently uses **expansions**, adding more information and/or more elaborated sentence structure to the child's utterance, and **expatiations**, where the adult adds new information or details, models inferences, evaluations, or predictions.

Adult: Right, we have to use a mixer because it would be too hard to get the butter and sugar creamy by just stirring it with the spoon.

> The adult suggests an actual hands-on test of this explanation to help the children understand the meaning of this inference and to engage in hypothesis testing.

Adult: Maybe we can try it with both.

The scaffolded interactions facilitated thinking and talking within the **Zone of Proximal Development** (ZPD) for the children, enabling them to talk using Discourse structures and Semantic displacement at levels higher than they would be able to independently apply to the situation. The oral language interactions also serve to rehearse and organize actions before they are actually performed, first by examining the recipe and then by orally planning actions immediately before performing them. Discussing the actions that had been performed and why in a follow-up discussion (a Decontextualized-Egocentered level on the Situational continuum) while the cookies baked would provide a third opportunity to translate the event into words. This creates the element of

redundancy needed for the process of both internalization of complex sequences of actions and the language used to talk about them to occur.

Contextualized-Symbolic Play

At a higher level on the Situational continuum, similar types of learning activities can be created using symbolically represented actors, objects, actions, or states instead of real objects. One such context is that of play, where miniature replicas of real objects, such as toy dishes, food, and appliances are available, or where the child substitutes an arbitrary object for one with no available replica, such as using a yellow crayon to represent butter. Play at the Contextualized-Symbolic level is an excellent context for facilitating development along the Expressive, Transactional, or Poetic Discourse dimensions. In the story *Soup* (Cowley, 1988e), the main character, Souperman, makes soup for the people in the factory each day. But one day a spark caused the factory to catch fire, and no one could put it out until Souperman arrived with great pots of soup. He doused the flames, but then had the problem of feeding the hungry mob. The day was saved by Souperwoman who brought a truck filled with soup ingredients. After reading the story as a means of modeling a simple *Complete narrative* with goals, attempts, and consequences, play could be initiated with miniature houses, dishes, trucks, and other props. The story serves to provide models and ideas for the play, but the play also is free to emerge collaboratively between participants with its own event structure.

Jeremy: I'm gonna put out the fire! (grabs firetruck and drives it over to the house, pretends to squirt flames with hose, then loses interest and begins to examine and perform actions with other trucks).

Tom: Here's the soup. It all goes on the house (pretends to dump a pot of soup on the house and then picks up the abandoned firetruck and begins to squirt at the flames).

The play exhibited by the boys parallels their oral storytelling, characterized by referring to one or two high-action events within Descriptive Lists, with no elaboration, relational terms connecting ideas, or elements of story structure evident in the play. To facilitate higher levels of Discourse and Semantic organization, the adult becomes a collaborator in the play.

Adult: Wait, let's play that someone started the fire. My people were just having an ordinary day. They were making really neat cars.

Jeremy: They were working, making cars and stuff.

> Many of the same scaffolding strategies, including cloze, prompts with relational terms, and reference to relevant objects are used to help the children establish the first element of story structure, or the "ordinary existence" of the characters.

Adult: (picking up a play person) He needs to finish making this _____

Jeremy: car

Adult: and so he _____ (pretends to plug in a cord)

Jeremy: plugs in the plug

Adult: and started to drill _____ (uses pretend drill on car door)

Jeremy: on the car door and make holes for the handle and the lock. He does it like this (pretends).

Adult: Oh oh, he wasn't paying attention, because he was looking at the door, and he didn't see _____

Jeremy: the fire start and catch everything on fire and all the people ran out screaming like this (screams).

> Additional scaffolding strategies are seen in this excerpt, including the use of **constituent questions**, or a question that asks for a specific person, action, state or other information to contribute to the dialogue, and questions, such as a request for a prediction or a motive.

Adult: Right, the plug caused a spark to shoot out and catch some _____; What did it catch on fire? (points to some paper)

Tom: some paper and stuff on fire and catch everything on fire.

Adult: So what should we make the people do?

Tom: The people ran out

Adult: because _____

Tom: they were scared

Jeremy: they were gonna burn up.

Adult: They were scared because they thought they might burn up! Well, then what happened?

Tom: The fire truck came.

Adult: (pretends to call) My man is going to call the fire truck.

Jeremy: The firemen saw the smoke and they got in the truck and came to the fire, to put out the fire.

Through the collaborative play, the adult helps the children to establish Discourse structure of the story. This is done by reenacting an event with the play characters and props. The ordinary existence was established, followed by adding an initiating event, or incident, that created the problem fire. The children spontaneously provided the reactions of the characters. The goal and beginning of an attempt to put out the fire were then incorporated. Through this scaffolded play, the children were enabled to participate in contextualized storytelling at the level of an Abbreviated Episode, a level far above what the children's independent abilities could support.

The scaffolding strategies are used to maintain the narrative nature of the interaction, with the adult and children often sharing the responsibility of completing a single, complex sentence across several turns. The children are immersed in the production of long, coherent sentences and units of discourse, thus functioning as collaborators who both initiate ideas and contribute to the formation of ideas initiated by the adult or peers. These ideas are expressed in a manner incorporating relational terms, complex grammatical structures, specific vocabulary, and elements of narrative discourse structure, or language that the child has difficulty independently coordinating and using without support. By actively participating in the construction of language at this level, the child begins to internalize the sentence and discourse patterns, and these more organized and complex patterns begin to appear in future play or conversation.

Contextualized-Symbolic Illustrations

These same types of interactions can be created when pictures serve as the representations, rather than replica or substituted objects. Pictures vary widely in regard to the amount and specificity of characters, actions, objects, and other features of the situation that are depicted. Generally, illustrated storybooks with lower levels of readability (preprimer or primer level of difficulty) will provide pictures that tell much of the story without words, because the written text and pictures generally maintain a close relationship (Golden, 1990). Often, each page or illustration represents a Abbreviated Episode and thus can be used in itself as a unit for generating a narrative. The same storybook can be used across several sessions, with each episode providing the child with experience in narrative discourse and the overall story functioning to help the child interpret Complete, Complex, or Interactive levels of Discourse context.

The first two facing pages of the story *The Donkey in the Lion's Skin* (Biro, 1986) shows a donkey examining the hide or skin of a lion lying in a field in one picture and the donkey wearing the skin with his own ears, nose, and hooves showing below the hide in the facing page. The facial expressions are detailed, providing many opportunities for interpretations of the donkey's motives and feelings, as well as descriptions of his actions. The interaction begins with the adult inviting the children to provide an interpretation of the illustrations.

Adult: Jeremy, what do you think the story is about? Look at the pictures and tell us a story.

Jeremy: Here, the um, donkey is smelling the lion (explanation: the donkey is examining the lion skin, but visually, the nose is located near the lion) and here the donkey has the lion thing on, I guess its a lion suit, and you can see his nose right there.

Tom: Well, the lion is on um is on the um grass or lying down, or maybe he's dead or something, and the er horse, or what is that called? [Jeremy: a donkey] Yeah, the donkey has on the lion thing.

Adult: The donkey might be smelling the donkey, but I think he's doing something else. Look at his eyes, what are his eyes doing?

Jeremy: kind of looking at the lion.

Adult: He's probably looking at the lion to see _____

Tom: the lion.

Adult: Right, to see him and to find out if what?

Tom: if he's sleeping or um, alive.

Adult: Jeremy, what do you think?

Jeremy: To see if he's sleeping 'cuz his eyes are closed.

Adult: So the _____

Jeremy: donkey is looking at the lion

Adult: to see if _____

Tom: he's sleeping or dead

Adult: and when he looks real close he finds out _____

Jeremy: he's sleeping.

Adult: Do you think he's sleeping? Let's look at the next picture. If the lion was sleeping, could the donkey wear his skin?

Jeremy: Oh, he wasn't sleeping, he was dead.
Adult: Yeah, he probably was dead, but was it the whole lion? Look at his body, it looks very flat (points to parts of the picture to attend to). What might it be, if it's not the whole lion?
Tom: Just the outside skin.
Adult: So, the donkey was walking along, through the _____
Tom: grass
Adult: when all of a sudden he stopped because _____
Jeremy: he saw a lion skin laying flat on the grass
Adult: and so he looked at it very carefully to see _____
Tom: if it was dead or asleep, but it wasn't asleep 'cuz it was flat.
Adult: Right, and so he knew it couldn't hurt him so he _____
Tom: put the lion skin on him, on the donkey, on him.
Jeremy: That's funny! He put the lion skin on *himself*
Tom: on himself.

> Following the scaffolded interaction, Jeremy's retelling indicated that he had internalized many of the ideas and events, and was able to express them at higher Discourse and Semantic levels.

Adult: So who would like to tell the story?
Jeremy: The donkey was just walking and um, and in the grass (pointing between donkey's eyes) he saw this lion and it was flat. **[Adult prompt:** so he stopped to _____) He stopped to look at it to see if it was dead and it was 'cuz it was just the skin, so the donkey put it on but he doesn't really look like a lion 'cuz you can see his mouth and feet and stuff.

Using the same type of collaborative dialogue and scaffolding strategies as seen in other contexts, the children's stories were elaborated to include more information establishing a setting, better interpretation of the actions, and levels of semantics that included interpretations of the donkey's motives and emotions, and story structure that went beyond simply describing the main event in each picture. Once again, sentences were longer, more complex, and more specific in word use. The redundancy that occurred by summarizing old parts of the story before adding new ideas enabled the children to state more of the ideas independently and with greater clarity.

Summary

Contextualized activities and scaffolding strategies can be used for a wide variety of purposes, including Expressive functions (example: using play figures or pictures to role play appropriate behaviors in a social situation), Poetic functions (telling stories about real or imaginary events), and Transactional functions (example: the cooking activity, or using objects to conduct experiments or to simulate some historical or cultural event). They allow for Discourse and Semantic dimensions of language to be learned and used in a context that is supported by the present and ongoing Situational events.

■ DECONTEXTUALIZED INTERVENTION ACTIVITIES

As the Situational context becomes increasingly decontextualized, fewer actors, actions, objects, states, or other elements are present within the environment and instead must be recreated symbolically, through language. If the situation that is re-created was an event personally experienced by the child, then at an earlier time the actual objects were present and manipulated, and the actual feelings were experienced by the child. This previously experienced event generally provides greater support for re-creating the context in language than one that was merely observed or only imagined. However, children with less flexible language systems often experience great difficulty in attempting to use language to create context and to establish reference to nonpresent objects and events. Without the visual input provided by the context, it is difficult for them to recall and organize a sufficient number of actions or states to linguistically recreate an experience.

Creation of Graphic Organizers

One strategy for bridging the transition from contextualized to decontextualized situations is to use flowcharts or other **graphic organizers**. Graphic organizers are visual representations of information consisting of the arrangement of key words or concepts in a visual array. The most basic type is a semantic web in which a key concept is entered into a circle, and then lines are drawn from the circle outward, like the legs of a spider. On each leg, categories of related concepts are listed, so that if the key concept is "weather" one leg might attach to a list of precipitation terms (rain, snow, hail, sleet), another a list of air temperatures (hot, cold, warm, humid, muggy, freezing), another sky conditions (sunny, cloudy, stormy, clear, overcast), and another a list of storms (hurricane, tornado, thunderstorm, cyclone, twister). Flowcharts are more complex, and are similar in their content and underlying organization to outlining. Flowcharts are structured in the format of a visual hierarchy, with the most superordinate concept placed at the top. Below this, the major subcategories are placed parallel to each other, each with a line connecting it to the main concept. Each of these subcategories may be similarly divided into subordinate categories or concepts, and so forth.

Flowcharts can be used to structure decontextualized experiences to enable the child to learn how to talk about an event with specific referents, organization, and completeness. The objective at this level might read:

Objective

Child will be able to recount a personal experience (i.e., Decontextualized-Egocentered) with Discourse structure at the Abbreviated level, and with 85% of the referents clearly specified.

Approximations to Goal	**Date Achieved**
a. When teacher assists in creating a Flowchart, child uses the chart to recount the experience.	
b. The child creates a Flowchart and uses it to recount the experience.	
c. The child mentally plans the main ideas and supporting details, and uses this mental plan to recount the experience.	

An example of the use of a Flowchart for this purpose is presented below as Christy, an 8 year old, attempted to talk about her ski trip (i.e., Expressive Discourse).

Christy: We um first I took ski lessons, lessons, and they had this little one, we had to walk up and when we were just learning how to ski, and it, it um, my hair was in my face and then my mom and dad came up, I was crying and I didn't want to do it, and then we went up the ski lift, you had to go up all by it, all by yourself and get off and stuff,

and we went and then when they, um, when we came
back, we said "I don't wanna go."

Through scaffolded interactions, Christy was helped to think about
how she might organize her ideas on the flowchart.

Adult: What is your story about?
Christy: About the ski lift and stuff.
Adult: Well, you told me about the ski lift, but you also told me
about lessons, and the lessons weren't on the ski lift, so what
can you say that the lessons and the ski lift were both about?
Christy: Skiing, my ski trip.
Adult: Okay, so that will be our topic and we will write it on
the top.

See Step A of Flowchart (Figure 4–1)

Adult: What are the main things that you did on your ski trip?
Christy: I got scared and I skied and I went on the lift and I
went down.
Adult: Is getting scared a main thing? Or did you get scared
when you were doing something?
Christy: When I had to um go down, not at the end, at first, when I
was um taking, I took lessons.
Adult: Okay, so one important thing that you did was take
lessons. Can you think of another?
Christy: um, rode the ski lift, went up the ski lift.
Adult: Okay, and then?
Christy: and then skied down.
Adult: Okay, put those ideas on the flowchart.

See Step B of Flowchart (Figure 4–1)

Adult: Okay, so let's think about the lessons for a minute. What
would you want your friends to know about lessons if
they had never been skiing?
Christy: um, you um learn how to ski.
Adult: How?

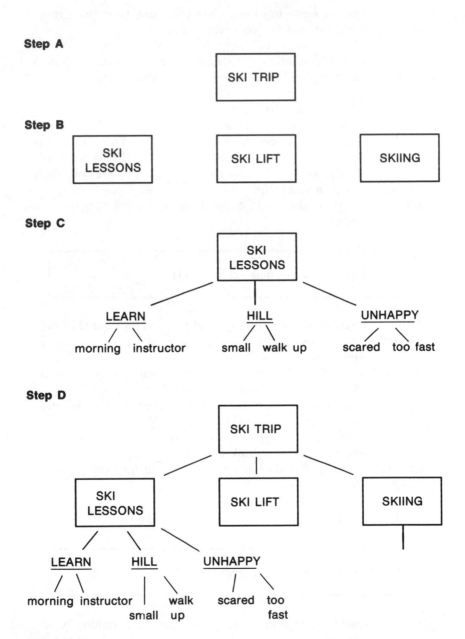

Figure 4-1
Creation of a flowchart used to structure a decontextualized experience.

Christy: The instructor helps you, and its in the um morning.
Adult: Where?
Christy: On the um hill, the um small hill that you um walk up
with no lift.

See Step C of Flowchart (Figure 4–1)

The topics of the ski lift, and the actual skiing were similarly developed. Once the flowchart is constructed, scaffolding strategies can be used to assist the child to talk about the experience with greater coherence, complex sentences, specific vocabulary, and topically organized discourse.

See Step D of Flowchart (Figure 4–1)

Adult: (pointing to various key concepts on the flowchart) One
day last _____
Christy: winter
Adult: you and your _____
Christy: family went on a ski trip, in the, in Colorado.
Adult: On the first day _____
Christy: I took ski lessons (adult points to "morning") in the
morning
Adult: with _____ (points to "instructor")
Christy: with the instructor and she taught us how to ski.
Adult: The lessons started on (points to "small," then "hill")
Christy: the small hill because the instructor didn't want us to
_____ (Christy uses the flowchart to help structure her
discourse, pointing to "too fast," and then "scared") go
too fast and get scared
Adult: but _____ (points to scared)
Christy: I got scared.
Adult: You got scared anyway! There was no _____ (points to
"ski lift," then "small" and "hill")
Christy: ski lift on the small hill so (points to "walk up," "small,"
and "hill") I had to walk up the small hill.

The interaction continued in this manner until the adult and child had collaboratively talked about the experience on the ski lift and the actual fun of skiing. Relationships within and across nodes on the flow-chart were pointed to and tied together using scaffolding strategies in many different ways to talk about different aspects of the trip. Initially, the adult's turn consisted of highly scaffolded input, but as the child began to understand how to organize her ideas using the flowchart and began to internalize the patterns for talking about the event, the adult's input was reduced to primarily acknowledgments or prompts with relational terms for another idea.

The experience of collaboratively thinking through the logic of determining which ideas are main events, what ideas are part of or support these events, and visually organizing them to represent the relationships on the graphic organizer serves to raise the child's awareness of the need to structure discourse. The use of the constructed graphic organizer to talk about events using different levels of Discourse structure further raises awareness and provides the child with direct experience using word, sentence, and discourse patterns to express this structure. It provides for the redundancy needed for the child to abstract out both the patterns of language and the specific content information that are important to the development of a flexible and well organized language system.

Multiple Uses of Graphic Organizers

Flowcharts and other types of graphic organizers can be similarly used with other levels of Decontextualization within the Situational context, such as **Decentered** (i.e., talking about experiences that were only observed but not directly experienced), **Relational** (e.g., organizing a daily schedule, or understanding classroom rules, as in Figure 4–2a), **Symbolic** (i.e., creating experience completely from words, as in listening to a lecture in science or geography, as in Figure 4–2b), or **Logical** (i.e., logically created events or concepts, such as the composition of an atom, or the greenhouse effect of the atmosphere). A word or picture symbol placed on a flowchart provides a graphic context that has many advantages compared to an unsupported oral discussion. These advantages include:

- Words or symbols can be used to keep a new or difficult concept visually available to the sensory system so that it can be reexamined.
- Concepts on the graphic organizer can be viewed in relationship to their superordinate and subordinate concepts.

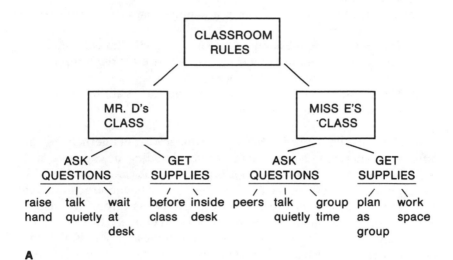

A

B

Figure 4-2. A. Example of a flowchart used to teach classroom rules.
B. Example of a flowchart used to teach a science lesson.

◼ Concepts can be held in focus long enough to be compared and placed in relationships with other new and old concepts and events.

◼ A topic can be talked about in a manner that maintains order and coherence.

◼ The topic can be reexamined across time, so that new information acquired later in a theme cycle can be used to reinterpret or elaborate on the old information.

◼ The graphic organizer can be reviewed for recall, or used to structure an oral monologue.

All of these uses function to facilitate the process of internalizing the language patterns and the content, or the building of cognitive networks. Flowcharts and other graphic organizers also can be used to facilitate various levels of Transactional, Expressive, or Poetic structure, such as the structures found in levels from Descriptive Lists, through the highly integrated episodes and interwoven topics found in Interactive structures.

Using a similar format, the main idea or topic of any unit of narration or exposition, such as the concept behind a story, or element of story structure, or story episode can be placed in the highest node. For example, in the story *The Discontented Pig* (Butterworth, 1986a) Percy the young pig was discontented with his life and wanted to see the world. He crept away from home and in his travels met many animals that he admired, including the giraffe for his long neck, the elephant for his ears, and the peacock for her tail. He looked at himself in a pool and made a series of wishes, each asking for a body part like those of the animals he admired, which were granted. However, when he returned home, his family did not recognize him and chased him away, causing him to become so sad that he ran back to the pond to make another wish to return to being himself. When it was granted, he returned to his home where he was wanted and missed, and he was no longer discontented.

The overall story could be placed on a flowchart, with "PERCY'S WISH" at the superordinate position, and "PIG" "MET" "CHANGE" "CONSEQUENCES" placed at the next level, representing important main components of the wish. Under PIG, key concepts such as "discontented," "see the world," and "be like others" could be entered; under MET, the word giraffe could be entered with itself having the subordinate words "neck" and "see forever" displayed; the other animals encountered could be similarly represented on the chart. Key ideas under CHANGE and CONSEQUENCES would be filled in to complete the flowchart. The *act* of constructing the flowchart through collaborative scaffolded interactions would involve the child in active problem solving and categorizing events into topics, thus developing many critical thinking and language skills. Once created, the flowchart also could be used for many purposes, including:

- helping the child learn how to retell or summarize a story
- structuring ideas into Poetic discourse at various levels of story structure
- combining ideas into complex relationships of time, space, causality, intention, and so forth
- learning to use grammatical structures and cohesive ties
- metalinguistically examining story structure to see how authors create stories that inform a listener.

Use of Role Playing and Drama

Another strategy for bridging the transition from contextualized to decontextualized situations is the use of role playing and drama. Children progress through different qualitative stages of role playing and drama from the preschool state of *being* a character, to the middle childhood stage of *playing* a character, or pretending to do and act like some fictional or actual person or animal, then returning to the notion of *being* a character at adolescence, but at a higher level that incorporates all of the discoveries about characters, their motives, intentions, reactions, actions, and beliefs acquired at earlier stages (Colby, 1988). Young children primarily reenact real-world scripts or everyday events, while older children play progressively more imaginative events and roles that are very different from their own real-world roles.

Drama and role playing can be used to reenact experiences, to retell a story, to view a situation from another person's perspective, to express personal ideas, or a wide variety of other purposes along the Situational and Discourse dimensions. They may be enacted at any level of formality, on a continuum from written scripts to completely spontaneous actions and dialogue. They are highly facilitative to the process of decontextualization because they engage children in a form of conscious symbolization, where language must be used to represent absent objects, transform people into characters with roles, and use real actions to perform pretense functions (Pellegrini, 1985). They place demands on the child to use a literate form of language, where roles and props are delineated precisely at the beginning of play episodes, topics are explicitly introduced, ambiguous roles are clarified, and specific language is used to create the physical and affective context (Pellegrini, 1984).

For example, a story can be introduced using an illustrated book or a play, such as *The Goats and the Troll* (Ciantar, 1988). The script can either be read by or to the children, depending on their age and reading ability (this text is written at a grade 2 readability level). The illustrations can be examined and discussed to gain additional insights into the characters, their attitudes, and responses to events. The sequence of events can be logically examined so that the children understand why some events necessarily occur before others and the effect that one action has on another action or state.

In this story, the goats' peaceful existence is disrupted by a bare field of grass on their side of the river and a bad tempered troll living under the bridge. In past crossings, the big goat had usually done all of the fighting with the troll, but during the last fight, he bent and broke his horns. On this occasion, he crossed the bridge first, convincing the troll not to fight him because the weaker, middle-size goat would be along next. The middle-size goat crossed second and convinced the troll that the small goat would be far easier to fight. The little goat used his wits to dodge the troll's first attempt to hit him, crashing his fist into the brick wall of the bridge instead. The little goat goads the troll, telling him not to let the bridge get away with such a thing, so the troll punches it harder; the scenario is repeated once again, until the troll knocks himself out and the little goat passes over the bridge.

The children can be helped to reenact the story at different levels of decontextualization. Costumes made in art, props such as the bridge can be used, and each illustrated page of the play can be shown at the time that the children act out that event to provide a visual context in which to embed the dialogue. The adult can scaffold the dialogue in the same manner modeled in the examples of play and illustrated narratives above. As the children begin to internalize the story, the play can be reenacted without the support of the pictures, with some children functioning in the narrator's role to set the stage and talk about changes in time and location, while others play the roles of the characters. At an even higher level of decontextualization, the costumes and props can be eliminated, with the characters and bridge created exclusively through language.

While some children perform as narrators and characters, other children can function as drama critics, providing feedback to the actors on whether they are capturing the appropriate affect or providing sufficient information to the listeners. This role engages the children in Metalinguistic analysis of an event. Thus, language for many meaningful purposes at numerous interacting levels of Situational, Discourse, and Semantic context simultaneously is used by the children, with decreasing levels of environmental support and adult scaffolding. These literate uses of language are important to reading and writing. The language of drama and reading share the same types of decontextualized functions and metalinguistic processes (Vygotsky, 1967). It is not surprising that comprehension of literature, reading achievement, understanding of cause and effect, motivations, and emotional responses to literature, and the organization of written compositions are correlated with the ability to represent narratives in drama (Wagner, 1991) and that the use of drama in turn helps to refine each of these abilities.

Use of Retelling to Multiple Listeners

Repeated tellings of the same information, story, or procedure to different listeners is another strategy that can serve to bridge the transition from contextualized to decontextualized situations. Listeners vary in their degree of familiarity to the child, thus there will be differences in presuppositions, or the level of knowledge that can be assumed without explicit mention. The child must be able to take the conversational perspective of the listener and determine what information must be provided and the level of language that the listener can comprehend. Listeners who share experiences with and/or who are familiar with the language patterns used by the child will require less explicit information, while those who have no known shared background will require specific language and sufficient information to recreate the context talked about by the child.

Similarly, even familiar listeners will vary in the amount of information that they share with the child about an event or topic. As children move beyond the preschool years, they increasingly go places with their peers and acquire experiences independently of their parents. The child must use language to carry the information from the context in which it was experienced to the context in which it is reported.

Repeated opportunities to retell the same information or to report on the same event provide the child with the redundancy needed to learn to recount the information with greater organization and specificity. For example, a parent and child might have taken a trip to the zoo and learned about jungle animals. The first telling should occur with the informed participant, in this case the parent, as the listener who was also present when the experience occurred. The interventionist collaborates with the child to tell the information to the informed listener. The information may be rehearsed prior to the telling, using flowcharts and scaffolding to determine what is important to communicate and how it might be organized. As the child tells the information to the informed listener, the adult may use scaffolding strategies to prompt important ideas or to help the child structure the language when false starts and linguistic nonfluencies begin to occur. The informed listener can provide feedback to the child, indicating when insufficient information has been given or events are inaccurate or out of order. The adult can provide prompts or other assists to this participant also (e.g., Did he forget to tell you something important about the elephant?) Thus, both speaker and listener are actively engaged in reconstructing the event using language and monitoring the accuracy of content and form used in telling about it.

The second telling should occur with a participant who is familiar with the child but not the event, such as a friend, grandparent, or teacher. This telling will require more specific reference to be established since less background knowledge can be presupposed and the listener will be less able to fill in unclear or missing bits of information. The listener should be instructed to signal a communication breakdown when the content is unclear or the form of the language is difficult to follow. The adult provides scaffolded assistance, including expansions and expatiations to model the greater detail and specificity needed by an uninformed listener.

A third telling should involve a listener who is only casually familiar with the child and not familiar with the event, thus requiring an ever greater degree of decontextualized language style; a fourth listener may be a stranger to both the child and the situation.

With each telling, the amount of scaffolding necessary to present the most critical information should diminish, as the child begins to internalize both the content and the form for communicating the event. The scaffolding should shift toward helping the child to include more detail, higher levels of semantic interpretations, more elaborated sentence and discourse structures, and greater fluency of expression. The retellings to different listeners provide the child with opportunities to adjust the message to meet the needs of different listeners, including adjusting the style of speech for the intended audience and purposes, recognizing different points of view or perspectives, and considering the differences in background and information between listeners (Strickland et al., 1989). The retellings also serve to internalize the patterns of language that are appropriate for use in such contexts, or a generalized script that can be applied to other situations or content.

Parents who receive training in the use of this type of scaffolded reporting also can serve as facilitators. The flowchart generated during the rehearsal phase can be sent home to provide the parents with key ideas and context to expect and to prompt for as the child tells the information. The parent can then help the child report the information to siblings, the other parent, grandparents, friends, and other relatives, both in face-to-face encounters and over the telephone. The parent can provide the necessary scaffolding to enable the child to successfully communicate the information to the various listeners, and provide the child with feedback on the needs of a particular participant or setting. Particularly for the low language ability child, this strategy provides the child with something that can be successfully talked about in conversation with a variety of people, and thus serves a social as well as a language learning function.

Summary

There are many additional contexts of language intervention, strategies of language facilitation, materials for language stimulation, and methods of providing scaffolding to children, as well as variations of the ones presented here that are consistent with Whole Language philosophy and principles. They have in common thematic organization within complex contexts; redundancy in experiences focused on topics or events; whole-to-part refinement of language at all levels of Situational, Discourse, and Semantic contexts; and the use of social collaboration as a primary means of facilitating this refinement. They emphasize learning language by making sense or meaning out of experience within communicative contexts, rather than meaningless drills or worksheet activities They allow language to emerge from the interactions rather than attempting to target and teach specific elements of language.

The scaffolded interactions are designed to be used in the context of intervention or teaching. They provide the child with guided experiences where strategies, discourse structures, mental planning, classroom rules, conversational patterns, abstract modes of thought, sensitivity to listener needs, distinctions between fact and fiction, and a wide variety of concepts and information can be internalized and used. An ideal Whole Language classroom would additionally provide many small group and collaborative situations where the child could apply these abilities in a more independent manner with the support of peers.

■❏ PROVIDING INTERVENTION IN THE CONTEXT OF READING

Written language, including the use of illustrated books, written plays, recipes, flowcharts and other graphic organizers were used in the context of oral language intervention as described in the above examples. Written language is useful in facilitating oral language because the print provides a visual, and therefore more Contextualized, level of input that the child can use to organize oral language. But the relationship between oral and written language is far more complex than written language simply providing a visual representation of a language system formed through oral experience. Rather, oral and written language represent two *modes* of language, each of which has its own developmental sequence beginning at infancy, and each of which contributes to the creation of the *language system* as it exists within the child's mental network of logical patterns or "rules," and concepts representing the physical and mental world. The two modes do not function independently, but rather in an overlapping relationship, with insights or discoveries in each mode informing the other and facilitating development from the earliest stages of language development.

◼◻ EARLY DEVELOPMENT OF WRITTEN LANGUAGE

Storybook reading has been shown to be the single most important activity for building the skills and knowledge required for reading. This activity helps children to become acquainted with the language and the conventions of books as well as the reading process. Storybook reading also benefits young children's language development. Parents facilitate both vocabulary acquisition and the patterns of language by expanding nonverbal responses, labeling characters and objects, describing actions, asking questions, providing feedback related to the child's comments, and in many other ways facilitating understanding and use of language (Anderson, Heibert, Scott, & Wilkinson, 1985; Altwerger, Diehl-Faxon, & Dockstader-Anderson, 1985; Cazden, 1983; Sulzby, 1985, 1986; Teale & Sulzby, 1986).

Repeatedly reading the same storybook is a common practice in many homes, particularly at bedtime. Children often request that the same book be read each night for several days, weeks, and even months. This practice appears to be important to the learning process. During initial readings, children primarily name pictured items, respond to adult questions, and repeat or restate the text read by the adult. Having thus established the names and simple actions presented, the child's focus changes to more complex aspects of meaning and story content. The child's questions and comments occur more frequently and become more interpretive and evaluative with repeated readings of the same story. The child tells more of the story independently, with improvements in the organization and completeness of the story emerging over time. More aspects of the pictures and text are discussed with greater detail, elaboration, and interpretation of issues. When the meaning and language of the story are well understood, the child then beings to focus on the print and ask questions about letters and words. Eventually, "reading" of the story emerges by shifting focus from the picture in early readings to the print in later readings (Bloome, 1985; Martinez & Rozer, 1985; Morrow, 1988; Snow & Goldfield, 1983; Sulzby, 1985; Yaden, 1988; Yaden, Smolkin, & Conlon, 1989).

The social interactions that occur between adult and child during storybook reading are instrumental in facilitating these developments. Numerous studies have revealed a highly interactive process in which both participants actively construct meaning based on the text and mutual feedback (Bloome, 1985; Morrow, 1988; Morrow & Smith, 1990; Ninio & Bruner, 1978). Parents establish storybook reading routines in which they help children to focus on important elements of the book through use of attention-getting dialogue, questions, naming or describing salient characters, objects, or events, and by providing informative feedback to children's questions and comments. These strategies direct a child to expect meaning from the book and the pictures, and maintain a child's attention on the most important aspects of the story.

Adults' Roles That Facilitate Learning

Within the storybook reading routine, adults assume different roles, each of which facilitates different aspects of development. These roles are the same as those that should be assumed by adults in intervention with school-age children.

First, adults assume the role of *co-respondents* by initiating discussions, recounting parts of the story, sharing personal reactions to characters or events, relating the experiences depicted in the book to real life experiences, and inviting children to produce similar types of responses.

Second, adults serve as *informers/monitors,* explaining events depicted or read, providing information that is important to understand the event, and asking questions to determine what a child understands about the story as they go along.

Third, adults function as *directors* who help the child learn the conventions of storybook reading and narrative language. They introduce the story, attending to titles, characters, and settings, and highlight conclusions, often with formal codas such as "The End." They lead the child to anticipate elements of story structure with comments such as "What do you think will happen next?" And they direct the child's attention back to the theme of the story when the child engages in off-task behaviors (Heath, 1982; Roser & Martinez, 1985).

Children's Roles as Active Learners

Children are not passive participants in storybook reading. The role of the school-age child should also be that of an active participant. As active learners, children listen attentively to the information read by parents, particularly the first few times that a story is read. They imitate the labels and descriptions provided by adults and ask for the names of characters and objects depicted, even when they already know the information. Numerous questions about the events in the story are asked, particularly during initial readings (Roser & Martinez, 1985). Comments are made regarding information that is familiar or known.

The interaction between adult and child results in changes in both participants across time. Adults modify their interactions to correspond to the child's changing needs and abilities (Heath, 1982; Morrow, 1988; Morrow & Smith, 1990; Yaden, Smolkin, & Conlon, 1989). As the child establishes more basic information, the adult asks questions on higher levels of semantic displacement, including predicting future events, providing motives or causes for events, making inferences, evaluating the quality and/or the events of the story, and associating the story events with personal experience. Gradually, the adult shifts from talking about the pictures and the story to more actual reading of the text, until all text alteration has been eliminated (Altwerger, Diehl-Faxon, & Dockstader-Anderson, 1985).

Children similarly change in their storybook behaviors. With successive readings, they attend to and comment on story elements highlighted by the adult in earlier readings, as well as elements that the child had pointed out or commented on in earlier readings. The child's comments closely mirror those modeled by the adult in both topic selection and information provided. The child also begins to attend to new and less literal information with repeated exposure to the same events. The child's questions shift from a focus on naming and specifying single actions, to requesting feedback on predictions or evaluations. The child talks more as the story becomes familiar, with decreasing questions and increasing comments (Martinez & Roser, 1985; Morrow & Smith, 1990, Snow, Nathan, & Perlman, 1985; Yadin, Smolkin, & Conlon, 1989). These increasing comments include many connections between events described in the book and the child's own life experiences (Mason & Allen, 1986).

Repeated readings of the same book allow for this development to occur. As more basic information becomes known to the child, more attention can be directed to details, similarities, elaborations, abstractions, and the language used to talk about them. This same type of learning is critically important to the school-age child who has failed to learn language with elaboration and flexibility and thus has the job of acquiring fluency in both oral and written language to succeed academically.

■□ INCREASING THE FOCUS ON PRINT

Children's awareness of written language increases Semantically along the Metalinguistic dimension, initially during the preschool years, and increasingly throughout the early elementary years. From an emerging awareness that the adult attends more to the print than to the picture during storybook reading, the child develops an increasing curiosity about the letters and words in the text. This emerging concept of word-ness, or metalinguistic awareness (i.e., Metalanguage-Erudite), is different from the child's use of language for communication, spoken without effort or reflection (Metalanguage-Experiential). Instead, meta-awareness reflects a conscious examination of written words. The printed words begin to acquire a status of object permanence, wherein the same words are recognized as referring to the same concept in different contexts. Metalinguistic awareness also is reflected in an increasingly more sophisticated understanding of the correspondence between letters and sounds, both independently of and within meaningful words.

This level of print awareness occurs simultaneously with other levels of print knowledge. Prior to fluent reading, children engage in reading-like behaviors. They generate a story from picture cues or from previous hearings of the story and then "read" the text with intonation characteristic of oral reading. They match their text to the story event, read from left to right, top to bottom, and change their intonation to match punctuation marks such as exclamation points or question marks. They self-correct their "reading" in attempts to try to recreate the actual story, and they use a more complex and formal literate language style. They engage in explorations of various aspects of print, at times showing a great curiosity in identifying and writing letters, and at other times concentrating on creating a meaningful message or story. They touch the printed words as they read, demonstrating an increasing correspondence between the words spoken and those separated by white spaces in the text. They begin to make judgments about the length of the printed words and the corresponding syllabic structure of the oral word, expecting long words to have many letters (Clay, 1991; Downing & Valtin, 1984; Sulzby, 1985).

The transition to fluent reading requires that all language processes must be coordinated for children to recognize and comprehend print. They must read the words in relationships of meaning within the sentences and across sentences to form Discourse structure, they must process the multiple embedding of ideas within one sentence as they are expressed through complex sentences and embedded clauses, they must understand how prefixes and suffixes function to modify the meaning of a word or to change its interpretation to reflect modulations in time or number, they must understand the vocabulary, and the vocabulary must exist within a flexible network so that multiple levels of meaning and interpretation can be activated simultaneously. Fluent readers must activate the correct background information and make the correct inferences to derive the author's intended meaning, they must be aware of strategies in the language that reorganize information into different spatial and temporal orders, and they must be able to change perspective to that of each character within a dialogue or each person referred to by the narrator. These and many other processes must be coordinated in integration with knowledge of print for fluent reading to result (Goodman, 1985; Norris, 1991; Smith, 1985).

Unfortunately for children with less flexible language systems, many of these processes of language are not well developed or refined, or if present are not activated with flexibility and generalizability in a variety of contexts. They are not available to facilitate the process of learning to read and, in turn, are not further refined during the process of reading. The vocabulary acquisition, mastery over multiply embedded sentences, development of complex and interactive levels of discourse structure, knowledge of how cohesive ties operate in long and convoluted text, and metaphoric and metalinguistic uses of language that normally result from reading and writing experiences are not stimulated for these children. Thus, the language system is not refined, so the child experiences continuing difficulties in both oral and written uses of language at school age.

■▢ FACILITATING ORAL AND WRITTEN LANGUAGE DEVELOPMENT

The principles of language facilitation shown to occur in the context of storybook reading can be used to facilitate language development in both oral and written modes in the older child as well. Book reading for the older child provides a potentially rich context for learning for all children, but in particular for those with less flexible language systems who have failed to acquire language at a level comparable to their peers. A book provides a repeatable context for observing and commenting on the same people, objects, and events across time. It allows for flexibility in interaction, because the same elements can be talked about at different levels of complexity or with a changing focus as more of the information becomes old or given. It provides a context in which the child with limited flexibility in language can function as an active participant in processing complex text by examining and using these patterns of language presented in print, which can then be commented on by the adult. Book reading provides the adult with a forum for talking about the same topic for an extended period, for asking picture and text related questions that are near the upper limits of the child's ZPD, and for providing the child with salient information and feedback (Norris, 1988, 1989, 1991, 1992).

Written language is the ideal context for facilitating refinement of the language system. Written language presents a stable expression of language that can be examined to create an awareness of its various components and levels without isolating any element from a context of use. The permanence of a written message allows the same information to be repeatedly examined or compared across sentence, paragraph, or story contexts, and difficult information to be reexamined or reorganized without the constraints on memory that limit oral language. Written text allows for the development of either narrative-centered or topic-centered *theme cycles,* provides for *redundancy* through repeated readings and integrated curriculum, enables the child to examine the language to discover how text maintains unity and *cohesion* through language. Whole-to part learning occurs as smaller elements of language are parsed and examined from within the whole text, and active learning occurs through the *social collaboration* provided by peers and the facilitative adult.

The use of written language in intervention to refine the language system is referred to as **Communicative Reading Strategies** (Norris, 1988, 1989, 1991). In this intervention, reading is conducted as a meaning-making process, where all cuing systems are simultaneously available and contribute to the child's processing of the written text and underlying language. Oral and written language are paired, so that the adult uses oral scaffolding and reference to specific aspects of print to enable the child to effectively reconstruct the author's written message. The amount of scaffolding used depends on the needs of the child, so that when more difficult text is encountered the adult may parse the sentence into constituent phrases or words and mediate the child's recognition of the meaning and form of these elements. When the text is easier to process, the adult's mediation may consist of modeling inferences, evaluations, or other higher levels of language interpretation.

Using Communicative Reading Strategies with the Nonreader

Many children with less flexible language systems remain essentially nonreaders even though they appear to have mastered prerequisites to reading. They guess at most of the words attempted and often refuse to read or skip over words or guess at words based on the pictures. They have difficulty decoding words, even though they appear to be able to associate sounds with letters in nonreading contexts. Many letters are only inconsistently recognized, or recognized only within the context of a familiar word, such as a name of a person, a toy, or a food logo. They struggle with each word, or rapidly call out best guesses without monitoring for meaning or sense. Punctuation is ignored, and comprehension is based primarily on background knowledge that the child may already have for the topic and can associate with the few words accurately read.

Selecting Text For the Nonreader

■ Pictures and Text should present similar information
■ Simple levels of Discourse structure
■ Semantically Descriptive text
■ Limited Interpretations or Inferences required
■ Topic that is interesting to the reader
■ Short and simple sentences
■ Predictable and redundant text

To facilitate the ability to process the written text, the print should be contextualized through illustrations that closely match the content of the story, or a **Contextualized-Symbolic** level. The **Discourse** structure should be simple, at levels of Descriptive Lists, Ordered Sequences, or perhaps Reactive Sequences. The **Semantic** context should be largely Descriptive with minimal demands for Interpretations or Inferencing. One story that can be effectively used with the older child because of the ageless topic of the story is *The Big Toe* (Melser & Cowley, 1980). The story illustrations depict a rather rough looking old woman who rides a motorcycle and wears a large floppy hat. She discovers a large toe lying in an overgrown cluster of plants, examines it with a magnifying glass, and puts it in the basket of her motorcycle with her groceries and takes it home. In the distance, a voice starts calling for its big toe, becoming progressively closer and louder with each page until the disembodied voice enters the old woman's house and demands its toe. The first five pages of the text read:

> An old woman found a big toe,
> and she took it home.
> Then something in the hall said,
> "Who's got my big toe?"

In Communicative Reading Strategies (Norris, 1988, 1989, 1991), the adult uses scaffolding strategies that parallel those used by adults to facilitate storybook reading in young children. These strategies enable children to simultaneously use multiple cuing systems when they process the written words, including the meaning suggested by the pictures, the contextual information activated by the adult's statements, the ideas communicated in previous sentences, predictions based on the Discourse structure, knowledge of probable words based on grammatical structure, knowledge of probable words based on semantic context, and knowledge of probable words based on phonemic structure and its relationship to letters.

The steps that are used to facilitate fluent reading and options for cues and feedback that can be provided in context are profiled in Figure 4–3. A transcript of an interaction is described below to provide a model of how the strategies are communicatively used to simultaneously assist the child to acquire more advanced language and reading abilities. [The interaction begins with a **preparatory set** that is specifically related to the idea communicated in the print. It is designed to activate the correct background knowledge needed to interpret the words and draw an association between the most important elements depicted in the illustration and the text.]

Adult: Jeremy, I wonder what the woman found in the flower bed? (points to the text which reads "THE BIG TOE")
Jeremy: A toe.

[The adult acknowledges the child's correct interpretation by verbally confirming it and then showing the child where that information is stated in the text. The adult then directs the child through a second preparatory set to consider another element of the sentence, or the size of the toe, and then models the reading of the sentence through an expansion.]

Adult: Right, a toe (points to the word "toe" in print). There is something unusual about it, something about its size.

(text continues on page 236)

Figure 4-3
Communicative Reading Strategies: Steps and optional strategies that can be used to simultaneously facilitate language and literacy development.

STEP 1

Provide the child with a *Preparatory Set*. This should activate very specific background information that suggests to the child what the meaning of the text will be. Any level of Preparatory Set can be provided, depending on the needs of the child and the purposes for the reading event.

Sentence to be read: **An old woman found a big toe**

The Preparatory Set can refer to a sentence.

> Prep Set: I wonder what she noticed?

OR

The Preparatory Set can be used to parse a difficult sentence into shorter phrases or ideas.

> Prep Set: This person (pointing to the old woman) noticed something
>
> Prep Set: and this is what she saw.

OR

The Preparatory Set can be used to unify larger units of meaning, such as a paragraph, particularly when the text is familiar or easy for the child to read.

> Prep Set: Find out why it's not smart to take things that don't belong to you

OR

The Preparatory Set can be used to become Metalinguistically aware of the structure of the discourse.

> Prep Set: Read about the initiating event, or the thing that changed the old woman's ordinary existence.

STEP 2

The child should be given the opportunity to read a unit of text that roughly corresponds to the Preparatory Set, or slightly more if the child maintains fluency and success.

STEP 3

IF

the child reads the text fluently

THEN

Acknowledge the communicative value of what was read by responding as if the child had orally told the information in conversation.

> Acknowledgment: She really is old!

OR

Expand the complexity of the sentence to include more markers of time, location, state, or attribution.

> Expansion: There was a very old woman!

OR

Expatiate by adding information that elaborates on the information communicated by the text.

> Expatiation: An old woman with wrinkles and warts!

OR

Extend the idea by linking the next phrase or sentence with an additional Preparatory Set.

(continued)

233

Figure 4-3 *(continued)*

> Extension: I wonder what that old woman found?

OR

Add *Semantic Displacement* by modeling an Interpretation, Inference, or Evaluation, including Erudite meanings.

> Semantic Displacement: She should have left that toe
> where she found it!

OR

Associate the information presented in the text with previously read or discussed information.

> Association: Oh, the old woman who was riding the
> motorcycle.

OR

Generalize the information to relevant situations or events that are familiar to the child or that would model an appropriate generalization.

> Generalization: She's just like the adventurous older lady
> that lives in our town!

BUT
IF

the child miscues when reading the text

THEN

Provide a *Semantic Cue*, such as a synonym or defining characteristics to assist the child to retrieve the word.

> Semantic Cue: An old "lady," older than a girl . . .

OR

Model a *Fluent Reading* so that the child can hear and see the word as it is used in context. Point to the miscued word as it is read.

Fluent Reading: An old *woman* found a big toe

OR

Divide the segment read into *smaller units*, such as phrases or words if the child's reading showed poor fluency, inappropriate phrasing, or drops in volume.

Smaller Units: This is what was found (*a big toe*)
And this is who found it (*an old woman*)

OR

Paraphrase the text to make the meaning clearer or more evident to the child, followed by reading it using the author's wording.

Paraphrase: This old woman saw a big toe in the garden, and so she picked it up. "An old woman . . .

OR

Remind the child of some previously read, discussed, or relevant *"Old Information"* that will help the child associate the print with meaning.

Old Information: Remember — How did we describe the person on the motorcycle?

OR

Reinforce the word, building a *Network* of information related to it using Expansion, Extension, Expatiation, Semantic Displacement, Association, Generalization, and so forth.

(continued)

Figure 4-3 *(continued)*

STEP 4

Following the reading of the passage, Metalinguistically *Analyze* the words that were difficult for the child, beginning with information already known by the child about its orthographic structure. See the text for a description of strategies for refining the child's analysis.

> Analysis: As a writer, how would you spell the word
> "woman"?

Jeremy: It's a big toe.
Adult: Right, it's The Big Toe (pointing to each word in the text).

[The children are then provided opportunities to read the text independently, which they are able to do in part because of immediate recall, but also because they are becoming Metalinguistically aware of the words as referents for the ideas in the story. The reading is referred to as a meaningful act, by asking the children to explain the story "by reading".]

Adult: Tom, you explain to us by reading what the woman found.
Tom: She found "The big toe" (points to the words as they are read).

[After the association of the print to language is established at the level of Description (i.e., what the woman found), the interaction then shifts to discussing the text at higher levels of Semantic displacement. The children are helped to think about where the toe came from (Inference), what the woman should do (Evaluation), and to derive a moral.]

Adult: Sarah, where do you think that toe came from?
Sarah: Maybe from someone who had an accident.
Jeremy: I think it looks like a giant's toe.
Tom: Yeah, a giant's toe, and it was cut off in a fight.
Adult: Do you think that she should take that toe, or just leave it there?
Tom: She should leave it there.
Adult: because . . .?

Tom: because the thing might want it back.

Sarah: Yeah, it belongs to the giant and not her.

Adult: So you think that it's not wise or right to take things that don't belong to you?

Tom: Yeah, you can get in trouble.

[The text is then examined at the level of Metalinguistics.]

Adult: As a reader, how do you know which word is "toe"?

Tom: Its this word (points to the word "big").

Adult: Well, that word tells my mouth to say "big" because of this letter "b" at the beginning. That is information that I use as a reader to help me read the author's message. What about the word "toe"?

Jeremy: (points to the word "toe") This is toe 'cuz it starts with "t."

Adult: Right, watch my mouth (exaggerates the production of the word) — the letters make my mouth say "toe." What other letters in the word help you to know what the word says?

Sarah: (points to the letter "e")

Adult: When we look at the vowels, we need to look at both of them together (covers the letter "t," leaving the "oe" visible). These two letters together show me to make the "o" sound.

The child is provided with purposeful reasons for establishing meaningful contrasts between letters and for associating letters with something that a reader *does* with the information that they provide. The adult begins by asking the child what he or she already knows and then provides feedback to the child regarding what additional information should be attended to and how conventions operate. In this manner, all levels of language are examined in a whole-to-part manner, beginning with the whole event and then parsing out elements to attend to, and by focusing on the lowest levels of displacement first within the semantic context, then systematically moving the focus to higher levels, with metalinguistics comprising the last level of discussion. In this manner, a context of meaning expressed through words, sentence structure, contextual cues, discourse structure, and background knowledge is activated and serves as a foundation for embedding the abstract metalinguistic aspects of language.

[Longer sentences in the text, such as "An old woman found a big toe and she took it home" are **parsed** into their constituents through the adult scaffolding. This strategy enables the child to successfully read the sentence even though it is above the independent level of reading ability, thus helping the child to process written language at upper levels of the zone of proximal development.]

Adult:	Sarah, tell us *who* found something.
Sarah:	The old woman . . .
Adult:	Right, "an" old woman (pointing to the word in the sentence), and now tell us *what* she found.
Sarah:	found a big toe
Adult:	And then tell us where she *took* it (pointing to the word "took" in the sentence to be read).
Sarah:	She took it hum, hom
Adult:	She's on her motorcycle and she's done with her grocery shopping (points to the groceries in the basket) so she's probably going _____
Sarah:	home!
Adult:	Right, so first she *found* the big toe (pointing to that word) *and* (pointing to the word) next she _____
Sarah:	took it home!
Adult:	I'm not sure that I would want it in my home! Jeremy, you tell us by reading about the woman and what did she . . .

The interaction continues with each child "telling" the story, locating words in the text that communicate various parts of the message, discussing the meaning at increasing levels of semantic displacement, then analyzing and comparing words for their Metalinguistic, or orthographic structure.

Following the reading of this episode, the children would engage in writing and exploration of key concepts through other media (art, drama) and related content areas (examining fingerprints under a magnifying glass; studying anthropological techniques for determining the species, size, and appearance of an animal from fossil remains). During the next intervention session, the old pages would be reread, this time requiring less scaffolding from the adult to read the words or prompt basic ideas, focusing instead on using language to specify a more elaborate setting or background for the event, predicting things that could happen next, and examining words Metalinguistically to discover more about the properties and patterns found in written words. The next episode of the story then would be communicatively read and discussed at all levels of language.

At the level of Discourse structure, the function of the first episode (i.e., establishing the setting and the initiating event) could be compared to the second episode (i.e., the faint voice calling out for its toe, or the consequence of the old woman's actions). The adult could help the children talk about how the author creates a story, the kind of information that he must give the reader first, and how it creates a problem that must be solved.

Thus, through careful examination of the same story over an extended period of time, with repeated readings and discussions occurring at many levels of Situational, Discourse, and Semantic context, the reader is helped to make an array of discoveries about reading and how it is done. The child is provided the time, the redundancy, the social collaboration, and the meaningful basis needed to internalize the information, including the logical patterns used in written language and the content needed to comprehend the story at different levels of abstraction. The oral and the written modes of language are simultaneously refined, and the flexibility of the language system is increased because the contextualized analysis of the language helps to facilitate an integrated network of knowledge.

If the time is taken to examine the text repeatedly and in detail, teaching to all levels of language, only one or two stories at this level of readability need to be examined before the child will have internalized sufficient knowledge about the orthographic patterns of written language in coordination with other levels of language to move to more complex text.

Using Communicative Reading Strategies with the Nonfluent Reader

Many children with less flexible language systems acquire rudimentary word recognition and decoding abilities, but are not able to coordinate this knowledge with the many other levels of language processing that must be integrated for fluent reading to occur. They read in a manner that is word-by-word, with frequent miscues and poor intonation. They miscue on words in one context that may have been correctly identified in the preceding sentence, and decode without also cuing on the meaningful and grammatical nature of the word in context, resulting in the production of nonwords such as "hoose" for "house." Some children at this level of fluency are able to get enough information if the topic is simple and familiar to comprehend the basic meaning of the text, but most children expend so much effort and attention on decoding that they attach little meaning to anything that is read. Often, the text that is read requires the child to make Interpretations and to draw Inferences from the context to understand the author's message, but the child may instead be processing the meaning primarily at the level of Description. Thus, the child may be able to answer factual questions or even retell major events, but fail to understand what the story is about.

To facilitate the ability to process the written text at this level, the print should be accompanied by illustrations that provide many aspects of meaning. Facial expressions, the actions related to the main ideas, and other significant cues should be depicted, although there will be many ideas that are presented in the text alone without corresponding illustration. The text itself will consist of longer sentences than that designed for a nonreader, with more difficult vocabulary words, more multisyllabic word patterns, and more sentences per page of text. One story that is humorous and motivating to children is *The Secret of Spooky House* (Cowley, 1990o). In this story, a monster family is eating supper in their castle when the baby monster begins protesting and tantruming. She is tired of monster food, such as boiled beetles, fried mice, and caterpillar juice, and demands popcorn. The monster parents cannot imagine where she gets her strange tastes from because monsters have *never* eaten popcorn, but the father eventually gives in, disguises himself and goes to a store to buy some. While popping it for the baby, he sneaks one little piece and then convinces his wife to "Dig your fangs into this!" It becomes a regular part of their evening meal, which they eat in secret so that the monster neighbors do not find out.

In Communicative Reading Strategies (Norris, 1988, 1989, 1991) the adult provides as much scaffolding as the reader requires to attain a level of fluency. When miscues occur, the adult uses these as an indication that some element of language is not understood and that the child is in need of more information to process the vocabulary or the grammar of the sentence or the meaning of that word or phrase in context. Thus, the child is helped to establish the meaning and intention of the author's communication first, then the Metalinguistic elements of the words are examined, if necessary. The adult behaves as if the child is communicating meaningful and interesting information, even when miscues occur, and provides feedback to the child that essentially "pushes meaning into" difficult words or phrases. The miscue is used to make decisions about what information the child is failing to process, rather than viewed as a error to be corrected. The steps and strategies profiled on Figure 4–3 are used, but the Preparatory Sets and feedback strategies correspond to the longer text and more sophisticated ideas compared to those for the nonreader. An example of an interaction is presented below.

> In Spooky House, the Monster family was at the table. Mr. and Mrs. Monster were having supper. The Monster child was having a tantrum. "Beetles! Beetles! Beetles!" she screamed. "I'm sick of boiled beetles! I want popcorn!" "Stop!" said Mr. Monster. "You're making my blood curdle."

The interaction begins by **parsing** the complex sentence, which begins with a prepositional phrase that had been transformationally moved, into its more basic constituents. A **preparatory set** for the idea communicated in the first constituent is provided to help the child achieve simultaneous fluency and meaning.

Adult: This describes the Monster family's home (pointing to the first phrase).
Andy: In Spooky House ...

[The child reads the phrase, and the adult responds with an enthusiastic comment about that spooky house, indicating to the child that what was read was meaningful and interesting to the listener. This is a very different type of **feedback** than what is typically given to readers, who often receive remarks such as "good reading." This latter type of remark tells the child that what is important is "getting the words right" and leaves the child's act of reading devoid of any communicative value, meaning, or purpose. The adult also uses feedback as an opportunity to **expatiate**, or model, an interpretation of the spooky house derived from the words and the pictures.]

Adult: It is spooky — it looks like an old castle.

[The **preparatory sets** that are provided are highly conversational, since Communicative Reading is treated as a dialogue occurring between the author, the child, and the facilitative adult. They ask the child to "describe," "find out," or help to answer the queries "I wonder why," or "What were they doing?"]

Adult: Find out what they were doing in that spooky house.
Andy: The Mans ..., the Munser

[When miscues occur, the adult's first goal is to help the child to establish the meaning of the idea, since this level of information is critical to communication. The adult may provide the child with **synonyms, explanations, contradictory evidence**, or activate relevant **background knowledge**, as in "They're not people, its a different kind of family who would live in a spooky house."?]

Adult:	They're not people, its a different kind of family who would live in a spooky house.
Andy:	The Monster family was (pause)
Adult:	(points to the monsters seated at the table)
Andy:	at the table.
Adult:	They were sitting at that table, wearing their bibs and holding their spoons. I wonder why Emily, what were they doing? (pointing to the next sentence)
Emily:	Mer and . . .
Adult:	This is the word that people use to talk about men, they don't call them by their first name, they call them _____
Emily:	Mr. Mr. Monster.

[Immediately after the meaning has been established, as in the discussion of the abbreviation for "Mr.," but preferably later, after the paragraph or episode is read and discussed, the adult may choose to examine miscued words for their orthographic structure and their similarity to other words or spelling patterns (see the example below). The metalinguistic level of discussion is different in purpose and form than the level of processing that is focused on maintaining the communicative nature and coherence of the passage. If a metalinguistic analysis occurs with high frequency, it often interrupts the child's attempts at reconstructing meaning and attaining fluent expression.]

Adult:	Right, lets look at that word. You may not have seen it in print before. It is really an abbreviation for the long word "mister." See the period at the end of the letters Mr. — that tells me its an abbreviation. So what were the parents doing?
Emily:	Mr. and Mrs. Monster were having supper.

[When a miscue occurs on a word that may not be in the child's vocabulary or may not be readily retrieved, even with cues, the adult may behave as if the child read the word correctly (as in "tantrum") and then support the word with **expansions** (i.e., he is having a *temper tantrum*) and **expatiations** that serve to "push" meaning into the word.]

Adult:	They were; I can see them eating supper. But Jim, look, it doesn't look like the baby is eating his supper. What is he doing instead?

Jim: The Monster child is having a tan ... tanterm
Adult: Right, he is having a *tantrum*.

[In this case, the children were helped to generate expatiations through the adult's use of **comprehension questions** [i.e., How can you tell he is throwing a temper tantrum?], thus allowing them to make **interpretations** and use language at higher levels of semantic displacement. The adult also helps the child to attend to relevant contextual cues by using pointing and other gestures that highlight actions, facial expressions, or other details that inform the reader.]

Adult: Look at the picture. How can you tell that he is throwing a temper tantrum?
Emily: His mouth is open real wide like he's yelling or something.
Adult: I bet he's really yelling loudly! What else?
Andy: He's throwing his hands like this (demonstrates) and the bugs are flying everywhere.

The adult may also use **cloze**, beginning a sentence or phrase and then letting the child complete the idea by contributing relevant words. This strategy is particularly useful if a very difficult sentence is encountered in a story and the child begins to show signs of anxiety or frustration.

Understanding Written Language Conventions

Elements of written language convention are discussed as they are encountered during the reading process. The adult talks to the children as though they were **collaborators** in the process of making sense of the author's code. Thus, quotation marks and punctuation points are shown to the children in context, accompanied by an **explanation** of how and why a reader might use them. In the Communicatively Read passage below, each child is then given opportunities to take the role of the speakers within the dialogue of the text, and is provided feedback on the success in capturing the affect and intentions of the character's lines. Also modeled in this passage is attention to **cohesive ties**. When the text indicates that the baby monster is a girl through the use of the pronoun "she," the adult **points** to the word in the text that shows where she is getting the information about the referent and associates it with **old information**, or previously established facts or concepts, by pointing back and forth between the pronoun and the original referent.

Adult: Now we will find out exactly what the baby monster was yelling during that tantrum. See these quotation marks

	(points to the punctuation)? This tells us as readers that someone is talking. And look (points to exclamation marks), this tells us that they are saying something *very* loudly. Jim, pretend you are the baby monster and tell us what he said.
Jim:	"Beetles! Beetles! Beetles! she skeem.
Adult:	Oh, its a little girl monster, and she (points to word in text, and then points back and forth between the pronoun and the words "Monster child" found earlier) didn't just quietly say Beetles! She opened her mouth wide and made a lot of noise, she _____
Jim:	screamed!
Adult:	Yes, she is saying "Yuk, I don't want beetles, I'm sick of beetles, beetles are disgusting" She says the word "Beetles!" like she is very disgusted. Emily, you be the little monster and scream about the beetles to show the parents that you do not want anymore beetles (each child role plays the dialogue several times for both the little monster's tantrum, and the father's reply).

In the context of role playing, the adult can make the children aware of the difference between narration and dialogue by discussing the "instructions from" the author (i.e., the author is telling you as a reader that you need to scream [pointing to "she screamed"]), or information "given by" the author (i.e., "In Spooky House, the Monster family was at the table"), versus the "characters lines" or "actual speech" used by the characters. The children can take turns functioning within the narrator's role and the characters' roles by having some of the group members read the narration while others are assigned to a character's part. This helps the children to understand that there are many levels of discourse occurring within a story and more than one perspective that must be simultaneously considered (Bruce, 1981). Several stories and books can be examined and compared for their relative use of dialogue versus narration, from plays that primarily consist of dialogue to narratives and exposition that vary widely in the amount of dialogue used.

Creating an Understanding of Conventions

■ Collaborate to make sense of the author's code
■ Introduce punctuation in context while reading
■ Role play to differentiate dialogue from narration

(continued)

> ■ Refer to author's intention or purpose behind the use of conventions of form and style
> ■ Change roles and talk about perspective taking
> ■ Read for "hidden meaning"
> ■ Subject difficult words to Metalinguistic analysis

As always, the information communicated in the episode can be discussed at progressively more abstract levels of **Semantic displacement**. Questions can be used to help the children infer why the little monster does not want beetles and what the parents should do and why. The metaphor "You're making my blood curdle" can be examined, and the children can be helped to decide what it means through reference to **context cues** (pointing back to old information, such as the screaming, the tantrum, and Mr. Monster's command for this to stop) and a discussion of how the children feel when somebody is annoying them or will not stop doing some aversive behavior. The children can be helped to retell the story by **summarizing** the most important events (van Dijk & Kintsch, 1983). This process helps the children to decide what information constitutes main ideas versus supporting details, and it provides them opportunities to logically organize and express ideas at varying levels of **Discourse structure**, especially as more episodes are added to the story. Thus, the children are provided opportunities to examine the story at levels of Metalanguage.

During the oral reading, the adult should either record or mentally note the words that elicited miscues or that were difficult for the child to rapidly recognize or decode. Several of these words should then be subjected to **Metalinguistic analysis**. This may occur on several occasions during the reading, such as at the end of each paragraph, or conducted only after that day's reading is completed, or may even occur in the context of the first reading if a word is particularly problematic or unfamiliar to a child. This analysis should be conducted as a **collaborative process**, where the children are engaged in active problem solving under conditions of guidance and feedback from a facilitative adult. The purpose is not to teach the child orthographic rules, but rather to enable the child to *deduce* the regularities and patterns in syllable structure and orthographic representation. The analysis is approached from the perspective of meaningful and purposeful communication between authors and readers, rather than as skills to learn. The interaction begins with what the **children understand,** or their belief about the representation of the word, and refines the representation in accordance with the information that they are failing to consider or cannot yet coordinate.

```
┌─────────────────────────────┐
│                             │
│   Metalinguistic Analysis   │
│                             │
│       of the word           │
│                             │
│        scream               │
│                             │
└─────────────────────────────┘
```

Adult: Let's look at a few of the words (takes out a white board and marker). If you were the author and wanted the reader to say the word "screamed," how would you spell it Jim?

Jim: s-k-e-m-d

Adult: (writes the spelling and then points to the letters in sequence) That tells my mouth to say "skemed" instead of "screamed". Listen to the beginning of the word, I think I hear more sounds at the beginning.

Andy: s-r-k-e-m

Adult: (writes word and provides feedback) That tells my mouth to say "serkem." Listen again, sc-ream (exaggerates production).

Emily: Oh! s-k-r-e-m

Adult: Okay, that helps me as a reader. Now it tells me to say skrem. But something about the vowel in the word is still different from what I am expecting. Listen to the difference, "screm" — "scream". What two letters could I use to make the vowel an /i/ sound?

Jim: An "e" on the end

Adult: That's one way (writes it), but it is not the way that the reader expects the word "scream" to look. There must be another way of using two vowels together.

Andy: "ee"

Adult: Let's try it (writes it). That's kind of what the reader expects, but not quite. Some other vowel besides this second "e."

Jim: Try "ea"

Adult: There you go (writes it). Now the vowels are what the reader expects. But there is one more difference, some other letter besides "k" that can make that /kʌ/sound.

Emily: A "c."

Adult: Okay, so tell me how to write it now.

Unison: s-c-r-e-a-m

Adult: Now we are telling the reader that there was a scream, but the author told us that the baby already screamed. What do we need to add?

Andy: Add "ed."

Adult: Let's see if that's how the author spelled it (retrieves the book and the children find the word in context and make comparisons to their spelling).

Summary

Too often in school, book reading is treated as something that must be hurried through, to get on to the next book and to cover all of the stories dictated by some arbitrary curriculum or lesson plans. Children are discouraged from rereading favorite selections because it is believed that they are not learning anything new or covering enough material. Discussions, if they occur at all, are cursory and often consist of "comprehension checks," rather than explorations of intentions, background information, or evaluations of characters and their actions. No one learns very much from such trivialized treatment of a story, and children with less flexible language systems learn the least of all. Research has shown us that literacy and language emerge in a context of repeated readings conducted over time with a facilitative collaborator helping the child to increasingly coordinate more elements of the text and the reading process at higher levels of linguistic sophistication and with greater independence. It is this supportive type of learning environment that intervention must seek to emulate.

Common Mistakes to Avoid When Using CRS

- Fail to activate background using Preparatory Sets
- Fail to parse complex sentences into constituents
- Focus on the form of a miscued word (i.e., sounding it out) before meaning has been established
- Allow the child to quickly read multiple sentences despite miscues and poor intonation
- Ask comprehension questions instead of working together to construct the meaning of the text
- Fail to use print to teach complex aspects of syntax, morphology, semantics, or pragmatics
- Define unknown words, rather than deducing a meaning from context
- Quiz child for the meaning of concepts instead of using expansions, extensions, expatiations,

(continued)

---

associations, and generalizations to push meaning
into words
■ Use of noncommunicative statements such as "good
  reading" in the mistaken belief that they are
  reinforcing
■ Skipping over a child who doesn't know an answer
  instead of taking the opportunity to teach language
■ Discussing or asking questions only at the most
  explicit level of recall, instead of using open-ended
  statements and questions that encourage higher
  levels of Semantic interpretation.

Often when individuals are attempting to implement Communicative Reading Strategies with children, they fall into old patterns of
"teaching reading" that they encountered in school. They ask the child to
read before activating background knowledge with a preparatory set,
require the child to read an entire sentence without parsing it into its
constituents, ask the child to "sound out" a word when a miscue occurs
without giving the child any clues as to what concept he might be trying
to retrieve, allow the child to quickly read multiple sentences without
providing expansions and expatiations that push meaning into the
words, even when the child's reading is monotone or the phrasing is not
appropriate to the meaning, and then ask a series of comprehension
questions (e.g., Who was the story about? Where did they live? What
were they getting ready to eat? What did the little monster do? Why was
he screaming?) and so on, ad nauseam.

The child quickly gets the message that oral reading has no communicative value and is done only to get information that can be used to
answer questions that are asked for no purpose, that are boring, and that
contribute essentially nothing to the interpretation of the story or the
language. When a child cannot answer a question, he is often skipped
over in favor of a child who can, and so *no one* learns anything because
the child who could not answer still has no information that can be used
to find out **where in the language** that information was communicated,
and the one who can answer already knew the information and is provided no expansions or expatiations of existing knowledge.

More is accomplished when one or two stories at a given level of
readability are read slowly and examined at multiple levels of situational,
discourse, and semantic structure than when ten times as many stories
are read on a superficial level, or when children are not even allowed to
experience print in the context of a story because they "can't read well

enough yet" or "haven't mastered prerequisites." All of the skills that they need to know can be mastered in the context of reading, just as all of the language behaviors that children need to know are learned in the context of speaking during the preschool years and beyond. If the time is taken to comprehensively help the child to internalize a wide range of information regarding the patterns of language and the content networked within themes and topics, then the child will have the foundation to move on to more complex levels of readability and to deal with higher levels of Decontextualization, Discourse structure, and Semantic displacement. The social collaboration and familiarity of the topic provided for through facilitated repeated readings of the same book enable this process to occur at an accelerated rate.

■ PROVIDING INTERVENTION IN THE CONTEXT OF WRITING

Reading well written stories and expository text provides the child with opportunities to learn how language communicates meaning through the use of words, cohesive ties, complex sentences and their strategies for embedding and establishing relationships between ideas, Discourse structures at all levels of Transactional-Expressive-Poetic context, literary style, and levels of Semantic displacement. By reading as a *language learner* rather than a word decoder, the child begins to internalize these many levels of language and to coordinate them into networks of interconnected knowledge. But learning to actively reconstruct an author's message is not the same as coordinating these multiple levels of language to be an effective communicator of one's own ideas and information. Children need facilitative experiences using written language to express their own experiences and concepts of the world to refine language at levels that support effective communication.

■ EARLY DEVELOPMENT OF WRITING

During the preschool years, children view writing as a holistic process, done for purposes of communicating a message. A few marks written on a paper represent an entire message or story, in much the same way that single words stand for whole events in early language development. Writing at this level is primarily at the highly personal **Expressive Discourse** level, used to investigate the patterns of letters and organization, to play with, and to use in personally satisfying ways. Many discoveries about writing are made through these explorations, including the directionality and arrangement of writing on a page, the formation of letters, the phonetic and syllabic aspects of word representations discussed in Chapter 3, and the types of messages that can be written for different purposes and audiences (Clay, 1991; Ferreiro & Teberosky, 1982).

Each dimension of writing develops in coordination with the others, each with its own progression but each interacting with and informing other aspects. A child in one instance of writing may compose an entire story, but this complex discourse structure may be represented using the child's least sophisticated encoding procedure, such as a series of random scribbles and marks. In another instance of writing, the child may carefully make letters that maintain many of the features of conventional letters for purposes of exploring graphic features and representations. In this case, no message may be intended, although after making a letter it may remind the child of a person's name or other referent, and it may be pointed to while declaring "That says Rachel." Through these different types of experiences engaged in for different purposes, the many facets of writing begin to refine and interconnect.

As the child becomes more aware of the need to coordinate both the meaning of the message and the conventions of the form, writing may be perceived as more difficult by many children. The child may be less willing to compose by putting down random letters or initial sounds, but instead shows concern that the letters correspond to the intended words in some conventional manner and that the writing tells a real story. They begin to rely on other more mature writers and models of writing for support as they attempt to simultaneously coordinate the different aspects of writing (Calkins, 1991; Clay, 1991).

■□ FACILITATING WRITING IN THE SCHOOL-AGE CHILD

The reliance on models and more mature writers during the writing process provides many opportunities for scaffolded interactions to occur. The amount and type of scaffolding provided will depend on the purpose for writing, the independent abilities of the child, the amount of contextualization provided by the situation, the topic of the composition, and the type of discourse structure used.

Often, children are expected to write spontaneously on a topic, with minimal attention devoted to developing ideas and rehearsing the information to be included. They are provided with a specified, frequently minimal amount of time to complete the composition, and once the first draft is on paper the paper is considered finished. Thus, writing is treated as an activity, rather than as a means of communication. The object becomes "getting done" rather than expressing ideas with completeness and clarity. The results of this unplanned and unsupported writing is static, unelaborated, and impersonal writing that lacks creativity and style. A worse result is a child who believes that writing is a difficult, boring, and nonproductive activity. To prevent these negative attitudes and poor products of writing, children must be assisted to develop interesting ideas that are motivating to them and to organize much of the content and form before information is actually encoded into print.

Using Communicative Strategies with the Nonwriter

Many children with less flexible language systems remain essentially nonwriters even though they appear to have mastered many aspects of writing as separate skills. They may be willing to dictate a story to someone who will act as a scribe and encode it into writing, or they may be willing to copy some already completed work, or punctuate lists of sentences in the context of a worksheet. But when they attempt to coordinate these separate processes into an integrated composition, the results may be a few poorly spelled words ordered in ungrammatical strings that communicate a simple label or comment. Conventions of punctuation or capitalization are not observed; therefore, a random combination of capital and lower case letters may be used within the same word, based on which form of the letter is most easily retrieved, easiest to make, or thought of first, with no attention to the meaningful purposes of capitalization or punctuation.

Writing strategies should be chosen by the adult to assist children to attend to and incorporate the elements of writing that they presently cannot coordinate. The Situational-Discourse-Semantic model can be used for this purpose. For example, by reducing complexity along the Situational dimension by writing about personal experiences (Decontextualized-Egocentric) or about topics represented through objects or pictures (Contextualized-Symbolic), the child can attain experience with planning a message with more complex Discourse structure, or greater Semantic displacement. Similarly, by reducing complexity along the Discourse dimension (see the suggestions presented within the levels of the Discourse Context presented in Chapter 2), greater attention can be directed at the Metalinguistic level of the Semantic Context, including spelling, punctuation, and handwriting.

The following are strategies that can be used to immerse the very beginning and/or very reluctant nonwriter in writing about meaningful, communicative topics.

Modeled Dictation

If a child is to compose like a writer, then it must be understood what a writer does and thinks about during the composing process. Modeling the writing process in response to the children's dictation is one method for helping them to learn how to think like a writer (Lee & Allen, 1963). Often, this is conducted by engaging in an experience, such as going on a field trip, or doing an in-class experiment, followed by dictated writing about the experience. Many excellent resources are available for learning more about dictated writing experiences (McGee & Richgels, 1990; Temple, Nathan, Burris, & Temple, 1988). However, many children with less flexible language systems lack the Semantic and Discourse abilities to move beyond simple Collections or Descriptive Lists in their writing. They dictate ideas such as:

I saw elephants.
I saw a giraffe.
I saw a monkey.

When they try to dictate something more complex, the ideas lack coherence, are poorly structured in form, and lack creativity. The interventionist is left trying to help the child refine or reorganize text that the child considers to be already finished. This usually results in frustration for all participants. Instead of trying to repair completed text, the adult needs to help the child to rehearse and organize ideas before they are dictated. The scaffolded use of flowcharts described previously in this chapter can be used to organize the ideas from the field trip, experiment, or other experience. A second strategy is to use a picture. The actions and ideas depicted can help the child to learn to organize ideas and talk about interesting things at higher levels of Discourse and Semantic context.

Pictures can depict events similar to an actual experience (e.g., the field trip to the zoo), a procedure (e.g., a classroom experiment), or an event. The children can select a picture for discussion and writing that is related to the topic. The event depicted should be familiar to the child so that background information can be easily activated, but should also have something unusual or interesting to talk about. For example, one illustration in the book *Busy Baby* (Cowley, 1989b) shows a baby sitting on the floor chewing on an empty bag of flour, while his older brother (looking quite angry) is busily sweeping the white powder. The cabinet where the flour had been stored is wide open and messy. The older sister is using a feather duster and cloth to wipe off the curtains, sink, and other areas coated in the flour.

Scaffolded interactions should be used to discuss the picture, beginning with a comment generated by a child and then elaborated on in a topic-centered manner. For example, the child might offer:

Child: The boy is sweeping the floor.
Adult: You're right, he is, probably because _____ (pointing to the baby and flour sack)
Child: the baby has the sack.
Adult: Well, the sack *used* to have flour in it, but now _____ (points to places where the flour is scattered)
Child: Oh, that's funny. The flour is all over the room!
Adult: because the baby opened _____
Child: the sack and spilled it all over everything.
Adult: The boy is _____ (points to the boy's face, then to the flour all over the room)
Child: mad because the flour is all over the room, on the floor and the cabinet and sink.
Adult: The boy and his sister were *supposed* to be watching the baby but _____
Child: they forgot 'cuz they were playing.

After collaboratively structuring an interpretation of the event with logical relationships between actions, states, and characters, the children are encouraged to discuss and develop the oral story further.

The adult then asks for a sentence to be written down. This is now an easy request, because the children have many well organized and relevant ideas that they can share. For example, one child may dictate "The baby spilled the flour and made a big mess." The adult begins the writing process, talking metacognitively about what she is thinking about as she engages in the writing process.

> "I'm going to start in the middle of the paper because I want to leave room for my illustration. A writer always begins on the left side of the paper, and so I will put my first letter right here. Let me think, "the," it makes my mouth say /ð/ and so I will use the letters "th" to help the reader make that sound. It is the first word in the sentence, and that is important information to give readers so I will capitalize the "T" — The. I'm done with that word and so I will leave a
>
> *(continued)*

> white space and then try the word "baby." I need to tell the reader to make the /bʌ/ sound — do you have any ideas what letter I should use?"

Similar metacognitive "thinking out loud" occurs while the adult is writing. The children then are asked to help choose a way to illustrate the story in a manner that matches the story. The adult draws in response to the child's instructions. After one or two modeled dictations of sentences, the children are encouraged to write and illustrate their favorite part of the story.

Writing in response to modeled dictation can be used as one easy method of documenting change and maintaining records for purposes of accountability. Observing children in the process of this writing also provides the adult with insights into the aspects of writing that are developing versus those that are not yet emerging. For example, judgments can be made regarding whether the child approaches the writing task with an idea to communicate, as reflected by the oral dictation and rehearsal, the illustration, and/or the actual text written. Observations can be made to determine what information was picked up from the metacognitive talk, such as letters that are capitalized, left to right or top to bottom directionality in the writing, and white spaces between words. The spelling can be evaluated for the types of patterns that are evidenced, from prephonemic through conventional, as well as the phonological processes found in semiphonetic approximations. The amount of additional encouragement and scaffolding required to engage and maintain the writing also is noted. All of these judgments are viewed as baseline data, or the present upper end of the ZPD. These observations reflect the amount of complexity and conventionality that is achieved under conditions of strong Contextual support. Progress is measured relative to these initial observations, and refinement is facilitated from these baseline levels.

Writing From Illustrations

Some children will reject attempting to write, even following modeled dictation, but they will orally rehearse a story and/or draw an illustration. Scaffolded interactions should be used to help the child put the story into pictures with more complexity and detail. Drawing and speech are considered to be first-order symbol systems, or modes of expression that a child learns to control before second-order systems like writing (Dyson, 1988). When assisted by scaffolding, children can learn to translate between speech and writing when the ideas are first represented in drawing. For example, if the child draws the big brother sweeping as a primitive stick figure, the adult could prompt refinement by saying, "But I really can't tell if you're character is happy or mad about having to sweep. As an illustrator, how could you communicate that information to your reader?" or "But I really can't tell what he is sweeping or where the mess came from. What could you put in your illustration to help the reader understand that part of the story?"

Once a fairly elaborated picture is drawn, the child can be encouraged to write a few words about one element of the picture. The adult can help the child think about ways to represent these words, using the same types of collaborative interactions used to derive a spelling for the word "scream" in the example above. At a later time or another day, a second element of the picture can be represented, and so on. Within a short period, even a very reluctant writer will have composed a fairly lengthy and coherent passage (Calkins, 1986, 1991; Dyson, 1988). The child gains confidence and independence because of the redundancy of the topic and context of the writing and the words that appear redundantly across sentences (i.e., flour, baby, mess, clean). The illustration provides a visual scaffold from which to write, and oral interactions can be used to scaffold possible word choices and sentence structures to explain parts of the illustrated story. These multiple sources of contextual support reduce the amount of processing that must be expended on higher level language processes so that the child can focus attention and efforts on gaining control over the use of print to encode the message.

Writing Through Alteration

Alteration can be used at a variety of different levels of writing complexity and for different purposes. It is often successful with the poor or reluctant writer who will not attempt to write sentences in response to modeled dictation or drawing. Alteration may begin with a photocopy of a page or episode from a story that had been read and discussed using Communicative Reading Strategies (Norris, 1988, 1989, 1991). For example, Chapter 3 of *Busy Baby* (Cowley, 1989b) reads:

> We took Vanessa out into the yard. She crawled over the grass and laughed at us. "Don't let her eat any worms," I said to Peter. "Will they make her sick?" Peter asked. "No, but it'll make me sick to watch," I replied. (p. 16)

The child can be provided with a bottle of liquid paper, or the white correction fluid used by typists. The child can then change as many or as few elements of the story as she chooses to reflect her own ideas. The names of the characters can be changed, the location can be moved from the yard to the garden, the item eaten changed to dirt instead of worms (children are *much* more creative at this than we are with our examples).

By only attempting to encode single words that reflect the child's own ideas, the child can create a unique story that is meaningful and creative, that has sentence and discourse structure, and for which punctuation and spelling are largely supplied by the existing text. This is highly reinforcing to children who struggle to put words on paper, but have only illegible writing with undecipherable spelling as a result. Other types of alterations can be encouraged, such as adding embellishments to the existing ideas using adverb, adjective, or prepositional phrases, or adding extensions or expatiations through use of a conjoined clause, or appending another sentence to a paragraph. These alterations can be collaboratively facilitated, as in the following dialogue:

Adult: As readers, we really don't know very much about Vanessa. You could give the reader more information about her personality if you used an adjective in front of her name (draws a caret ˆ in front of the name on the text) like "naughty Vanessa" or "adventuresome Vanessa" or "baby Vanessa." What adjective would you choose to let the reader know something important about her?"

Child: I think she's cute, so I'll put cute — cute and bad.

Through these types of scaffolded alterations, the child learns to add detail and creativity to writing; begins to gain control over encoding ideas in print; engages in repeated rereading of the passages as decisions about modifications are made; begins to develop a self-concept of a creative and successful writer; and learns about grammatical analysis of sentences and parts of speech in a meaningful, contextualized manner. Critical thinking, activation of background knowledge, and explorations of spelling, as well as many other skills, are engaged in as the child chooses and conducts alterations.

A variation of this alteration process can be used in the context of dictated stories. Rather than writing all of the words dictated by the child, the scribe can leave blank spaces to accommodate important words or words that the adult believes to be within the child's independent level of writing. The child then completes the composition. One advantage of this use of alteration is that the child's own ideas comprise all of the composition, but the responsibility for encoding the ideas into writing is shared. Thus, ideas that the child could not independently put into writing are communicated through collaborative efforts with an adult or a peer who has better control over the writing process.

Using Communicative Strategies with the Nonfluid Writer

Fluid writing requires the author to choose a purpose for writing, decide who the audience will be, evaluate the needs and sophistication of the audience, select a topic, develop the topic, organize it in an appropriate Discourse structure for the purposes of the composition, choose the appropriate Semantic level to express the ideas, use syntactic and morphological strategies to order the ideas in the most appropriate semantic relationships, Metalinguistically represent the sound and intonational patterns of the words in orthographic patterns and punctuation, and coordinate the fine motor movements needed for handwriting.

Rehearsal strategies help the child to do many of these steps prior to writing and enable the ideas to be placed into words orally first. Rehearsal strategies provide a scaffold that reduces the number of processes that must be conducted at the time of writing. The result is a more creative, better organized composition that is more likely to have spelling attempts at the child's upper level of the ZPD. Two types of graphic organizers that can be used in the process of rehearsal are semantic webs and flowcharts.

Writing From Semantic Webs

As children gain more control over the writing process, less comprehensive scaffolds can be provided. One strategy is the use of semantic webs or other graphic organizers. They may be used with spontaneously generated stories or expository text, or they may be used to parallel the story from a book. For example, for a beginning writer a book such as *Who Will Be My Mother?* (Cowley, 1983b) can be used. In this story, a lamb's mother died and so he searched from animal to animal looking for someone to be his mother. First he approached the horse and asked "Horse, Horse, will you be my mother?", then the bull, the rabbit, the hen, and finally a boy. He was told by each that they could not be his mother. A semantic web can be drawn (see diagram), with a space for the baby animal of the child's choice in the center. On one leg of the web, the names for potential baby animals can be generated by the group, such as puppy, kitten, calf, or piglet. On another leg, zoo animals that the baby animal could ask to be its mother could be listed, farm animals on a third leg, people in different occupations on a fourth, and so on. One leg could have reasons for the baby animal's orphaned status: The mother died, moved, disappeared, was sick, and so forth. As the web is being constructed, the children could help generate the spellings for some of the words, as exemplified for the word "screamed."

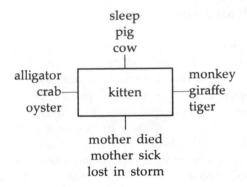

Using the web, the children then could generate a story that paralleled the book version, substituting a baby animal of the child's choice for the lamb and other animals for those encountered. The context provided by the text in the original book, the words organized on the semantic map, and the oral discussion would reduce the information processing load sufficiently for many children to write a well structured composition, including success with the encoding process. Some children would rely to varying degrees on copying the text from the book and integrating concepts from the semantic map, while others would only use these visual representations as references or scaffolds for stories that vary creatively from the original. This enables children with a wide range of writing abilities to participate in the same oral discussions prior to writing, but compose at their own level of independence.

For a more advanced writer, the same principles could be applied at a level of greater complexity, by using a book such as *Crocodile! Crocodile!* (Mahy, 1990) to organize a story. The text on the first page begins:

> There was once a crocodile who lived in the middle of a deep, dark, dismal, dripping swamp. For years, he had lived on nothing but swamp fish. "I'm sick of swamp fish," the crocodile said one day. "Other crocodiles eat all sorts of things. I shall go to town and eat everyone I catch."

As the story progresses he crawls under a hedge, frightens a man away, and eats his deck chair and paper; he then climbs over a wall, terrifies the mail carriers, and eats their bags of letters; he crawls down main street, chases off a patron and eats her overdue library books, and so forth. This level of Complex Poetic structure presents a series of parallel episodes in which there are changes in location, action, characters, and objects, and yet the basic plot remains the same throughout. The text models complex sentence structures, but is composed of easy words and provides opportunities for the child to use the author's model to experiment with adjective phrases and other relational language in a manner that is humorous and creative. Once again, the center of the semantic web can be reserved for the child's choice of creature, and each leg can be used to brainstorm potential places where the animal could roam, people and animals he could scare, verbs used to describe the creature's actions, verbs used to describe the victim's responses, and so forth.

Writing From Flowcharts

Flowcharts can be used to help the child generate a well structured story or exposition with relative independence. They provide a visual map of both obligatory and optional elements that may be included in the child's composition and, when completed, provide a method for orally rehearsing the word choices and sentence structures that can be used to communicate the ideas before the first draft is written. Original stories, historical accounts, scientific comparisons, experimental procedures, and categories such as geographic landmarks, may be organized on the flowchart, using procedures discussed under examples of Intervention in Oral Language Contexts presented previously in this chapter.

Flowcharts also may be used to enable children to use a well composed story to write a parallel one of their own. In the story *The Giraffe Who Could Not Walk* (Butterworth, 1986b) a giraffe is sitting in the middle of the forest because he has hurt his leg. He asks himself what he will do, since he cannot walk on his leg. This page thus establishes the setting and the initiating event of the story. The text can be collaboratively examined, as the adult helps the children to determine how the author informs the reader about who the character is, where the character lives or is found, and where this information is located in a well formed story. Similarly, the manner in which the author uses both narration and dialogue to introduce the problem can be discussed.

One child's idea for a story can then be flowcharted, using the style of the story presented in the book as a model. By referring to the strategies used by the author to provide key information to the reader, the children can generate parallel ideas for their stories, and these key words can be entered on the flowchart. For example, the child may choose as elements of setting a character (e g., a bird), a location (e.g., a sky-scraper), and a time period (e.g., last week). Elements of the problem can then be charted, including the goal (e.g., feeding baby birds), the road-block (e.g., too windy to fly), and the internal response (e.g., worried about the nest and the babies). Oral scaffolding then can be used to rehearse strategies for putting the information into words. The child can use the key words to spontaneously generate sentences, or if the child needs assistance the adult can point to a sequence of ideas on the flow-chart and use scaffolding strategies such as prompting with relational terms, cloze, constituent questions, and so forth to help the children put ideas into words.

Summary

Often the task of writing is overwhelming for children with less flexible language systems and the results of their attempts are short, unelabo-rated compositions that fail to focus on a topic, exhibit little more than rudimentary Discourse structure, or reflect poor spelling and punctua-tion. Attempts to refine the composition once it is already in writing are sabotaged by the child, who considers the written product to be com-pleted, and who lacks the Metalinguistic skills needed to analyze the content or form for purposes of editing. Many of these problems can be eliminated by spending time in the rehearsal process, before ideas are committed to print. Variations of the suggestions provided here enable children to be successful creative writers who use collaborative editing to refine their compositions, rather than to criticize and completely re-structure their work. The scaffolding procedures facilitate the child's progress along the continuum from maximum reliance on visual context and socially mediated assistance, to independence at decontextualized levels of writing.

◼️ SUMMARY

This chapter has provided an overview of language intervention as viewed from a Whole Language perspective. The goal of intervention is to facilitate participation in language experiences near the upper limits of a child's Zone of Proximal Development (ZPD), as defined by Vygot-sky (1978). Intervention occurring at upper limits of the zone serves to guide development along paths of greater complexity and abstraction. The use of language in the context of social mediation, or scaffolding, has been shown to be critical to this process. Numerous suggestions for providing contextual support and verbal scaffolding in contexts of oral and written language were demonstrated. The strategies described in this chapter do not comprise a comprehensive overview of the techniques that can be used in intervention, but rather serve as models for understanding how holistic interactions might proceed and how they can be implemented. The strategies and methods are merely interpretations of the Whole Language philosophy; the number of potential interpretations is infinite.

Different types of theme units and cycles that can be established to meet the varying needs and purposes of the group members, the interventionist, and the setting in which intervention is provided were discussed. There is no one best way for establishing thematic contexts for learning, but it is important that these contexts are established. They provide a natural setting for networks of interrelated knowledge to emerge; and they are conducive to the integration of the curriculum; redundancy in topics and contexts of learning; parsing of increasingly more refined, abstract, and complex elements of knowledge from within a whole event; and the social collaboration needed for the processes of parsing, scaffolding, and refining to occur.

Developing Implicit Understanding of Language: Intervention for the Higher Academic Level Child

The upper-elementary and middle school child faces new challenges that increase with each grade level. The decontextualized demands imposed by lectures, the abstract concepts and complex language found in content area textbooks, the increasingly metaphoric expressions found in literature, and the social interactions of adolescence all require that the child understand and use language at the highest levels of the Situational-Discourse-Semantic continua. Unfortunately, many children with less integrated and flexible language systems have not mastered the linguistic strategies needed to organize ideas into complex relationships of meaning within discourse. The language problems exhibited by these children can affect all aspects of academic achievement and social interactions. This chapter will discuss

■ Increasing language demands encountered in literature
■ Increasing language demands encountered in expository text
■ Increasing language demands encountered in the classroom
■ Characteristics of facilitative learning environments
■ Models of service delivery
■ Intensive intervention theme cycles
■ Examples of language-learning activities

Research during the past decade has increased knowledge about language, its development, and its use by normally developing children, as well as those with delays or disorders. As we have seen, these findings are causing a reevaluation of methods of assessment and intervention toward more holistic and meaning-based approaches. This research also is leading to changes in views on prognosis and expectations regarding the efficacy of intervention. When language was viewed from the discrete skill perspective (i.e., the acquisition of a finite system of syntactic rules, morphological markers, phonological processes, and vocabulary words), then it was possible to think in terms of what can be called a "fix the problem" model of language intervention. The deficits, such as sounds incorrectly articulated, grammatical errors produced within sentences, morphological markers omitted, or limited vocabulary, could be targeted and taught, with some finite endpoint to language intervention. Once these forms were acquired, the language problems were thought to not exist anymore. This discrete and narrow view of language has resulted in a failure to meet the language learning needs of many school-age children. Research has shown that children identified as exhibiting language disorders at the preschool or early elementary level are relabeled as exhibiting learning disabilities or dyslexia by the third grade, with little or no attention directed at language (Maxwell & Wallach, 1984).

The relabeling does not mean that the child no longer experiences difficulties with language. For example, Gibbs and Cooper (1989) found that of 242 children between the ages of 8½ years and 12½ years who had been classified as learning disabled and placed in LD classes, 90.5% were found to have language deficits on the basis of standardized test score results. None of these children were receiving services provided by speech-language pathologists, except for a small percentage (6%) who also presented articulation disorders, and then only the superficial speech problems were addressed in therapy. As the child diagnosed as dyslexic profiled in Chapter 3 demonstrates, standardized tests may completely fail to identify the language deficits exhibited by this population of children, so the percentage of students classified as learning disabled, dyslexic, or low achievers who in fact exhibit language deficits as the primary problem is probably higher than 90%.

■□ INCREASING LANGUAGE DEMANDS WITH INCREASING AGE

Because of findings demonstrating continuing language problems across age and grade levels, it is increasingly recognized that language disorders are not outgrown, nor are they "cured" or "prevented" through intervention, but rather that they manifest themselves differently at various points of development and under different Situational, Discourse, and Semantic context conditions. This view would indicate that children exhibiting language related learning problems will require long-term monitoring and management of language learning and use throughout the school years. This monitoring and management could involve ongoing consultation with classroom teachers to make them aware of the child's learning needs and strategies for facilitating learning, paired with periodic episodes of intensive direct intervention to increase language abilities. This is particularly critical at points in the school curriculum when major changes occur in goals and teacher expectations that correspond with increased language demands. Third grade is one such critical point in that most children in a classroom are fluent readers and have mastered the basic principles of writing. The classroom curriculum changes from a focus on "how to" read and write to a focus on using reading and writing to explore scientific and world knowledge.

The transition to middle school is another critical point of change. The educational demands imposed by the physical and social environment of middle school require a sophisticated level of language ability. Students are expected to coordinate many levels of knowledge, discourse structure, classroom rules and procedures, abstract vocabulary, and multiply embedded sentence structures when engaging in school discourse. These middle years of sixth, seventh, and eighth grades are critical points in the school curriculum, when changes in academic goals and teacher expectations correspond with increased language demands. Curriculum design and teacher expectations are based on assumptions about children's personal and world knowledge, as it has been facilitated, used, and internalized through language and previous experiences during the preschool and elementary school years. Children are expected to be independent learners and to have a sophisticated foundation of language and content knowledge to use for problem solving in academic and social situations.

Facility with a wide range of language skills is needed to successfully participate and learn in a middle-school classroom. The child must be able to change language registers and discourse patterns to be appropriate to the situation. The language that is used within a situation depends on many interacting factors, such as what is being talked about, to whom, and for what purpose. By the middle-school grades, when teachers and students converse, it is usually in academic settings during classroom routines, such as oral lectures or instruction, where little nonverbal support is provided to aid comprehension. All of the information must be understood, remembered, and organized using language. In assigned readings, the pictures in expository text and literature selections are minimal, and the written text is lengthy and complex. The curriculum expects children to evaluate information relative to sophisticated personal and world experiences and simultaneously interpret information on literal and nonliteral levels of meaning.

Unfortunately, for many students with less integrated and flexible language systems, these assumptions often are not consistent with the actual knowledge and language levels of the children. As expectations increasingly change from learning oral and written language skills to applying these abilities to learn about hypothetical scientific constructs and understanding the world through literature, these children lack the academic and language skills needed to succeed. Because these language demands imposed on older elementary and middle-school students escalate in complexity and abstractness with each passing year, it is important to know about these children, their language, and their curriculum.

■□ INCREASING LANGUAGE DEMANDS IN LITERATURE

Literature reflects the world and culture that it is designed to comment on. It is used to interpret our lives or to impart the values of the culture to others. It may use humor as a means of simultaneously informing and entertaining or use drama to impose a sense of crisis and pathos in order to make a point. It constitutes a context of shared meaning, where the author uses language to create an event that must be reconstructed by the listener or reader. To accomplish the goal of shared meaning, the author makes certain presuppositions about the knowledge, background, and linguistic competence of the reader, and chooses the type and amount of information, expressed within a level of vocabulary and discourse structure, accordingly (Norris, 1991). Presuppositions are made on the basis of the age, gender, educational level, experiential level, and culture of the reader for whom the text is written (Bruce, 1981).

The language demands associated with these presuppositions can be examined by evaluating the classroom curricula. By the third grade and increasing with each grade level thereafter, the curricula is highly Decontextualized. Pictures in expository text and literature selections are minimal, and the written text is lengthy and complex. The text uses language to create all of the Situational context, including moment-to-moment changes in location, time, characters, affect, physical appearance, reference to previous events, necessary background information, and actions. For example, in the story *Guher and Suher* (McLeish, 1986b), written for the upper grade level student, a beautiful girl was raised from infancy by songbirds in a tree. She was discovered by a Turkish ruler's son, Muvaffak, who decided to capture her and keep her in a cage. The text reads:

> "But you can't keep a girl in a cage..."
> "Oh yes I can. I want her, and I want her now!"
> shouted Muvaffak, and he stamped his foot and sulked like the selfish brat he was.
>
> His father sighed, and sent soldiers to open the cages and set all the songbirds free. After that they went to the forest to fetch Suher from her tree. But how were they to get her down? They wondered whether to chop down the whole tree, or to light a fire at the bottom and smoke her down; they swarmed up the tree with ropes and nets, and the rooks met them with such a storm of flapping wings and gouging beaks that they scrambled down again twice as fast as they went up. Each time they went back to the palace empty-handed, Muvaffak stamped his foot and sulked even harder than before. In the end, his father was forced to make a proclamation offering a thousand gold pieces to anyone who could bring Suher down from the tree without harming her.
>
> One of the people to try was a wrinkled, gnarled old woman who lived not far from the elm-tree, in a woodcutter's cottage beside a lake. (p. 16)

The following analysis of this sample of literature reveals a few of the linguistic challenges encountered by the child with a less flexible language system. For example, children with learning disabilities, mental retardation, specific language disorders, hearing impairments, and other delays have all been shown to exhibit difficulty with temporal and spatial aspects of language (Bernstein & Tiegerman, 1992). As preschoolers, this difficulty was related to the acquisition of morphological markers of time and of prepositions. By the upper grade levels, the amount of temporal and spatial information that not only must be understood, but also coordinated, transcends sentences, paragraphs, and episodes. Similarly, these same children exhibit difficulty understanding roles and taking the perspective of others within an interaction. Literature at this grade level requires perspective shifts that change continuously and interact with temporal-spatial changes.

Coordination of Temporal and Spatial Changes

In the story above, the changes in spatial location are quite complex. The dialogue between the ruler and his son took place in the palace, a fact that is stated 13 sentences earlier. The location then changes to the cages within the palace (their location established 20 sentences earlier), followed in the next sentence to a tree in the forest, and then by recursive trips between the palace and the tree. The fact that there were multiple trips can only be recognized if the reader uses the phrase "Each time they went back to the palace empty-handed" to reinterpret the series of earlier attempts to fetch Suher as not occurring on one occasion, but rather as repeated trips. It is only implied that the father's proclamation was made from the palace and that it was sent throughout Turkey. The introduction of the old woman yields yet another change in location, with three spatial relationships that must be coordinated: The location is a cottage, the cottage is by a lake, and both are very near Suher's tree (a fact that is only established by recognizing that the article "the" means that it is the previously established elm tree, rather than any one in the forest).

Coordination of Multiple Perspectives

Multiple perspectives must be coordinated, each character with goals and reactions that are in opposition to those of the other characters. In the dialogue, the father indicates that a girl cannot be kept in a cage (one perspective), but in the next line the son insists that she can (an opposite perspective). Neither of these perspectives represents that of the child who is reading, even though the pronoun used in the text says "I," as in "I can. I want her . . . ." In a contextualized situation, "I" would refer to the child herself but, in reading, this pronoun must be read from the character's perspective. By the end of that same sentence, the perspective changes to that of the narrator, and the son is referred to as "he" instead of "I." In that phrase, the pronouns "he" and "his" are used three times to refer to Muvaffak (i.e., and *he* stamped *his* foot and sulked like the selfish brat *he* was), but in the next phrase the pronoun "his" is part of a noun phrase referring not to Muvaffak but to his father (i.e., *His* father sighed).

The perspective then changes to that of the soldiers, who were introduced as the object of one sentence (i.e., His father sighed, and sent soldiers . . .), but then become the subject of the next, referenced only by the pronoun "they" (i.e., After that *they* went to the forest). A child who fails to process the shifts in perspective would interpret that Muvaffak and his father went to the forest. The perspectives of the soldiers and the birds are then coordinated in different phrases within the same sentence, one trying to capture the girl and the other trying to protect her, but even this is only implied and never explicitly stated.

The next three sentences require the perspective to shift back to Muvaffak, then to his father, and finally to the narrator who refers to the old woman. This short excerpt is embedded within a longer story, all of which is replete with similar difficulty. Children with poorly integrated and inflexible language systems are often hopelessly lost in all of the changes in time, location, and perspective in this type of story, written at the highest Poetic-Interactive level of Discourse and presented at the Decontextualized-Symbolic level of Situational context. At best, the child may understand some of the events at the Descriptive level, but will fail to establish the necessary background and implicature to process the higher levels of the Semantic context.

■□ INCREASING LANGUAGE DEMANDS IN EXPOSITORY TEXT

The language demands encountered in the context of expository text are equally challenging. In the Situational context, the level of discussion is primarily that of hypothetical constructs that must be created out of logic and coordinated with many other hypothetical constructs within a Transactional-Interactive level of Discourse structure. For example, in *Our Changing Atmosphere* (Walker, 1992d) many issues related to the atmosphere are simultaneously considered. The text begins:

> Over four billion years ago, the earth was a very hot ball of molten rock. There was no air or *atmosphere* around it. There was no life on earth — it was just too hot! As the earth began to cool, gases from the surface and from volcanoes started to form the atmosphere that surrounds the earth.
>
> *(continued)*

Violent natural events gave the earth an atmosphere very different to the one we breathe today. The atmosphere today is made up of layers of gases. The atmosphere next to the surface of the earth is called the *troposphere.* Above that is the *stratosphere.* Within the stratosphere is a natural layer of gases which form the *ozone layer.*

Ozone is a form of oxygen that is made when the sun's rays alter the oxygen near the top of the troposphere.

The atmosphere has been constantly changing since it was first formed — but volcanoes and natural events are not the only things to make fast, dramatic changes in our air.

[The text then introduces the concept of ultraviolet rays in relationship to the ozone layer, the hole in the ozone layer, the effects of chlorofluorocarbons, their uses in our culture, legal bans and limitations, and the greenhouse effect.]

The following analysis of this sample of expository text reveals a few of the linguistic challenges encountered by the child with a less flexible language system. For example, children with learning disabilities, mental retardation, specific language disorders, hearing impairments, and other delays have all been shown to exhibit difficulty with metalinguistic aspects of language (Bernstein & Tiegerman, 1992). As young children, this difficulty was related to the acquisition of print awareness and word analysis skills related to concrete words. By the upper grade levels, the concepts that must be metalinguistically considered are themselves metalinguistically created. These abstract concepts also must be coordinated within temporal and spatial changes that transcend hypothetical time periods.

Metalinguistic Creation of Concepts

To understand this text, the child would have to understand the Semantic context at the level of Metalinguistic definitions to *create* most of the objects (i.e., atmosphere = natural layer of gases; ozone = form of oxygen made by sun rays altering oxygen near top of troposphere; troposphere = atmosphere next to surface of the earth, and so forth) that are organized in relationships of cause-effect, time, location, and state, to form the Situational context (i.e., the relative location of the gases in the atmosphere, the changes over a four billion year period, the state of oxygen lower in the atmosphere versus near the top of the troposphere, and so forth). The language itself is the primary means for creating the concepts and the context and integrating them in complex relationships for comparison and problem solving. Thus, understanding this text is at the highest levels for Situational, Discourse, and Semantic contexts.

Coordination of Temporal and Spatial Frames

Children with less flexible language systems will struggle to form concepts from definitions, create a context across time frames that are so vast as to have no practical meaning, and use language to establish the correct relationships. For example, in the sentence *"As* the earth *began* to cool, gases *from* the surface *and from* volcanoes *started* to form the atmosphere that *surrounds* our earth," the relational terms and syntactic word order must be interpreted to recognize that the cooling of the earth and the gases emitting from both the surface of the earth and volcanoes were occurring at the same time and that this simultaneous action took place continuously over billions of years. That continuing past time frame must be interpreted relative to the present time frame where the resulting atmosphere now spatially surrounds the earth. The only two words that have any concrete visible referents are "earth" and "volcano," the first of which is never seen except in pictures as an identifiable whole object, and the second of which is directly seen only by people in specific geographical areas. The majority of the words in this sentence are *function* words, or those that establish relationships between ideas (i.e., as, the, to, began, from, and, started, that, and our).

Activation of Erudite Knowledge

Background knowledge from the domains of world geography, earth sciences, the sun and its relationship to sunburn, cancer, sunblocks, and plants, the relationship of insects to plants, manufacturing, refrigeration, economics, and chemistry must be combined with the words or ideas provided by the text to understand the multidimensional problems and issues involved in protecting the atmosphere that are developed within the first five pages of the book. Children with inflexible language systems have difficulty activating the appropriate information, even when this knowledge is possessed, and often are more limited in exposure to this world and scientific knowledge because of their poor reading abilities and difficulty processing information presented through oral lectures.

The difficulties encountered by older children with poorly integrated and inflexible language systems in the classroom are compounded many times compared to those of younger children. They remain delayed compared to their peers in the acquisition of basic word ordering strategies for expressing meaning, and struggle to organize ideas using higher level Discourse structures (Loban, 1976). Their language remains concrete, at a time when classroom curricula introduce new concepts Metalinguistically. The child increasingly must rely on language to function successfully in school, but much of the information presented is above the child's Zone of Proximal Development (ZPD) and no longer serves to help the child to refine language further. Unfortunately, at a time when the child needs scaffolding the most, the classroom is set up in a manner that minimizes opportunities for such assistance, as exemplified by lectures.

■□ INCREASING LANGUAGE DEMANDS IN CLASSROOM LECTURES

Children with reading problems often learn equally poorly by listening as by reading. The underlying difficulty comprehending language and quickly reconstructing the meaning is related to a general inflexibility in language and is not specific to written language. Thus, hearing information through lectures and oral discussions is not a more satisfactory mode of learning for children with language-based reading disabilities. The rapid and temporary transmission of information presented orally requires that lengthy, complex, abstract, and highly transformed linguistic signals be converted and interpreted into meaning simultaneously with hearing the sound. These characteristics of the auditory signal make the process of comprehending through listening even more difficult than through reading for some children (Elliott & Hammer, 1988; Pearson & Fielding, 1982; Sinatra, 1990).

Contexts of Passive Listening

The ability to listen to classroom discourse is an acquired ability. Listening in this context is different from listening in the home or other settings. In nonschool settings, much of the discourse takes place in Contextualized situations, with considerable use of Expressive functions of language. The discourse participants are relatively equal, with both contributing to the topic and meaning of the interaction. Parents expand on whatever children say, thus providing opportunities to use and elaborate on language. In classroom settings, children spend the majority of the school day in passive listening, with some estimates showing less than 2 minutes of talking time per child in a typical school day. The meanings generated by children are considered incorrect if they do not match those of the teacher, and rather than being expanded on, the child's ideas are ignored and another child with the "correct" information is asked to respond. The topics are frequently highly decontextualized and abstract, primarily presented as Transactional monologues. When a child does not understand a concept, there is little richness or depth in the dialogue to assist the child to establish a clearer interpretation (Wells, 1985, 1986).

Contexts of Restricted Discourse

Whole class, teacher-led "discussions" are the most common form of discourse in the classroom. Unfortunately, they provide limited opportunities for explorations through language. Three distinct types of whole-class discussion are typically found, each with their own kind of conversational control. The most common, occurring for about 60% of classroom lessons, is comprised of closed questions that are initiated by the teacher and that can be answered with single words or brief answers. The goal of the teacher is to transmit information and then to periodically quiz the students to measure whether targeted facts are recalled. The students' responses are evaluated for correctness, with no opportunity to examine quality or depth of understanding. The second most common type of discussion, comprising 30% of interactions, occurs when the teacher asks open-ended questions and responds to children's replies. This provides the students with opportunities to participate in exploratory talk. The third type, occurring with low frequency, allows for student-initiated questions, and interactions that are channeled to peers as well as to the teacher. Questions within these discussions tend to be open-ended and facilitate critical thinking about a topic (Watson, 1987).

Children with less flexible language systems experience increasing difficulty with classroom discourse as the grade level increases. More of the content in areas such as science, math, and social studies occurs at the highest levels of Situational, Discourse, and Semantic context, presented in lecture format as an oral monologue that students must process in a passive manner, with little or no visual or other sensorimotor support. Thus, on every dimension of language and learning, the task of listening places maximum demands on the child's language system.

Since the child can only understand what he possesses a mental representation for, children who lack an internalized structure for the highest levels of Transactional or Poetic discourse, who do not have an extensive interwoven network of background knowledge for a wide variety of topics, who have difficulty creating concepts at abstract levels of Semantic context and who rely on contextual support to interpret and organize events, will comprehend and organize only disconnected bits of information and are soon frustrated by the classroom experience.

◨ INCREASING LANGUAGE DEMANDS FOR CLASSROOM SCRIPTS

Many children experience difficulty understanding classroom discourse because they fail to recognize and use the discourse patterns or generic structures needed to function within a particular content area. In the early elementary grades, teachers structure the classroom routines for children and provide many explicit cues and instructions for changing activities or completing tasks. Frequent reminders or cues, such as asking the child what needs to be done next, are provided to assist the child to internalize classroom scripts or routines. With increasing age and grade level, children are expected to abstract these patterns without explicit instructions. Often, different content areas are taught by different teachers, so the scripts will differ from one class period to the next. For each content area, success is dependent on learning not only the vocabulary or terms specific to that subject, but also the discourse patterns that are characteristic of that domain, or those used by a particular teacher.

Violating Classroom Scripts

One generic pattern or "script" that children must learn is that of a three-part sequence of turns in which the teacher asks a question, the child responds, and the teacher evaluates or reformulates the child's response. Violation of the script is viewed as misbehavior or noncompliance. Additionally, children must learn the behaviors and language that teachers associate with successful students, in addition to the content and turn-taking scripts. Informal, everyday talk is not acceptable to many teachers. Rather, children must learn to use "elaborated codes" in which information is reconstructed and evaluated at higher levels of the **semantic context**, embedded within more complex monologues along the **discourse dimension**, and stated explicitly and succinctly. Teachers follow these scripts and codes when they prepare their lessons and plan the presentation of information and thus mentally expect the information in this format during classroom discussions (Bruner, 1983, 1978; Cazden, 1988; Shavelson & Stern, 1981).

The scripts that children must learn include both schemata, or sequential scripts or rules for participating within an event, and procedures, or knowledge of how to do something within a schemata. Knowledge of the classroom script or schemata enables the child to determine what is appropriate to do or say within an event, including the roles taken by different participants, the amount and type of information to provide, and the locations of the participants within the setting. Children must develop a general script for "What happens in a classroom and how I am supposed to behave," and then modify this script to accommodate specific classrooms, content areas, and teachers. A general script might be to

1. determine what books and materials will be needed in a class
2. collect those books and materials
3. arrive in the classroom before the bell
4. sit in an appropriate location or desk
5. listen for information or instructions regarding assignments or lectures
6. ask questions about assignments or content
7. recognize what needs to be done as homework or preparation for the next day.

Violating Classroom Procedures

Within the schemata, the child also must have scripts for procedures, or how to implement or conduct specific aspects of the script. For example, the procedures for asking questions in the classroom include determining at what time questions can be asked, if hands are to be raised or some other signal used, if questions can be directed to peers, how the teacher signals that it is alright to ask questions versus listening, and so forth. Similarly, the procedure for collecting materials must be organized, including where they are found, if permission must be sought, who may gather them, and at what times they may be procured. Many schemata and procedures are specific to content areas, such as a scheme for drawing a proportional figure and its component procedures for measuring, sketching, and calculating ratios. Both elements of scripts must be internalized and coordinated by the child to independently perform many requirements within the classroom.

Many children with less flexible language systems fail to organize the routines or patterns found within classrooms into scripts. Lacking the overall schemata, they arrive in class without necessary materials and assignments and do not accurately predict what will happen next in the classroom sequence, or what they should have completed in a given amount of time. They are surprised each day by events that would be predictable if associated with a script. Since procedures are not internalized, the child does not finish a task once begun. One or two steps in the procedure are completed before the child becomes distracted or switches to another task. The script for the procedure is not used to anticipate how much time will be required to complete the procedure, or to determine when the task is complete (Creaghead, 1992; Marzano, 1991).

Scripts, including schemata and procedures, are organized, marked, and reflected on through language. Language enables planning to occur within a specific implementation of a script. For example, as the child begins the procedure of gathering materials, decisions must be made regarding how many subject areas must be prepared for during one trip to the hall locker (i.e., at what times during the day opportunities will be afforded to be at that location and still make it to class before the bell), what specific materials are needed for each subject area (i.e., those materials which are generally required and those that are specific to that day's assignments), and which materials are available in each respective classroom. Each of these dimensions of time, location, and planning are conducted through language, at high levels of situational and semantic context (Graesser, Millis, & Long, 1986). The child must use language to exert metacognitive control over goals and steps in the procedure and schema, monitor progress toward reaching the goals, and provide self-evaluation or internal feedback on the success or need for modification in the script as implemented (Marzano, 1991). Children with less flexible language systems have difficulty using language in a manner that coordinates time, location, and intention, and thus fail to exert the required control until the task is completed.

■□ INTERVENTION AT HIGHER LEVELS OF LINGUISTIC CONTEXT

Many new language challenges face the older school-age child, beginning at third grade and increasing thereafter. The complexity of the language and the decontextualization encountered in literature, content area reading such as science or social studies, lectures, and language arts increases rapidly as children are no longer expected to focus on learning how to read, write, speak, and listen, but rather to apply these abilities independently to learn about the world at greater distances from personal experience. Most children with less flexible language systems will not be ready for this shift to the independent learning of decontextualized and abstract information without considerable scaffolding and situational support from the environment. If it is not received, then most of these children will not refine language at a level required to deal with content area reading at upper grade levels and will experience continuing failure in school.

■ CHARACTERISTICS OF HIGHER LANGUAGE LEVELS

In normal development, children enter school with oral language in advance of written language development. Young children tell fairly well developed narratives; use a series of adjectives to modify the same noun; specify complex time relationships between actions and events using the auxiliary verb system (i.e., could have been going to + Verb); coordinate multiple ideas within the same sentence using syntactic embedding; conjoin multiple sentences that maintain meaningful relationships expressed as "then," "so," "because," or "while"; subordinate the roles of different people or agents into both subject and object positions; and possess a vocabulary of approximately 2,000 words learned primarily through oral language experiences. In contrast, the sentences read and written in first and second grades are structurally simple in narrative form, discourse function, sentence length and grammatical order, and vocabulary selection (Baumann & Kameenui, 1991; French & Nelson, 1985). The children's oral language abilities are far in advance of the language that they are learning to read and write. Even children with inflexible language systems often have sufficient refinement to process the meaning, form, and function of language at this level.

However, by the end of second grade, the stories read by and written by children equal, and from that point forward begin to exceed, the structural complexity found in oral language. Exposure to written language and the formality in the grammar, discourse structure, and word choice serves to refine and guide language development in the school-age child. This process continues through grade 12 and beyond, as children become increasingly aware of literary strategies for creating different intentions and effects, and as vocabulary expands to reflect an increasing knowledge base in all content areas. It is not until the middle school years that students include detailed information about character's motivations and reactions in their stories, or provide elaborate accounts that are coordinated across perspectives of time and characters in their renditions of events (King & Rentel, 1981; Loban, 1976). Similarly, well developed arguments and problem/solution forms of Transactional writing are only well controlled by middle school age or later (Langer, 1986).

A sudden increase in the use of complex and infrequently used grammatical constructions appears in normal development between 10 and 14 years of age, particularly in the use of multiply embedded sentences that coordinate the subjects and predicates of the sentence. This accompanies the child's increasing ability to form logical and hierarchical links between ideas and to coordinate multiple perspectives of time, location, and states. Greater control over passive constructions and center embedded clauses also emerge during this time in both oral and written language (Loban, 1976; O'Donnell, Griffin, & Norris, 1967).

The ability to follow and produce pronoun shifts within and across sentences and paragraphs, or cohesion, develops rapidly but can remain problematic through adolescence, particularly for reflexive forms such as "himself," "herself," and "themselves." Greater command over derivational morphology is acquired, in which one part of speech (e.g., a verb) is converted to a different part of speech (e.g., a noun) through the addition of a suffix (e.g., run + er = runner). The full range of prefixes and suffixes is acquired gradually throughout the school years, often in the context of reading and writing (Wiig & Semel, 1980).

Vocabulary increases by a low estimate of 3,000 new words each year from third grade onward, so that by senior high, students should have a minimum vocabulary of 40,000 words. Nagy and Herman (1987) estimate that fifth-grade students who read only a moderate amount encounter approximately 10,000 different unknown words per year. While not all of these words are learned from one exposure through reading, between 25% and 50% of the new vocabulary words learned in a year are acquired through such incidental reading. Other words are acquired through lectures, vocabulary study, content area exploration, and oral conversations.

Children with less flexible language systems thus are disadvantaged from all perspectives. They enter school with less refined language systems that are less able to process information at higher levels of situational, discourse, and semantic context. This lack of refinement results in greater difficulty in learning written language patterns required for both reading and writing. Instead of learning more complex grammar, discourse structures, morphology, vocabulary, and content information from written language experiences that in turn will support greater refinement in language, the child struggles to process written language at the most basic levels. Therefore, the child falls further behind in language development and refinement, so that, for example, only 50% to 70% of the vocabulary words are learned by low achievers compared to high achieving peers (White, Graves, & Slater, 1989). To reverse this downward spiral, the best alternative for these children is placement in learning environments in which there is ample opportunity for language to develop through active problem solving and critical thinking using language. The passive listening and unscaffolded learning in a traditional setting is not conducive to such language learning.

◼◻ CHARACTERISTICS OF FACILITATIVE LEARNING ENVIRONMENTS

Whole Language classrooms provide one of the best potential learning environments for children with less flexible language systems. In Whole Language classrooms, all children are not expected to read or study from the same book, on the same page, at the same rate. Rather, a variety of materials is available on the theme or topic that is in focus within the classroom. Some of the materials, including books, might exhibit considerable contextual support, such as detailed illustrations or sequences of pictures that suggest a procedure or depict a story. Other available books would be more dependent on written language, with readability levels that range from very low to those that are challenging even for the highest achievers in the classroom. Information available through media such as film, audio recording, or computer software also might be present for the children to use to explore a topic.

Unlike many traditional classrooms where working together is forbidden or considered cheating, collaboration is not only allowed, but often required in a Whole Language classroom. Children working in groups, with guidance from the teacher, help to decide what topics will be explored within a theme. Plans for the daily activities and the final outcome to be produced by the group are negotiated, and group members choose individual aspects of the enterprise to begin to explore. Group membership is heterogeneous so that some members contribute fluent reading, good note-taking strategies, accurate spelling, good group organizational abilities, mathematical competence, or skill at drawing or illustrating. Thus, peers serve as teachers and facilitators for each other so that children with less written language facility can still access information through the group, and each member contributes to the group enterprise in accord with individual strengths.

A combination of whole group, small group, and individual activities occurs throughout the day. The curriculum is integrated so that the same topic is explored in all content areas, from reading and literature to science, social studies, mathematics, writing, and art. This provides for the redundancy and the time to explore a topic through a variety of sources and from many perspectives so that oral and written language can be refined, and information can be understood and networked in meaningful ways.

A speech-language pathologist can easily function in a consultative role and/or as a direct service provider within a Whole Language classroom. Almost any activity that the child is engaged in can be used as an opportunity to facilitate oral and written language development. Small groups of children can be met with for intervention sessions within the classroom using any of the strategies presented in Chapter 4, including scaffolded discussions, use of graphic organizers to support writing, use of flowcharts to become aware of classroom scripts and procedures, and use of Communicative Reading Strategies (Norris, 1988, 1989, 1991) to study literature or content information. Books that are consistent with the themes and goals of the classroom can be interactively read, during which time children are helped to learn to interpret text at the interactive levels of Poetic or Transactional discourse, to use implicature to increase depth of Semantic understanding of this information, and to internalize the complex grammatical and morphological structures encountered in text. Similarly, group writing can be used to develop the ability to produce more complex and elaborated expression and to refine metalinguistic abilities such as spelling and grammatical awareness.

The speech-language pathologist also can work with the children in the classroom to facilitate metacognitive awareness, helping them to observe peers who are successful to determine what scripts and procedures they use to function within the classroom setting. Once the children have begun to discover these patterns, the speech-language pathologist can help them to use language themselves to establish goals and to engage in self-monitoring of progress, first by placing them on flowcharts and then gradually internalizing the scripts and procedures. Learning how to evaluate successful learning and how to set and monitor goals enables the child to generalize this knowledge to new situations with less support in the future.

Goals of Whole Language Versus Traditional Classrooms

Many individuals seek Whole Language strategies that can be used to teach the products of traditional curricular goals. Their objective is to enable children to perform at a higher level on tasks such as completing worksheets or responding to multiple-choice tests. These efforts will be frustrated, because the two types of curriculum are derived from opposite philosophies of learning. Since the underlying philosophies are opposite, the desire to use Whole Language strategies to teach children to memorize facts or to find the correct answers to teacher selected questions represents a contradiction in logic.

To understand the goals of a Whole Language classroom, a view of education based on the "real world" must be adopted. In the real world, people engage in goal-directed behavior. Learning is conducted for purposes of accomplishing those goals. For example, if a water faucet begins to leak, a book on plumbing or home repairs might be read to learn the appropriate procedure for fixing the leak, or a friend with knowledge in this domain might be called for advice. If a vacation trip is planned to an unfamiliar place, a travel agency might be called for advice and information, and travel brochures and literature describing the characteristics of the climate, culture, and events might be studied. If some unexpected money is inherited, procedures, risks, and potential benefits accruing from investing in the stock market might be explored. Because of the goals, people engage in learning activities in subject areas that they would not ordinarily broach.

People also engage in goal-directed learning for the pleasure of discovery. People become aware of an unfamiliar topic that interests them, or of some new information related to a familiar topic, and pursue an investigation of that topic because it is pleasurable. This type of learning occurs in the context of a hobby or for purposes of self-improvement. The topic may be studied for a short time, such as the amount of time that it takes to learn basic cake decorating, or it may become a long-term avocation.

Many different types of learning occur in the pursuit of goals. For example, in the context of learning how to fix a water faucet, the most obvious learning will involve the procedures for shutting off the water, replacing the necessary parts, and creating a water-tight seal. But other knowledge also can be acquired, such as learning how to use a wrench, how to read and order from a parts manual, how to clean tools, or how to find home improvement books in the reference section of the library.

Like adults, children engage in goal-directed learning. They learn how to ride a bike and in the process learn about balance, traffic dangers and patterns, the relationship between speed and distance, names for parts such as "pedals," "brakes," and "grips," and rules for where they can ride and for what purposes. Learning for purposes of accomplishing goals and for pleasure surrounds children, as activities that are everyday routines for adults constitute new experiences for children, and thus are replete with learning. In the context of learning how to dress themselves, children learn how to discriminate and name colors, how to match, the names for items of clothing, contrasts such as "clean" versus "dirty," how to dress for different occasions, and how to perform a wide variety of fine motor actions.

While people in real life are continuously learning, people do *not* engage in learning for purposes of answering questions, filling in worksheets, or memorizing facts that have no obvious utility or relevance. They especially do not engage in this type of learning when the topic or content of the learning is selected by someone else. Adults are not employed in jobs that require them to learn an arbitrary list of facts for purposes of passing an exam and would never be paid for such activity. Family members do not quiz each other on the topic of the week as part of the family routine. This type of learning only occurs in the environment of the traditional classroom.

In the traditional classroom, some external curriculum, often generated by a textbook manufacturer, chooses what children will learn. The learning is not embedded within some purposeful goal, so a system of rewards and punishments must be established to motivate children to engage in such learning. Someone other than the child, such as the classroom teacher, decides *exactly* what will be learned, and if those specific facts or behaviors are not learned or demonstrated on a test, then the child is evaluated negatively and self-worth is diminished. Individual differences and creativity are discouraged in favor of conformity and knowing the single "right answer." The objectives of learning are to acquire facts or "**products.**"

In Whole Language classrooms, the objectives of learning are to develop strategies for learning how to learn, or engaging in the learning **process**. This type of learning refines what children already do in everyday experiences, but incorporates Erudite meaning that the child cannot acquire from concrete, personal experience. It emulates what children will need to do in the workplace or when managing a family and home as adults. A topic that is interesting to the participants is pursued in some context such as finding solutions to a problem, exploring a historical event, or interpreting a literature selection. Each participant is exposed to a wide range of information, but there is no agenda on the part of the adult or the child regarding what will be learned. Rather, a variety of different outcomes may result from the learning. One child might learn how to use an encyclopedia and how to integrate information from two different sources to build an argument, while another child might learn 20 new vocabulary words and internalize a more complex Discourse structure. A third child might learn how to draw Inferences from facts and learn 30 facts about a topic. Individual differences and creativity are encouraged, and the accomplishments of each child are valued.

Evaluations are based on changes in learning how to learn, such as demonstrating greater independence in using reference material or locating relevant facts, greater complexity and argument development in writing about a topic, or an increase in the level of meaning used to interpret a statement. These things cannot be chosen by the teacher ahead of time, or measured by some multiple-choice test. Instead, they are **outcomes** of learning, and will be evident in the behaviors exhibited by the child in such contexts as participating in an oral discussion, reading and interpreting a passage, or writing a composition. Thus, the *goals* of learning and the perceived *role of products* within learning (i.e., the objectives versus the outcomes of learning) are completely opposite in Traditional compared to Whole Language classrooms.

Whole Language intervention for the older school-age child is focused on improving the children's ability to learn how to learn. It is a goal designed to facilitate a child's ability to solve problems and to make sense of personal and indirect experience, both in the present and in the future. It recognizes that if children know how to use resources, how to seek information from these resources, how to integrate information into logical arguments or discussions, and how to apply information to solve problems or interpret situations, then they will be able to explore any content area, from plumbing to economics, when there is a need for this information. It recognizes that many products will be learned, but that these will be logical outcomes of learning and not the a priori goals, any more than learning colors was the goal for getting dressed for the younger child. It recognizes that the best way to learn how to learn is by being immersed in the process of learning, rather than being taught the "products" of learning (i.e., learn to dress yourself by participating in getting dressed rather than learning to pick out the appropriate picture on command).

If a child is in a traditional classroom, many strategies for completing class requirements can be taught, such as learning to take notes, learning to use the index and chapter headings or subheadings of a textbook, learning to use elimination strategies to take multiple-choice tests, attending to the topic sentences of paragraphs and summary passages, and answering study questions provided by the text. These are behaviors that are used in the process-seeking information to solve problems in real situations and thus will provide the child with coping strategies in the present as well as in the future. Furthermore, a topic consistent with one from the classroom curriculum can be used to develop a theme that is explored in intervention. But it is not the role of intervention to teach the specific products that a teacher chooses to place on a test, or to tutor a child through specific tasks. Rather, the focus of intervention must be on engaging the child in the process of active learning and on facilitating higher levels of language learning along the Situational-Discourse-Semantic dimensions.

Service Delivery Using
Intensive Cycle Scheduling

Special service providers, such as speech-language pathologists, often have large caseloads and limited time to commit to individual students, whether services are provided inside the classroom, as described above, or in pull-out services. Some schools are small and the children eligible for services may be scattered across classrooms and grade levels so that there is neither time nor sufficient numbers of children to provide direct services in class. Additionally, while many upper grade level classrooms across the country are beginning to incorporate principles of Whole Language, the traditional teacher-led pattern of lectures and listening is still the most prevalent instructional model, particularly for older children. Research has demonstrated that children have less than one minute of talking time in such situations, and even then only short answer responses to teacher-solicited questions are permitted (Cazden, 1988). Many teachers welcome a specialist, such as a speech-language pathologist, into the classroom to work with children exhibiting language and learning difficulties, but others are reluctant to embrace such close collaboration. One service delivery alternative that can provide meaningful intervention to children under these conditions is the practice of *Intensive Cycle Scheduling*, also called block scheduling (Neidecker, 1980).

The intensive cycle-scheduling model has been used most frequently in the schools in the context of articulation therapy, with good results. In this model, children are seen four or five times per week for a concentrated block of time, usually 4 to 6 weeks. A minimum of two cycles, and preferably three to four each year, are provided to participating students. The first block may need to be longer to accommodate testing and program organization. Longitudinal studies showed that, using this model, a greater number of children could be enrolled during the school year, the length of time children were seen until dismissal criterion was reached was reduced, closer relationships developed between classroom teachers and the speech-language pathologist, children sustained greater interest in therapy over the period of intervention, and less time was spent in reestablishing old information, because long periods of time did not separate intervention sessions. Studies conducted in our laboratory have shown that significant progress in oral and written language can occur when short, intensive periods or blocks of language intervention are provided.

If services are provided within the classroom, the speech-language pathologist can work for an intensive block of time with a heterogeneous group of children within the classroom, including children with identified needs and higher achieving peers. In this case the child is provided with services in the least restrictive program, benefits from the models provided by the peers, and learns to function as an integral member of the group. When children are placed in a collaborative setting, providing assistance to others becomes a naturally occurring part of the group dynamics. Therefore, group peers are likely to continue to provide scaffolding for the child after the concentrated block of intervention is ended. If services are provided outside the classroom, the disruption can be minimized by carefully discussing and planning the goals of the intervention with the child's classroom teacher. Understanding the long-term benefits to the child's oral and written language development, and consequently performance in the classroom, can help the teacher and special service providers work cooperatively to prioritize goals, objectives, and curriculum expectations for the duration of the block. Neidecker (1980) reviewed studies indicating that the majority of classroom teachers preferred this model to intermittent intervention schedules, because it fit better with other aspects of their daily schedules.

■□ EXAMPLE OF AN INTENSIVE INTERVENTION THEME CYCLE

Methods of establishing theme units and cycles were discussed in Chapter 4. One example theme cycle will be used here to demonstrate how many of the language needs presented by the older child can be addressed using many of the same strategies adapted to higher level needs. This type of theme can be established within the regular classroom, or if that is not a practical option, children from different classrooms and different grade levels who are close in their developmental abilities or level of achievement can be grouped. A 4- to 6-week theme cycle can be implemented to address a variety of oral and written language needs. This type of theme cycle can be developed and implemented for students in upper elementary, middle school, and high school grades using materials and topics that are appropriate to the needs of the group.

In each 1-hour session of the block, in general a minimum of two resources will be used to simultaneously develop oral and written language. This may include reading an episode from a literature selection, followed by exploring some concept introduced in the literature through expository text. Or the literature or expository selection may be followed by a writing activity. Some information may be read by the children, while other information is presented as an interactive discussion in which the children are helped to decide what facts are most relevant to the discussion and how they may be written down in notes or organized on a flowchart. Attempts to complete an assignment may be planned and evaluated metacognitively by group members to learn to use language to establish procedures and other scripts. The sessions themselves are conducted as highly scaffolded, collaborative efforts to provide children an intensive experience with language learning and use, for a variety of functional purposes, in a compressed amount of time.

■□ SELECTING A NARRATIVE-CENTERED THEME

A book should be selected that is within the ZPD for the group. That is, it should be more difficult than the group members could independently read, but not so difficult that every phrase would have to be explained in detail, every few words assisted in word recognition and meaning, or every sentence parsed into multiple phrases to reduce the grammatical complexity. The upper level of instructional reading, or the level just below frustration level on a reading inventory when assistance is provided, would be appropriate. In many cases, this will be several grade levels below the child's actual grade level.

In this example theme cycle, a book at the fifth-grade level of difficulty, *The Stranger from the Sea* (Burleigh, 1990) has been selected. On the first day of the theme cycle, the first element of story structure, or the *setting*, is read using Communicative Reading Strategies. The picture accompanying the text shows a man with a fishing net sitting in front of his home looking out into the ocean. The text reads:

> On the south coast of the island, Thomas lived alone. He loved to breathe the fresh salt air and to hear the gentle rhythm of the waves lapping the shore or breaking on the rocks. Sometimes he thought he would like to share his life with a wife, a wife who would want to live in his cottage, smelling the salt air and listening to the waves. But then Thomas would sigh, and put the matter out of his mind. (p. 2)

■□ EXAMPLES OF LANGUAGE-LEARNING ACTIVITIES

A variety of example activities will be described below. Each activity views language from a slightly different perspective and facilitates different clusters of language abilities. All of them reinforce the theme, serving to create a network of knowledge regarding the content of the thematic topic, the Discourse structures used to organize this knowledge to meet different purposes, and the words used to refer to this knowledge at all levels of the Semantic continuum. Each of these activities is designed to facilitate language learning, as well as the use of language to engage in learning. Content area learning will be an outcome, but not a goal or objective of the thematic unit.

Learning Language Through Discussion

An oral discussion could be used to establish a larger context for understanding the story before it is read, using information derived from the picture and activating background knowledge possessed by the children (Contextualized-Symbolic situation, Semantic levels of interpretation and inference required). Presuppositions about the man, his occupation, and the part of the country or world where he might live could be generated, beginning with the ideas spontaneously provided by the children and built on or elaborated through scaffolded interactions. The adult analyzes comments initiated by the students for their level of Semantic complexity and asks a question or prompts a comment to increase the student's level of abstraction in thought and language use.

John: He's holding a net (description).

Adult: Yes, he's holding a net because his job is probably what (interpretation)?

Steve: A fisherman, he's probably a fisherman (label).

Adult: And right now he is not fishing, but rather, he's somewhere else. What do you think he's doing?

John: At home fixing his fishing net (interpretation).

Adult: And looking out into _____

Carol: the ocean to see where he will go fishing (inference).

Adult: I wonder where his home is, what part of the country or the world (inference)?

Steve: Somewhere with an ocean, along a coast somewhere.
Carol: Yeah, maybe California.
Adult: What do you think, John?

This type of discussion, in which children are guided to make interpretations and inferences, leads them to *expect* more than superficial meaning from experiences. They learn to bring those expectations to new events, illustrations, and text. By learning how to evaluate a situation at levels beyond the obvious, children qualitatively change the manner in which they think about events. The use of discussion should occur with high frequency as part of all other activities.

Learning Language Through Reading

The reading can then begin. The older student should be made more explicitly aware of elements of structure and how they function to aide communication. In this case, the story is introduced with a statement about the Poetic structure to heighten the children's awareness and thus to internalize this structure. Once internalized, children begin to use Discourse structure to frame other stories and thus bring greater organization, comprehension, and prediction to reading and writing. The structure is explained in terms of the author's purpose for using it, and the categories of meaning that are expressed.

Adult: Today we are going to find out something about the setting of the story. The author always lets us know some interesting facts about the people and places in a story so that we know something about their ordinary existence. Let's find out what the author wants us to know about this man.

Similarly, syntactic structures exist for purposes of establishing the intended relationships of meaning between ideas. A brief perusal of the page from the story will show that there are numerous elements of syntax that can be addressed. The first sentence begins with a transformation in which the object clauses of the sentence (on the south coast — of the island) are moved to the initial position of the sentence, so that the subject "Thomas" and the verb of the sentence are not encountered until the end of the sentence. This type of transformation is characteristic of literate, rather than oral, uses of language and may be unfamiliar to some children, resulting in miscues or inappropriate intonation.

The second sentence, beginning "He loved," contains two infinitive clauses, two conjoined clauses signaled by "and" and "or," an embedded clause in the object position with an ellipsis of the relative pronoun "that" (i.e., ... of the waves that *were lapping* the shore), two prepositional phrases, plus the coordination of past tense, simple present, and present progressive tense between the verbs. The next sentence is even more grammatically complex. The language presents simple metaphors of waves "lapping" and "breaking" on the shore and rocks. The content of the ideas refers to the character's thoughts, a Decontextualized-Symbolic level. The syntactic structures are not explicitly taught, separating the form from their content and function. Rather, the students are shown in print how the highly embedded and transformed structures function to communicate meaning. Each example below provides an explanation of the type of ongoing interpretation that the adult must make regarding *why* the children experienced difficulty and the subsequent scaffold that was provided to help them learn the difficult language.

> **Adult:** Explain to us where this man lives (pointing to the first sentence)
> **Steve:** On the south coast of the island (read with incorrect intonation) Thomas lived alone.
> **Adult:** Right, so Thomas lived on an island, clear down on the south coast, where it was probably warm (pointing in turn to each constituent of the sentence).

[The intonation was a cue that something in the utterance was not understood, and so verbal language is used to reorder the ideas from the most basic sentence constituent, or the subject, to the object and then the specific location. The adult also modeled an inference, or the significance of the island's location on the south coast.]

> **Carol:** That's so he can fish all the time.
> **Adult:** Right, the climate, or weather would be good for fishing.

[Considerable difficulty is anticipated with the complex embedded structure of the next sentence, and so it is parsed to visually show the children how the many ideas can be organized in logical relationships. Seeing the logic of these grammatical structures can help children who have difficulty processing long strings of words heard rapidly through the auditory signal to internalize these patterns through the visual signal instead. Once learned, these grammatical structures will be recognized and processed more easily when heard or read, so a qualitative change is observed in the child's learning and functioning.]

> **Adult:** Tell us one thing that he loved about his island.
> **John:** He loved to bre-thee the fresh salt air.

Adult: (points to "breathe") Yes, the salt air smelled so good, he loved to inhale it, he loved to _____

John: breathe the fresh salt air.

Adult: That's one thing he loved, and he also loved _____

John: to hear the gently rhyme of the waves.

Adult: The waves didn't rhyme, but they went in and out in a regular pattern, not too fast and not too slow.

Carol: Oh, a gentle rhythm of the waves.

[The miscues on the words "breathe," "gentle," and "rhythm" are viewed as evidence that the child was not maintaining the meaning of the passage or was misinterpreting the author's intent. Information is provided to direct attention to the meaning intended within the context, rather than to superficial decoding. In the case of the miscue for "breathe," synonyms and explanations were provided, while in the case of "rhythm," contradictory information was highlighted to enable the child to generate a reinterpretation. In both cases, the child's repairs were reinforced with a meaning-expanding conversational remark that verified the accuracy of what the child had communicated and reflected the listener's interest in the child's ideas.]

Adult: Right, it wasn't a storm or bad weather, so the rhythm of the waves was very calm, so he loved _____ (points to beginning of clause)

John: to hear the gentle rhythm of the waves

Adult: and this is what the waves seemed to be doing . . .

Steve: *laping* the shore or breaking the rocks

Adult: just *lapping* the shore. Can you picture a kitten lapping water from a bowl, very gently, making little waves? That's how gently the waves were _____

[Steve miscued on the word because the concept of "lapping" was not predictable in this metaphoric context. The adult helps the children to create a visual image or analogy and at the same time helps them to recognize that meaning is to be expected from print, and that miscues call for a new interpretation.]

Carol: lapping the shore or breaking the rocks.

[Both children omitted the word "on" in their reading, indicating that they confused the agent and recipient of the action "break." The children are helped to think about the logical relationships expressed in the phrase.]

Adult: Right, were the waves hitting the shore hard enough to break any of the rocks?

Group: No!

Carol: They were just gently lapping on the shore and the rocks.

Adult: So I wonder what that means, when it says the waves were breaking *on* the rocks?

Group: No response.

Adult: What things were breaking, the rocks or the waves?

Steve: The rocks.

Adult: Let's look at it carefully. The waves (points to that noun in the previous clause) were lapping *or* _____

Steve: breaking, oh, the waves were breaking. It means they were breaking up, splashing all over and stuff.

Adult: So how do you think he feels about his life? What has the author told you about him?

John: He's happy 'cuz he loves the island and the, breathing the air and the waves, listening to them.

[The question asked for critical thinking and elicited an interpretation from one child. He used facts provided to attribute some feeling or attitude to the man. This knowledge of the man is important to the interpretation of the next sentence.]

Adult: So he's happy with *where* he lives, but maybe not with all aspects of his life. Find out what he may want to make him even happier.

John: Something he thought he would, he would like to share his life with a wife (read with fading volume and poor intonation).

[The miscues, drop in volume and poor intonation all indicate that the relationships of meaning are being lost, even though most of the words are correctly recognized. The adult adds clarification, pointing to the constituents.]

Adult: Right, not often, but *sometimes* he was lonely and wanted a wife to _____

John: share his life. (rereads) Sometimes he thought that he would like to share his life with a wife.

[The appropriate fluency, intonation, and insertion of the word "that" into the grammatical structure indicate that the sentence was read at a level of meaning this time. Insertions of words not actually appearing in print generally occur when children are simplifying sentences by including elements that the text omitted through ellipsis from the surface level of the sentence.]

> **Adult:** And this would be his ideal, or perfect wife . . .
> **Carol:** a wife how would went

[The child is losing the meaning and becoming confused by the embedded clause inserted into the noun phrase. The adult uses the visual input of the text to show her how this complex sentence is structured to communicate meaning.]

> **Adult:** Tell us some of the things this wife would want (points past the relative pronoun "who," and to the verb structure)
> **Carol:** would want to live in his cottage, smelling the salt air and listening to the waves.
> **Adult:** Right, and the wife (pointing to those words) would be the one *who* (pointing to relative pronoun) would like these things; she is *who* likes the cottage, and *who* smells the salt air, and *who* listens to the waves.

[A preparatory set is used to establish a frame for interpreting the last sentence.]

> **Adult:** He thought that way sometimes (pointing to the word in the earlier text) but not for long.
> **Steve:** But then Thomas would sigh and put the matter out of his mind.
> **Adult:** What does that mean, to "put the matter out of his mind"?
> **Steve:** To forget about it, not think about a wife.
> **Adult:** I wonder why? If he wanted a wife, why would he just put the thought out of his mind?
> **John:** Maybe he didn't know anyone.
> **Carol:** Yeah, cuz he lives kind of out in the desert, well, not a desert but a place *like* the desert where nobody lives, and there aren't any girls.

While many of the strategies used within Communicative Reading Strategies are the same at this level as they were for nonreaders or nonfluent readers (i.e., preparatory sets, expansions, expatiations, parsing sentences, open-ended comprehension questions, and so forth), the goals are established at higher levels of the Situational, Discourse, and Semantic continua. In this interaction, lasting 15 to 20 minutes, the children were immersed in the active processing of many aspects and levels of language. They were helped to see how many elements of grammar and vocabulary serve to organize ideas in complex relationships of time, location, causality, and state; see how the author uses discourse structure to establish a setting; how to go beyond descriptive meanings and make interpretations or inferences; how to expect meaning and to seek analogies if the literal meaning does not make sense; and how to take the perspective of the character and his environment when interpreting the actions and motives of people. They also learned how to use language to negotiate meaning within a group.

Conducting Metalinguistic Analyses

As the reading progressed, the adult could note (mentally or in writing) words for which miscues occurred. Following the reading of the passage, these words could be examined for their orthographic structure. Rather than teaching word analysis using arbitrary materials with no immediate relevance, word analysis is focused on using words that the students actually experienced difficulty with. Since they were selected from the meaningful text just read, they remain networked to meaning and purpose, even though the focus in this activity is on form.

Adult: Let's think about how we could spell some of the words used by the author to tell us the story. If you were the author, how would you spell "breathe"?

Child: B R E E Z E

Adult: (writes BREEZE on the board, and points to the Z) Your spelling tells my mouth to read breeze. The Z at the end of the word says the sound /z/, we need a different sound at the end.

Child: Oh, I know that word, it's BREATH.

Adult: (changes spelling to BREATH). Now, it spells the word breath. But the author wasn't talking about a breath. He was talking about someone who liked to breathe ocean air. So he needs a way to show the difference between a breath and to breathe. How could he do that?

Child: He could put an "e" on the end.

Adult: Yes, he could (changing spelling to BREATHE) and that changes the noun "breath" into a verb. "Breathe" is an action, something you do. But you can tell that both words mean to inhale air. How?

Child: Cuz they're both kind of spelled the same, except at the end.

Adult: Let's see if that's how the author spelled it (locates the word in the context of the story and compares).

Other words for which miscues occurred could be similarly analyzed to assist the children to discover the patterns and regularities in orthography. The miscues produced by the children determine which patterns will be examined, and at what level of frequency. Immediately associating them back to the context in which the miscue occurred enables the child to "read like a writer," or expect patterns to be encountered in words and actively processed while reading, as well as writing (Smith, 1983). Children at this level will often show patterns of transitional spelling, characterized by many strategies for creating long and short vowels or other phonic principles, but inappropriately applied to the conventional spelling of specific words. In addition, many phonological processes continue to appear in the misspellings produced.

Discussing Expository Text

The setting of the story established that the character was a fisherman. One concept that could be explored further on that day is the occupation of fishing, both in general and in relationship to modern times. To facilitate oral discussion, a level of contextualization can be achieved by using expository text accompanied by pictures. One source is the book *Oceans of Fish* (Walker, 1992c). Open-ended discussions can be used to facilitate comparisons, evaluations, and other elements of critical thinking about many of the issues presented. For example, the net used by Thomas in the story above can be compared to modern nets. When he dropped his net, Thomas went out in his boat where he believed fish to be, but today instruments such as sonar are used to locate fish. The children can be helped to consider the advantages versus the problems of this practice, first by discussing known information and then by exploring reference material.

The children each can be asked to read *Oceans of Fish* and report on different aspects of the problem, ranging from overfishing (p. 14), the needs of other fish and mammals for the same food in the food chain (p. 11), and the problem of drift nets and their random killing of fish and mammals (p. 2–3). Communicative Reading Strategies can be used to facilitate the reading of the text, as needed. Once the information is read, the adult can act as a facilitator to enable the children to engage in a true discussion. For example, if one child reported that many species of fish are becoming scarce due to overfishing, the adult can direct a second child to find out why this is occurring. The adult can help the child to generate questions regarding what the fish are used for, where the fishing is occurring, what expenses would result from different methods or locations of fishing, how that would affect cost at the grocery store, and so on. If children do not know the answers, the adult can help them to search for information in the text that provides insights.

John: Some fish are being overfished, there's hardly any left in some parts of the ocean.

Adult: There must be a reason for that. Carol, what could you ask him to find out why those parts of the ocean are overfished? Think of a specific question you could ask.

Carol: Um . . . I don't know.

Adult: Think about where most of the fishing would occur — would it be far out in the ocean, or closer to shore?

Carol: Oh, are there certain parts of the country, by the shore, um, which shores are being overfished?

These types of discussions help children to learn how to pose problems or issues and then to consider them from multiple perspectives. The facilitation from the adult assists the children initially to think about the types of questions or issues that can be raised and how to formulate questions to elicit needed information. Instead of asking the questions herself, the adult facilitates asking by the children, so that they must actively process and think about the information. This social mediation enables the child to internalize the process of questioning so that in the future the children will more spontaneously ask questions of others and of themselves. Expository text thus becomes more than descriptive facts to be memorized and regurgitated on adult request but rather meaningful information to be used in the context of posing and finding solutions for real problems and important issues.

These types of scaffolded oral discussions, accompanied by pictures or even props such as fishing nets, reduce the level of complexity, so that difficult concepts are created through a combination of definitions, pictures, examples, and elaborations, and not just metalinguistic definitions. In addition, discussion allows for each type of information to be subjected to clarification and feedback as needed. Necessary background information can be established when it is relevant. The discussion accompanying the reading of the text enables the children to understand complex sentences and abstract vocabulary that they would be unable to process through silent reading or independent study. The children are immersed in using language at the Interactive level of Transactional discourse and will have a more well developed schema for interpreting and producing this level of discourse in the future. By reducing the levels of complexity along some dimensions and providing highly scaffolded verbal mediation, children are enabled to learn the content and the form of domain-specific language.

The goal of this interaction is to learn *how to* learn and to internalize more complex Discourse, Situational, and Semantic structures of language that will generalize to new contexts of learning in the future. The ability to create integrated networks of information is exercised, facilitating the processes of accommodation and assimilation. Strategies and procedures for using text as a reference for finding information to answer questions are developed. The specific content that is learned is viewed as secondary, or one forum for refining language across many levels.

Learning Language Through Analysis and Summarization

Abstracting the most important information from a complex source and developing a summarization of the main ideas is a critical ability required for problem solving. Many older children have difficulty determining what is an important or main idea, what is a supporting fact or detail, and what can be eliminated in an analysis or summarization. Note taking for purposes of gathering information for an oral discussion or written paper on a topic such as the problems associated with the fishing industry provide a forum for developing this ability.

When students do not know how to begin the process of analyzing and summarizing, visual images help to make them aware of the most critical or salient ideas. For example, page 2 of *Oceans of Fish* (Walker, 1992c) shows a picture of a single large fish trapped and drowned in a net. By examining the picture, the adult can help them to decide what information to abstract from the picture and how to organize it in some logical manner for later use.

> **Adult:** If I wanted to remember something about this picture to use in my discussion about fishing, what would I say the picture is about?
>
> **Carol:** A big fish.
>
> **Adult:** Is that the most important thing about this fish? Would the message in the picture be the same, even if the fish was small?
>
> **Carol:** Oh, it's probably most important that its a dead fish.
>
> **Adult:** Alright, so I'll take notes on the white board while you take notes on your paper. What do you want me to write, and where should I put it?

John: Write "Dead fish" and put it at the top of the board.

Adult: (writes the words) Alright, now I want to remind myself later on about some of the things that were important about the dead fish. What do you see that is important?

Carol: It's caught in a net.

Adult: So *one* thing that is important is that it's caught in a net. How could I write that so I remember that *one* important idea about the dead fish is that it was caught in the net?

Carol: Put a number 1 (points to a place under the words "Dead fish" on the white board) and then write "caught in a net."

Adult: (writes the words) What else is important, or a *second* thing I want to remember?

John: Its mouth is open, like it couldn't breathe.

Adult: What do we call that, when you can't breathe under water? What happens to you?

John: Oh, you drown, so put a number 2, and then put "drown."

The interaction continues, as additional facts are written down about the fish. The topic of the net is developed next in a similar manner. The adult then reads the accompanying text, and the students fill in more details on their notes that were not obvious from the picture alone. The simple picture in which the most important information is obvious, combined with the active problem solving that the students engage in to invent a system for logically recording that information enables them to learn how to analyze and summarize. They are then better able to abstract the most important or relevant facts from the more complex presentation given by the text.

Once the students can easily analyze and take notes in response to a simple picture, increasingly more complex pictures can be used, such as one fishing boat depicted with several types of nets and other equipment in the water, while another boat is being unloaded at the dock. The students can be helped to determine the unifying topic, the two main ideas, and several important subtopics within each by examining the primary actions or potential actions depicted. Once again, active problem solving can be used to help the students discover how to organize the information in written notes so that it can be remembered or accessed in ways consistent with the pictured topics at a later time. Details under each subtopic can be added, first from information present in the picture, and then listened to when the text is read.

Over time, less emphasis can be placed on the pictures, and more on analyzing and summarizing information presented in the text. For example, using a book in which the picture and the text present overlapping information, the students can be asked to generate notes from text first. The picture then can be shown, and the students can examine their notes to see if they organized information into topics that were consistent with the visual images. Increasingly, books in which there is a more distanced relationship between the picture and the text, and finally few or no pictures, can be presented.

Once again, the goal of these interactions is to learn how to learn, or how to abstract and organize aspects of meaning from a complex whole. Once children begin to think in this manner, they are better predisposed to view complex information in an analyzed manner and to form a summary of the whole. This ability enables them to think more critically about events and to impose more organization and sense on experience, both academic and everyday.

Learning Language Through Critique

Text can be read for the information that it presents, but it also can be examined or critiqued for the power and effectiveness of the language used by the author. One book that is conducive to this function is *The Big Fish* (Boon, 1990). Rather than reading the text to the children, the book is read as an ongoing conversation between the adult and the group. The adult begins by reading with expression and sincerity.

> The rod jerked frantically. But the fish, which had been tearing at the bait like a hungry shark, let go as I lifted the line. It was frustrating. Despondently, I reeled the line in. The badly mauled bait was hanging by a thread.

The passage from the story can next be examined from the perspective of a critic. The adult might indicate that the story is interesting to listen to because of the way the author told it. The children can be asked to choose some of the interesting word choices or strategies that he used, and the story can be rewritten without them and the two versions compared.

Interesting	*versus*	*Plain*
The rod jerked frantically.		The rod moved up and down.
. . . tearing at the bait like a hungry shark		. . . eating the bait on the hook
Despondently, I reeled the line in		I reeled in the line

This critique provides naturally occurring opportunities for Meta-linguistic analysis of language to occur, such as noting the "adjectives" and "adverbs" that make the text interesting, the use of simile to help people visualize the hungry fish, and the choice of very specific vocabulary words to express feelings. Several other excerpts from the story can be similarly read, recounted, and examined.

One group member who has a fishing story to tell can then be placed in the storyteller's position, while other members serve as critical listeners. The storyteller has the goal of creating an interesting, well organized recounting of the event. The listeners provide feedback, guided by what they have learned about critiquing from the model story and by facilitative comments provided by the adult (i.e., Did she let you know how she felt? You might give her some feedback about what the listener knows about her reaction. Suggest some words that she might use). Thus, children in both roles learn to plan and to reflect on their oral language and to consider the needs of the audience. They learn to choose words and word order to create an effect, rather than to just describe an event in minimalist terms. They can compare their attempts to a model and evaluate their productions relative to the evaluation criteria used to examine the model. Oral language thus serves as a medium for developing and refining language at the upper limits of a child's ZPD.

Learning Language Through Writing

The oral recounting of a personal fishing experience can then be turned into written language. This same writing project can be worked on for an extended period of time, such as 1 to 2 weeks, with some days spent in planning and rehearsal phases, some in writing and evaluating, and some in editing and clarifying. Individual parts of the experience can be specifically focused on and written in an elaborated form, with new elements added until the story is complete, such as establishing the setting or describing the initiating event, or an overall summary of the entire event can be drafted, followed by elaborating on specific parts on succeeding days. Much of this will be determined by the writing skills already possessed by the group members and the amount of scaffolding needed. The strategies used and the amount of the story initially drafted will be dependent on the purposes for the writing and is likely to change across time as skill and confidence increase.

Many of the strategies described for use with the younger child can be used with the older student. For example, a semantic map can be made of potential concepts that the group members could use in their personal account. The group members can tell a summary of their experience and then make decisions about the types of words that would be needed to tell the story in an elaborated format. Suggestions for words can be spontaneously generated by the group, and resources such as a dictionary and a thesaurus can be available to enable them to explore additional choices. Positive feelings experienced during the event could be placed on one leg of the map, negative feelings on a second, words pertaining to the size of the fish on another, and a description of the fish on a fourth. Actions performed while fishing and relational terms such as "but," "when," "otherwise," "even though," and so forth can be placed on other legs. The map can be begun as a group endeavor and then completed by individuals to conform to their personal experiences.

A first draft of the personal experience then can be written. To eliminate the task of rewriting or the extensive erasing that often discourages reluctant writers, the ideas can be written on separate strips of paper, if word processors are not available for student use (Calkins, 1986). The ideas then can be easily reordered, or other ideas inserted into the text, or a single sentence rewritten with better choice of vocabulary or word order without rewriting the entire composition. The drafts can be shared with peers who provide feedback, applying the critical listening strategies practiced earlier, and then rewritten to accommodate suggestions or criticisms. Scissors and glue, or liquid paper, can be available for small edits within sentences.

On successive days, more passages from the model story can be read and discussed in regard to the structure of the story, the content of the event, word and sentence choices made by the author, and the effects on the audience. For example, on the second page of the story, an old woman explained to the child in the story why the bait he was using failed to catch fish and gave him the correct procedures for baiting his hook. The children can identify a place in their story where a procedure was conducted and can examine strategies used by the book author to gain insights into how they might communicate that part of their own story to the audience. The idea of providing sufficient steps and details to conduct the procedure from start to finish can be explored thus helping the students to engage in metacognitive analysis of a task. On the fourth page, the child took a fish that he caught home to his cat, who walked away with disinterest. This provides an opportunity to explore how to talk about disappointing or failed attempts to achieve a goal. An episode from the children's personal stories can then be developed using language to reflect disappointment or discouragement.

By the end of the writing project, children will have experience writing different parts of a story that conform to some level of discourse along the poetic/narrative dimension; using words and word order to affect an audience; critically evaluating their work and the work of others; using oral and written organizational strategies to rehearse and prepare for writing; developing reference skills for materials such as dictionaries; controlling language to create different moods; metacognitively reflecting on steps within procedures for temporal-spatial sequences; continuing to work on the same project until it is in an elaborated and clearly written form; and a myriad of other language skills at many levels of Situational, Discourse, and Semantic context.

Learning Orthographic Patterns of Language

One part of the ongoing writing cycle involves editing the spellings of words. The spellings that students spontaneously produce should constitute the starting place for refinement, rather than lists of conventionally spelled words preselected by the adult. The number of words examined and edited on any one day will depend on the individual child's tolerance for and interest in this process. The goal is not to assure that every word in the composition is correct at the end of each day, but rather that the children have experience with nonthreatening exploration of orthographic patterns. If a child has 20 misspelled words in a composition, perhaps only 3 or 4 will be examined on a given day. Other students with more confidence may want to refine most or all of the misspelled words.

Orthographic editing may be done as a group activity, or may be conducted with individuals. For example, the adult might say, "Let's examine some words from your writing that will affect the reader's ability to read and quickly process your stories. Here are some words I noticed . . . . Can you identify a few words in your own stories that you think may not be spelled conventionally?" The group can then engage in the type of metalinguistic analysis described above to refine the spellings. Similarly, the adult can circulate among the children and help them to individually identify and modify words from their compositions. Children who are done with their first draft can function as peer editors, identifying words that are misspelled and thus cause the reader to struggle with the intended message. This experience with thinking about word structure as an author leads to a higher percentage of words spelled with greater levels of sophistication across time, even though conventional spelling may not emerge immediately.

For example, below are samples of the spellings produced by learning-disabled children participating in a 6-week intensive cycle of intervention. The word list from the spelling subtest of the Wide Range Achievement Test (Jastak & Wilkinson, 1984) was administered at the end of each week to have a sampling of the patterns of spelling shown for the same child attempting the same words across time. These words were never targeted or taught and, therefore, reflect generalizations that occurred as a result of the child's emerging awareness of orthographic principles and patterns.

Example 1: WILL

Week 1	Week 2	Week 3	Week 4	Week 5	Week 6
wosrn	wowy	wow	wnw	wow	wel

This child's first week attempt to spell "will" was early phonemic, characterized by the first sound followed by random letters to represent the rest of the syllable structure. By the second week, the child was closer to the correct syllable structure, producing a Consonant-Vowel-Consonant syllable with the phonological process of diminuation at the end (also found in the speech of young children learning oral language syllabic structures, as in "doggie" or "blankie"). This had disappeared by the third week, but the phonological process of assimilation was still present, in that the child used the consonant found at the beginning of the word to also represent the consonant at the end.

By week four, the appearance of the /n/ reflected the emerging awareness of tongue tip elevation, which finally was recognized as an /l/, separate and independent from the vowel by week six. At that point the spelling is completely phonetic, since /e/ is the phonetic representation of the actual tongue placement for the short i sound, as discussed in Chapter 3. Thus, while not yet conventional in the use of vowels, in 6 weeks this word reflected a series of discoveries that the child had made regarding the orthographic representation of words.

Example 2: KITCHEN

	Week 1	Week 2	Week 3	Week 4	Week 5	Week 6
Child 1	kitech	kentch	ketchen	ktchen	ketchon	ketchen
Child 2	kenen	kinchn	kenche	kenchen	kench	kechen
Child 3	kittch	kitchen	kittich	kitt(en)ech	kitten	kichen

The changes in spelling approximations for three different children across time are shown for the word "kitchen." The first child initially demonstrates the phonological process of final consonant deletion; by the second week attempts are made to include final consonants, and the child uses the strategy of writing the first sound (i.e., /ke/) followed by the last sound (i.e., /ken/), and then begins to focus on the middle of the word, simply adding it to the end. By the third week the child is able to coordinate the phoneme and the syllabic position of the final sound and begins to explore patterns of vowel usage.

By the sixth week the word is phonetically correct, again with the correct phonemic but not the correct conventional representation for the short i vowel. The second child shows the opposite pattern, originally showing awareness of the final consonant and using the process of assimilation to repeat it to capture the syllable structure. The assimilation remains throughout the fourth week as the child attempts to coordinate the sounds present at the end and in the middle of the word with the syllable structure. The assimilation is dropped by the fifth week, although the child now uses the strategy of attending to first sound, then last, then middle. Both the sound and the syllabic position are coordinated by the last week.

The last child shows the variability that occurs as the child attempts to refine productions. By the second week the child changed from final consonant deletion to conventional spelling, but the third week reveals that this pattern was not stabilized within the child's system. The child continues to show patterns of final consonant deletion, hesitantly putting the /en/ sound within parentheses on week four to indicate knowledge of its existence but unsure of how to coordinate it with the middle sound. By the fifth week, the sound sequence was ordered correctly, but only at the expense of the phonemic structure of the middle sound which was reduced to the stop element of the /ch/ glide (recall that /ch/ starts like a /t/ but then glides to a continuant in production). Both phonemic and syllabic structure are coordinated by the sixth week.

Example 3: EXPLAIN

	Week 1	Week 2	Week 3	Week 4	Week 5	Week 6
Child 1:	explpon	ecsplane	eplan	ecsplan	ecsplan	explan
Child 2:	expland	elopen	explaplan	elxope	explan	expalan

The first child in this example initially uses the convention /x/ in his attempt, but as he becomes more aware of the phonemic structure of words he represents the sounds that he hears, rather than the letters that he sees. Thus, during week two, the /x/ is replaced with /cs/, the cluster is deleted in week three, reappears in weeks four and five, and then is represented conventionally once again in week six. While the /x/ appears in both week one and six, the intervening representations would suggest that they are qualitatively different in what they represent about the child's knowledge of word structure and sound representation. The second child shows considerable uncertainty with syllabic structure during the first four weeks. The first attempt is characterized by the phonological process of stopping, which is eliminated in the second week's attempt which shows metathesis and epenthesis, as does the fourth. By the third week, reduplication of the blend is shown as the child produces all of the sounds in order. The syllable structure and phonemic representations are correct for weeks five and six, with the exception of the insertion of the vowel as the child slowed the production of the word as it was being sounded out.

These examples demonstrate that as children attempt to spell words that are above their independent level of spelling, they engage in generative, productive attempts that are entirely consistent with the attempts shown in the speech patterns of younger children. Their changing attempts reflect the refinement process, as they learn more about phonemic representation, syllabic structure, and conventional orthography, and work to coordinate all three of these elements. If allowed to experiment with word structure under the guidance of a facilitative adult who provides feedback based on the child's current level of knowledge, rapid progress is made in the child's underlying knowledge of word representation. This knowledge generalizes to other words, since it is part of the child's mental representation system, in a way that memorized spellings cannot. Rather than teaching a child to "spell incorrectly," facilitated experiences with developmental spelling foster long-term improvements in spelling and understanding of the underlying principles of orthography (Gentry, 1989; Hoffman, 1990, Hoffman & Norris, 1989).

Learning Language Through Summarization and Generalization

Children with less flexible language systems often cannot select the most important or main ideas from the background or details. The repeated readings of narrative-based themes assist them in making these distinctions. The first day that a page was read in the thematic book, every word in the author's language is read; attached to meaning through preparatory sets, parsing, expansions, and expatiations; and commented on in relationship to the story. The second day that this information is encountered, children may be asked to read passages to reexamine the difficult language and to reestablish the ideas. Much of this occurs as a monologue as the child independently reads, with assistance provided only as needed. By the third or fourth day, the language should be familiar to the students, with less need to teach the syntactic patterns, vocabulary words, inferences, and so forth. At this point, the text is no longer read in its entirely, but rather only summarized.

The summarization can begin with a highly scaffolded interaction. The adult can model main ideas by generating the sentences while pointing to key concepts or words in the text, pausing to enable the children to participate in expressing the ideas. For example, the adult might say,

> **Adult:** In this story _____ (pointing to the character's name, Thomas) lived alone _____ (points to the words "south coast of the island") where he was peaceful and _____. But sometimes he was lonely and wished for a _____ (points to word "wife"). He knew it was impossible, so he _____ (points to the phrase "put the matter out of his mind").

Students then can be asked to independently summarize the story. Each day, old events are summarized, so that soon the students are explaining a summarized version of a long and complex story. The earliest parts of the story that have been summarized on several occasions can be independently recounted by the children, while more recently experienced parts of the story may require greater scaffolding. The attempts produced by the children provide insights to the adult as to the amount of support that should be provided for each element of the story.

The adult can heighten the children's awareness by attaching Metalinguistic terms to the retelling, such as "Kim, give us the main ideas in the setting of this story," or "summarize the important concepts in this story." In addition to summarization, the story also can be used to engage the children in generalization. Once the plot or ideas as presented by the author are understood, group discussions can be used to establish associations to similar events experienced by the group members, or similar plots or problems encountered in other books. The children thus begin to see the patterns in setting, problems, and solutions that are present in many situations, even though the specific locations, characters, and events may appear to be very different on the surface. They begin to think of stories as reflections on experiences, rather than merely descriptions of events. The poetic nature of stories thus begins to emerge in the children's consciousness.

Learning the Language of Metaphor

The emerging awareness of the poetic nature of stories can be facilitated by exposure to fables, legends, and other tales that explicitly reflect on experience in attempts to explain unknown phenomena. For example, in the theme book, *The Stranger from the Sea* (Burleigh, 1990), the man's life changes when a horrible storm hits the island and washes a woman ashore. An explanation of the nature of storms can be explored in the Chinese legend *How the Weather Gods Help* (Candappa, 1988a). In this story, phenomena such as rain, thunder, lightning, winds, and storm clouds are explained by the actions of the powerful storm gods who gathered in one spot in response to the Emperor of Heaven's command for rain. The return of sunshine was caused by "The Lady who Sweeps the Sky Clear," who brushed the storm clouds away to make room for the sun. The explanations provided by fables can be compared to explanations found in expository text.

The metaphoric explanations for phenomena, such as the "Mother of Lightnings" who held up enormous mirrors to catch the sun's reflections and create lightning, or "Madame Wind" who rides full speed on the back of a tiger and releases bags of wild, imprisoned winds can be discussed. Cross cultural explanations can be compared, as in *The North Wind* (Butterworth, 1988a), where the wind is represented as a giant tiger whose roaring creates the mighty wind. The characteristics of a tiger that might lead to his appearance in fables about the wind across cultures can be explored. Children can be helped to decide why people felt the need to create explanations, why they resorted to gods and other fanciful explanations, and why they did not use scientific knowledge as explanations. Opportunities to generate metaphors for something that the students do not understand can then be provided. This type of experience helps the children to compare fact with fantasy, to explore both the nature of and reason for metaphor, and to learn to deal with the highly formal and abstract language used in these tales.

Poetry is another medium that can be used to explore abstract language and metaphor. In *Hurricane* (Berry, 1986) the power of a tremendous storm is explored through the destruction it reaps. Each word must be used by the reader to conjure up an entire image, requiring a far greater contribution in background knowledge from the reader than is explicitly provided by the author. For example, the opening stanza states:

Under low black clouds
the wind was all
speedy feet, all horns and breath,
all bangs, howls, rattles,
in every hen house,
church hall and school.

The reader must use knowledge of storms and the behavior of people and animals under these circumstances to interpret who might exhibit speedy feet and why; what types of horns might blow and for what reason; and what a hen house, church hall, and school represent on an implicit level. A careful examination of a poem helps children to read for maximum interpretation from minimal language, thus facilitating the expectation that knowledge must be brought to words, and not merely found there.

Comparing Fact and Fiction

The woman washed ashore in the theme book, The *Stranger From the Sea* (Burleigh, 1990) is unable to walk, and there are rumors that perhaps she was a mermaid. The exploration of metaphors through fables can thus be continued using a story such as *Merpeople* (McLeish, 1986a), a legend from England. In this tale, a man using diving gear follows a mermaid deep into the bottom of the sea where he finds a kingdom rich in jewels and other treasures. His companions pulled him up before he retrieved any of the riches and refused to believe his story about the merpeople and their kingdom. They thought that he merely chased a seal or a fish and that he hallucinated the kingdom because of the weak oxygen supplied by the diving equipment. The story ends with speculation as to the existence of the kingdom and if it will ever be found again.

The sources of the legends regarding both mermaids and treasure-filled kingdoms below the sea can be explored by using expository text for potential sources. The book *Extremely Weird Frogs* (Lovett, 1992) shows the metamorphosis that a frog undergoes from a creature with a fish-like tail to one with the legs of a mammal. The parallels between the frog's change and the mermaid's attempts to adjust to living on land can be drawn. The differences in the metamorphosis as it is seen in a variety of frogs around the world can be explored and compared, providing children with an enriched background for understanding this phenomenon. Similarly, shipwrecks and other events leading to treasures buried beneath the sea can be explored.

These experiences enable children to establish the connections between fact and fiction, to make comparisons at abstract levels for qualities of similarities and differences, and to explore a process that occurs across time in a predictable sequence.

Learning the Language of Scripts

Children can become metacognitively aware of scripts that will enable them to function more independently and successfully within the classroom. In the most controlled context, a book such as *Shopping* (Young, 1988c) can be used to examine the nature of scripts in an entertaining context. The steps in the sequence of events involved in the shopping trip, the conscious thoughts of the characters as they plan and recall the things that need to be done to complete the task, and the visual images that the characters create to remember the elements of the trip can be examined. The students can be assisted to abstract the main points of the shopping script from the total story.

In this story, the children are asked to go to the store for their father and to buy specific items. The students can be asked to generate actions, locations, or states that are part of the event. These can be organized into lists, flowcharts, or other graphic organizers.

Step 1	**Step 2**	**Step 3**	**Step 4**
Know the goal	*Gather required materials*	*Plan route to store*	*Dress to go*
a. listen to instructions	a. take enough money	a. estimate time required	a. walking shoes
b. write shopping list	b. take basket to carry purchases	b. choose safe streets	b. bring a sweater
c. identify destination			

On their way, they encounter a series of people who also request that the children make specific purchases for them. Thus, the script becomes more complex, and finer discriminations must be made. The students can use the general script as a basis for generating the elaborated script.

The script generated with the support of the illustrated story can then be used to enable the children to generate similar scripts for classroom procedures. Principles such as thinking about the things that are needed for the shopping trip, organizing the series of tasks to be completed into a sequence, visualizing the objects or events, remembering all of the tasks that need to be performed, and evaluating each completed step can be generalized first to short, limited scripts such as completing a worksheet or looking up information in an index, then gradually to more complex and interactive scripts for functioning within the classroom. The scripts can be practiced in the intervention room, then they can be used to examine the behaviors of successful peers within the classroom, then implemented in specific classroom situations. The speech-language pathologist initially can sit with the child in the classroom and facilitate the implementation of the script until the scripts are internalized and independently implemented.

■□ SUMMARY

Whole Language is a philosophy of language learning and use that is based on what actually occurs in the process of normal language acquisition. These principles form the foundation for learning activities that are provided to children within the regular classroom and within specific learning contexts such as language intervention. The strategies described throughout this book can and have been used effectively with children at all ability levels and all contexts. Children with highly integrated and flexible language systems will require minimum scaffolding and will be able to engage in much independent exploration of a topic with guidance from adults and collaboration with peers. Children with poorly integrated and less flexible language systems will require a high level of scaffolding. Many will benefit from modifications in the learning environment, including participation in small groups, a minimally distracting setting, assistance attending to the most important or relevant information, a high level of feedback and clarification, more frequent opportunities to respond, and assistance generating responses.

The goal of intervention is to provide intensive intervention experiences over a relatively short time to help the child to internalize patterns of language and learning that have failed to be spontaneously learned. As the patterns of language and learning become internalized, the responsibility for the learning increasingly becomes the child's. The goal is *not* to teach outcomes, such as tutoring specific content, in an effort to help the child to pass an exam or complete a worksheet. Tutoring, without changing the underlying language and learning system only results in more dependence on others for further learning. There is a place for tutoring, and for many children it will be an important and necessary part of their total educational program. But this type of teaching-to-task should not be the goal of language intervention.

The suggestions provided in this book are neither comprehensive nor the only methods and strategies for implementing Whole Language intervention with school-age children. Rather, they represent examples of how numerous goals and objectives can be simultaneously met across multiple levels of Situational, Discourse, and Semantic contexts of language use. The intervention is highly relevant to the written and oral language demands placed on the child in school. This type of intervention makes use of materials consistent with school curriculum, such as literature and expository text, but for purposes of facilitating actual language development to abstract greater meaning from the words and to accomplish more complex goals.

Many behaviors can be evaluated for evidence of change in the child's language. For example, the grade levels of independent, instructional, and frustration reading should increase to correspond with the child's greater ability to deal with the complexities of vocabulary, sentence structure, discourse structure, implicature, and decontextualization. The organization and complexity of writing should increase to reflect greater internalization of the patterns and content of both Poetic and Transactional discourse. The stories written and told should increasingly reflect on experience rather than just describing it, so that a greater percentage of comments are at higher levels along the semantic continuum. Spelling patterns should change to reflect greater awareness and coordination of phonemic structure, syllable structure, and orthographic patterns. Pronouns, articles, and other cohesive ties should establish referents with greater clarity within and across sentences embedded within longer discourse episodes.

The child should be able to metacognitively reflect on the steps and procedures involved in scripts and use language to complete more of a classroom task with fewer specific reminders. A broader background of world and cultural knowledge should be activated when interpreting a picture or story so that an event presented to the child in illustrated or oral form would elicit more relevant interpretations and inferences, rather than merely descriptions of contextually present information. Fables and legends should be evaluated for their relevance to real-world situations, with a greater understanding of metaphors and figurative expressions. A greater ability to identify metalinguistic elements of language, such as nouns versus verbs, the setting versus the problem found in story structure, and main ideas should be apparent. In other words, a wide variety of behaviors should begin to emerge and refine if the whole language system is addressed in the context of language intervention.

To recognize what is appropriate for a child at a given age or grade level, writing, reading, or language samples can be elicited from children who are achieving at an average or above level in the classroom. Either age/grade peer comparisons, or comparisons to younger but developmentally comparable children can be made. The complexity of the language along the Situational, Discourse, and Semantic contexts can be examined in these samples to obtain a frame of reference for what is "normal" language for the community in which the child resides, as shown in Chapter 3. Similarly, the language found in the curriculum can be examined to ascertain the level of complexity that the child is expected to process. Examples of this type of analysis can be found throughout this book.

The language system that must be acquired during the school years is far too complex to be mastered one discrete skill at a time. Rather, numerous abilities must be simultaneously acquired and integrated by both normally developing children and by children with less flexible language systems. Whole Language provides a theoretical framework for understanding how and why these language processes can be facilitated and for developing strategies to maximize every child's ability to learn and use language.

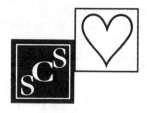

Epilogue

The language problems that seemed to disappear following kinder- garten language intervention began to resurface by the middle of first grade. The stress caused by the demands to understand and inter- pret text, instead of just recognizing the words, resulted in an increase in behaviors such as finger knotting and making noises. When Tommy's teacher told his parents that his peculiar behaviors were distracting to the other children, they sought the help of a speech-language patholo- gist (SLP) who ascribed to the Whole Language philosophy. She assess- ed his use of language in a number of contexts, including oral reading, summarization of the reading material, and narrative construction with and without pictures.

Tommy was asked to tell a story in response to a picture from the Apricot I series (Arwood, 1985) depicting a birthday party, where a mother brings a cake, a boy opens presents, two children hand the boy other presents, and another child points to the arrival of the cake. Tom- my's story was as follows:

> **Tommy:** This little boy bringing presents. Give him . . . the birth-
> day boy . . . and um . . . And the taking off the rib . . . the
> wrapper . . . That's all.

The story revealed no inclusion of the script for events that occur at a birthday party and a simple description of the most concrete actions depicted told from the child's perspective as an observer. This level of narration was inconsistent with the expectations required for reading comprehension.

This lack of prerequisite displacement and organization of language was confirmed when Tommy was asked to read an illustrated page from a first-grade reader. His reading was as follows:

> **Tommy:** Lucy was a buzzy working . . . she paint a lot of nice . . . pictures. She was . . . a good reader and she liked to put things away but Lucy . . . had . . . a problem she did not listen.

This reading was characterized by some word substitutions that Tommy did not recognize as problematic. For example, the text stated that Lucy was a "busy worker," not a "buzzy working." His incorrect phrasing, omission of verb tense markers, and monotone reading indicated that meaning was not attached to the words as they were read. When Tommy was asked what he knew about Lucy, he said he could not think of anything.

Intervention was initiated to enable Tommy to attach meaning to the words he read. Oral language was used to prepare him for the concepts he was about to read, to give him feedback about what his reading actually communicated, to elaborate on the ideas in the reading, and to relate the written words to his experiences. His classroom teacher noticed almost immediate improvement in Tommy's reading and asked the SLP how she worked with Tommy.

The SLP found that the teacher viewed good reading as "accurate and rapid word recognition," and thus had placed Tommy in the top reading group, called the "Sharks." The girls in this group were fluent readers with excellent comprehension, while Tommy and a second boy required considerable oral scaffolding to maintain comprehension. The SLP asked if the composition of the group could be changed to include nonfluent readers who also required assistance for comprehension during reading. Good reading from this Whole Language perspective was viewed as "accurate reconstruction of the author's meaning." The teacher agreed hesitantly, although with less reluctance than one of the girls reassigned to another group who huffed, "I guess this means we don't get to be 'Sharks' anymore!"

During the remainder of the year, Tommy's reading comprehension improved. The SLP was pleased with his progress and suggested her regular meetings with Tommy be terminated. She demonstrated to his parents how they could read with Tommy, and they set aside 30 minutes almost every day as "reading" time. Sometimes they would read with Tommy, and sometimes they would just ask him to explain the events of the story. However, the SLP left Tommy's parents with an unsettling pre-diction. She told them that Tommy's problem in organizing language was not gone. Difficulties were likely to recur when the language in his books became more complex, and the teacher's expectations for written language included more composing and less filling in slots on worksheets.

Tommy's problem reappeared in the second semester of third grade. In his social studies class, he had difficulty organizing expository information about times and cultures different from his own. In reading class, he was unable to follow narratives with complex time relationships and internal motives attributed to characters. He was spending hours at night finishing work he had not completed in school. His handwriting became illegible as he struggled to keep up, causing him to make errors in one of his better areas, arithmetic. He frequently forgot assignments.

Tommy's parents enrolled him in a Whole Language, after-school program. His language showed greater refinement at this time, with stories recounted in the form of an abbreviated episode. He described a problem presented to characters and the execution of plans to resolve the problem, but the resolution of the story was rarely reached. Semantically, he provided interpretations of underlying motives or causes and coordinated events within a temporal frame. However, when asked to tell what the characters would do next, he was unable to make logical predictions. Tommy was highly dependent on visual cues to organize his ideas. He struggled to use language to create the context.

When reading material included complex sentence structures, Tommy's oral reading rate decreased, his intonation became flat, and he read past punctuation marks. He was able to answer questions about facts that were literally stated in the text, but he failed to appropriately interpret metalanguage such as sarcasm, humor, and metaphor and was not comprehending the implied meanings of the text.

The after-school program sought to help the children develop strategies for learning from decontextualized learning situations and to use language within this context. The SLP presented pictures from expository texts that were discussed orally to help the children focus on main ideas and supporting details. The adult helped the children to generate questions about the topic that were important to understanding the overall event and the supporting details. The adult then presented an oral lecture while the children took notes. One of the children's notes then would be critiqued by the group, who would determine if sufficient and appropriate information was recorded. The adult aided in restructuring the information using semantic webs and flow charts. The children then would write their own expository texts about the information.

At the end of the 8-week intervention block, Tommy's expository writing contained more detailed information and was structured at higher levels of discourse organization. Topics were established and elaborated on at a descriptive level of semantic context. He most often comprehended and used language at a literal level, rather than using inference, or making statements about causality and motives.

The SLP counseled Tommy's parents to be aware of these deficits, and taught them how to provide information to Tommy during his home reading and homework times. Now in middle school, he maintains a B+ average and performs between the 75–95th percentile on group achievement tests, with the exception of oral listening and comprehension subtests which remain below average. Intervention has helped him to use written language to learn, interpret, and reorganize information that he is not able to grasp when it is presented through the rapid and temporary auditory signal.

Although Tommy scores well above average on tests of language ability, in reality he always will exhibit an inflexible language system. His language problems did not disappear when he learned to handle conversational rules or syntactic-semantic forms in his kindergarten speech therapy sessions, or when he learned to read for meaning in the first grade, or when he learned about school discourse in third grade. Whole Language intervention does not purport to provide a cure for language-learning problems. Rather, it provides a framework for developing teaching and intervention strategies that present information to children at levels of Situational, Discourse, and Semantic context at which successful learning can occur. As children learn more language, they function more independently at higher levels of context.

Tommy is aware of his language-processing problems and knows that he must work harder to learn information that is easily understood by his friends. At the end of the sixth grade, one of his teachers asked him to write 10 endings for the sentence fragment "I wish I could . . . ." His first was "I wish I could go to Chicago to meet Michael Jordon." His seventh was "I wish I could understand everything I can read."

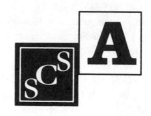

Appendix A: Suggested Materials for Assessment, Intervention, and Accountability

Arwood, E. L. (1985). *Apricot I language kit.* Portland, OR: Apricot.

Burns, P., & Roe, B. D. (1989). *Burns/Roe informal reading inventory: Preprimer to twelfth grade* (3rd ed.). Boston: Houghton Mifflin.

Eggleton, J. (1990). *Whole language evaluation: Reading, writing and spelling.* Bothell, WA: The Wright Group.

Eggleton, J. (1992). *Whole language evaluation: Reading, writing and spelling for the intermediate grades.* Bothell, WA: The Wright Group.

Ekwall, Eldon E. (1986). *Ekwall reading inventory* (2nd ed.). Boston: Allyn and Bacon.

Goodman, K. S., Goodman, Y. M., & Burke, C. L. (1987). *Reading miscue inventory: Alternative procedures.* New York: Richard C. Owen.

Goodman, K. S., Goodman, Y. M., & Hood, W. J. (1988). *The whole language evaluation book.* Portsmouth, NH: Heinemann.

Grill, J. J., & Kirwin, M. M. (1990). *Written language assessment.* Novato, CA: Academic Therapy Publications.

Kemp, M. (1987). *Watching children read and write: Observational records for children with special needs.* Portsmouth, NH: Heinemann.

Johns, J. L. (1988). *Basic reading inventory: Pre-primer-grade eight* (4th ed.). Dubuque, IA: Kendall/Hunt.

Loban, W. (1976). *Language development: Kindergarten through grade twelve.* Urbana, IL: National Council of Teachers of English.

Secord, W. A., & Damico, J. S. (Eds.). (1992). *Best practices in school speech-language pathology: Descriptive/nonstandardized language assessment.* San Antonio, TX: The Psychological Corporation.

Silvarali, N. (1989). *Classroom reading inventory* (6th ed.). Dubuque, IA: William C. Brown.

Stieglitz, E. L. (1992). *The Stieglitz informal reading inventory: Assessing reading behaviors from emergent to advanced levels.* Boston: Allyn and Bacon.

Wiederholt, J. L., & Bryant, B. R. (1986). *Gray oral reading tests-Revised.* Austin, TX: Pro-Ed.

Woods, M. L., & Alden, M. (1989). *Analytic reading inventory* (4th ed.). Columbus, OH: Merrill.

Zakaluk, B. L., & Samuels, S. J. (1988). *Readability: Its past, present, and future.* Newark, DE: International Reading Association.

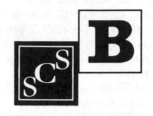

Appendix B: Recommended Resources for Intervention for the Lower Academic Level Child

Brown, H., & Mathie, V. (1991). *Inside whole language: A classroom view.* Portsmouth, NH: Heinemann.

Calkins, L. M. (1986). *The art of teaching writing.* Portsmouth, NH: Heinemann.

Calkins, L. M. (1991). *Living between the lines.* Portsmouth, NH: Heinemann.

Goodman, K. (1986). *What's whole in whole language?* Portsmouth, NH: Heinemann.

McGee, L. M., & Richgels, D. J. (1990). *Literacy's beginnings: Supporting young readers and writers.* Boston: Allyn and Bacon.

Pehrsson, R. S., & Robinson, H. A. (1985). *The semantic organizer approach to writing and reading instruction.* Rockville, MD: Aspen.

Secord, W. A. (Ed.). (1990). *Best practices in school speech-language pathology: Collaborative programs in the schools: Concepts, models, and procedures.* San Antonio, TX: The Psychological Corporation.

Temple, C., Nathan, R., Burris, N., & Temple, F. (1988). *The beginnings of writing.* Boston: Allyn and Bacon.

Westby, C. E. (1991). A scale for assessing children's pretend play. In C. E. Schaefer, K. Gitlin, & A. Sandgrund (Eds.), *Play diagnosis and assessment* (pp. 131–161). New York: John Wiley and Sons.

Wright Group. (1987). *Language is fun: Teachers' book, level one.* Bothell, WA: The Wright Group.

Wright Group. (1989). *Language is fun: Teachers' book, level two.* Bothell, WA: The Wright Group.

Wright Group. (1991). *Language is fun: Teachers' book, level three.* Bothell, WA: The Wright Group.

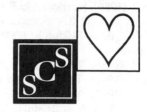

References

Allington, R. L. (1989). Coherence or chaos? Qualitative dimensions of literacy instruction provided to low achievement children. In A. Gartner & D. Lipsky (Eds.), *Beyond separate education* (pp. 75–99). New York: Brooles.

Altwerger, A., Diehl-Faxon, J., & Dockstader-Anderson, K. (1985). Read-aloud events as meaning construction. *Language Arts, 62,* 476–484.

Anderson, R. C., Hiebert, E. H., Scott, J. A., & Wilkinson, I. A. G. (1985). *Becoming a nation of readers.* Champaign, IL: University of Illinois, Center for the Study of Reading.

Applebee, A. N. (1978). *A child's concept of story: Ages 2–17.* Chicago: University of Chicago Press.

Applebee, A. N. (1991). Environments for language teaching and learning: Contemporary issues and future directions. In J. Flood, J. M. Jensen, D. Lapp, & J. R. Squire (Eds.), *Handbook of research on teaching the English language arts* (pp. 549–558), New York: Macmillan.

Aram, D. M., Ekelman, B. L., & Nation, J. E. (1984). Preschoolers with language disorders: Ten years later. *Journal of Speech and Hearing Disorders, 27,* 232–244.

Arwood, E. L. (1985). *Apricot I language kit.* Portland, OR: Apricot.

ASHA, Committee on Language Learning Disabilities. (1989). Issues in determining eligibility for language intervention. *ASHA, 31*(3), 113–118.

Baumann, J. F., & Kameenui, E. J. (1991). Research on vocabulary instruction: Ode to Voltaire. In J. Flood, J. M. Jensen, D. Lapp, & J. R. Squire (Eds.), *Handbook of research on teaching the English language arts* (pp. 604–632), New York: Macmillan.

Beasley, M. (1988). *The gingerbread man.* Bothell, WA: The Wright Group.

Bernstein, D. K. (1992). *Language and communication disorders in children* (3rd ed.). New York: Macmillan.

Berry, J. (1986). Hurricane. In E. Jones (Ed.), *Tales of the Caribbean: the beginnings of things* (pp. 32–33). Bothell, WA: The Wright Group.

Biddulph, F., & Biddulph, J. (1992). *What will float?* Bothell, WA: The Wright Group.

Biro, V. (1986). *The donkey in the lion's skin.* Bothell, WA: The Wright Group.

Biro, V. (1990). *The farmer and his sons.* Bothell, WA: The Wright Group.

Biro, V. (1991). *The fox and the crow.* Bothell, WA: The Wright Group.

Blank, M., Rose, S., & Berlin, L. (1978). *The language of learning: The preschool years.* New York: Grune & Stratton.

Bloome, D. (1985). Bedtime story reading as a social process. In J. A. Niles & R. V. Lalik (Eds.), Issues in literacy: A research respective. *Thirty-fourth Yearbook of the National Reading Conference* (pp. 287–294). Rochester, NY: National Reading Conference.

Boon, K. (1990). *The big fish.* Bothell, WA: The Wright Group.

Bowey, J. (1986). Syntactic awareness and verbal performance from preschool to fifth grade. *Journal of Psycholinguistic Research, 15,* 285–308.

Brewer, W. R., & Lichtenstein, E. H. (1981). Event schemas, story schemas, and story grammars. In A. D. Buddely & J. D. Lang (Eds.), *Attention and performance IX* (pp. 160–189). Hillsdale, NJ: Lawrence Erlbaum.

Bridwell, N. (1966). *Clifford takes a trip.* New York: Scholastic.

Britton, J. (1982). Writing to learn and learning to write. In G. M. Pradl (Ed.), *Prospect and retrospect: Selected essays of James Britton* (pp. 94–111). Montclair, NJ: Boynton/Cook.

Brown, R. (1973). *A first language: The early stages.* Cambridge, MA: Harvard University Press.

Brown, G., & Yule, G. (1983). *Discourse analysis.* London: Cambridge University Press.

Bruce, B. (1981). A social interaction model of reading. *Discourse Processes, 4,* 273–309.

Bruner, J. (1978). The role of dialogue in language acquisition. In A. Sinclair, R. J. Jarvella, & W. J. M. Levelt (Eds.), *The child's conception of language: Springer series in language and communication* (pp. 242–256). New York: Springer-Verlag.

Bruner, J. (1983). *Child's talk.* New York: Norton.

Bruner, J. (1986). *Actual minds, possible worlds.* Cambridge, MA: Harvard University Press.

Bryan, T. (1986). A review of studies on learning disabled children's communicative competence. In R. L. Schiefelbusch (Ed.), *Language competence: Assessment and intervention* (pp. 227–260). San Diego, CA: College-Hill Press.

Burleigh, L. (1990). *The stranger from the sea.* Bothell, WA: The Wright Group.

Butterworth, B. (1986a). *The discontented pig.* Bothell, WA: The Wright Group.

Butterworth, B. (1986b). *The giraffe who could not walk.* Bothell, WA: The Wright Group.

Butterworth, B. (1988a). *The north wind.* Bothell, WA: The Wright Group.

Butterworth, B. (1988b). *The two windmills.* Bothell, WA: The Wright Group.

Calfee, R., & Curley, R. (1984). Structure of prose in the content areas. In J. Flood

(Ed.), *Understanding reading comprehension* (pp. 161–180). Newark, DE: International Reading Association.

Calkins, L. M. (1986). *The art of teaching writing.* Portsmouth, NH: Heinemann.

Calkins, L. M. (1991). *Living between the lines.* Portsmouth, NH: Heinemann.

Candappa, B. (1986). The three dragon eggs. In *Tales of south Asia: How things began* (pp. 24–32). Bothell, WA: The Wright Group.

Candappa, B. (1988a). How the weather gods help. In *Tales of the Far East: Listen to grandmother* (pp. 22–27). Bothell, WA: The Wright Group.

Candappa, B. (1988b). Something strange for sale. In *Tales of the Far East: Daring deeds* (pp. 4–10). Bothell, WA: The Wright Group.

Carey, S. (1982). Semantic development: The state of the art. In E. Wanner & L. R. Gleitman (Eds.), *Language acquisition: The state of the art* (pp. 347–489). New York: Cambridge University Press.

Cazden, C. (1983). Adult assistance to language development: Scaffolds, models, and direct instruction. In C. Cazden (Ed.), *Developing literacy: Young children's use of language* (pp. 3–18). Newark, DE: International Reading Association.

Cazden, C. (1988). *Classroom discourse.* Portsmouth, NH: Heinemann.

Chomsky, C. (1971). Write first, read later. *Childhood Education, 47,* 296–299.

Chomsky, C. (1979). Approaching reading through invented spelling. In L. C. Resnick & P. A. Werner (Eds.), *Theory and practice of early reading, 2* (pp. 43–65). Hillsdale, NJ: Lawrence Erlbaum.

Chomsky, C. (1980). Reading, writing, and phonology. In M. Wolf, M. McQuillan, & F. Radwin (Eds.), *Thought and language/Language and reading* (pp. 51–71). Cambridge, MA: Harvard Educational Review.

Ciantar, G. (1988). *The goats and the troll.* Bothell, WA: The Wright Group.

Clay, M. M. (1991). *Becoming literate: The construction of inner control.* Portsmouth, NH: Heinemann.

Clymer, T. (1963). The utility of phonic generalizations in the primary grades. *The Reading Teacher, 16,* 252–258.

Colby, R. W. (1988). On the nature of dramatic intelligence: A study of developmental differences in the process of characterization by adolescents. Unpublished doctoral dissertation, Harvard University. *Dissertation Abstracts International, 49/06B,* 239.

Collins, A. (1986). *A sample dialogue based on a theory of inquiry reading.* Technical Report No. 367. Urbana, IL: Center for the Study of Reading.

Cowley, J. (1983a). *To town.* Bothell, WA: The Wright Group.

Cowley, J. (1983b). *Who will be my mother?* Bothell, WA: The Wright Group.

Cowley, J. (1987). *Just this once.* Bothell, WA: The Wright Group.

Cowley, J. (1988a). *Cousin Kira.* Bothell, WA: The Wright Group.

Cowley, J. (1988b). *Dragon with a cold.* Bothell, WA: The Wright Group.

Cowley, J. (1988c). *I love my family.* Bothell, WA: The Wright Group.

Cowley, J. (1988d). *Road robber.* Bothell, WA: The Wright Group.

Cowley, J. (1988e). *Soup.* Bothell, WA: The Wright Group.

Cowley, J. (1989a). *Bogle's feet.* Bothell, WA: The Wright Group.

Cowley, J. (1989b). *Busy baby.* Bothell, WA: The Wright Group.

Cowley, J. (1990a). *The big hill.* Bothell, WA: The Wright Group.

Cowley, J. (1990b). *Grumpy elephant.* Bothell, WA: The Wright Group.

Cowley, J. (1990c). *Hairy bear.* Bothell, WA: The Wright Group.

Cowley, J. (1990d). *Houses.* Bothell, WA: The Wright Group.

Cowley, J. (1990e). *Huggles' breakfast.* Bothell, WA: The Wright Group.

Cowley, J. (1990f). *The hungry giant.* Bothell, WA: The Wright Group.

Cowley, J. (1990g). *I want ice cream.* Bothell, WA: The Wright Group.

Cowley, J. (1990h). *If you meet a dragon.* Bothell, WA: The Wright Group.

Cowley, J. (1990i). *In the mirror.* Bothell, WA: The Wright Group.

Cowley, J. (1990j). *The jigaree.* Bothell, WA: The Wright Group.

Cowley, J. (1990k). *Little brother.* Bothell, WA: The Wright Group.

Cowley, J. (1990l). *A monster sandwich.* Bothell, WA: The Wright Group.

Cowley, J. (1990m). *On a chair.* Bothell, WA: The Wright Group.

Cowley, J. (1990n). *The red rose.* Bothell, WA: The Wright Group.

Cowley, J. (1990o). *The secret of spooky house.* Bothell, WA: The Wright Group.

Cowley, J. (1990p). *Stop!* Bothell, WA: The Wright Group.

Cowley, J. (1990q). *Water is my friend.* Bothell, WA: The Wright Group.

Crais, E. R., & Chapman, R. S. (1987). Story recall and inferencing skills in language/learning-disabled and nondisabled children. *Journal of Speech and Hearing Research, 52,* 50–55.

Creaghead, N. A. (1992). Classroom interactional analysis/script analysis. In W. A. Secord & J. S. Damico (Eds.), *Best practices in school speech-language pathology* (pp. 65–72). San Antonio, TX: Psychological Corp.

Cutting, B., & Cutting, J. (1988a). *Captain B's boat.* Bothell, WA: The Wright Group.

Cutting, B., & Cutting, J. (1988b). *The dandelion.* Bothell, WA: The Wright Group.

Cutting, B., & Cutting, J. (1988c). *Dreams.* Bothell, WA: The Wright Group.

Cutting, B., & Cutting, J. (1988d). *It takes time to grow.* Bothell, WA: The Wright Group.

Cutting, B., & Cutting, J. (1988e). *The new building.* Bothell, WA: The Wright Group.

Cutting, B., & Cutting, J. (1988f). *Space.* Bothell, WA: The Wright Group.

Cutting, B., & Cutting, J. (1988g). *Together.* Bothell, WA: The Wright Group.

Cutting, B., & Cutting, J. (1988h). *The tree.* Bothell, WA: The Wright Group.

Cutting, B., & Cutting, J. (1988i). *Underwater journey.* Bothell, WA: The Wright Group.

Cutting, B., & Cutting, J. (1988j). *What am I?* Bothell, WA: The Wright Group.

Cutting, J. (1988). *Come on!* Bothell, WA: The Wright Group.

Cutting, J. (1990). *To school.* Bothell, WA: The Wright Group.

Damico, J. S. (1985). Clinical discourse analysis: A functional language assessment technique. In C. S. Simon (Ed.), *Communication skills and classroom success: Assessment of language-learning disabled students* (pp.165–206). San Diego, CA: College-Hill Press.

Damico, J. S. (1992). Systematic observation of communicative interaction: A valid and practical descriptive assessment technique. In W. A. Secord & J. S. Damico (Eds.), *Best practices in school speech-language pathology* (pp. 133–144). San Antonio, TX: Psychological Corp.

Downing, J., & Valtin, R. (1984). *Language awareness and learning to read.* New York: Springer-Verlag.

Dyson, A. H. (1988). Unintentional helping in the primary grades: Writing in the children's world. In B. A. Rafoth & D. L. Rubin (Eds.), *The social construction of written communication* (pp. 218–248). Norwood, NJ: Ablex.

Edelsky, C., Altwerger, B., & Flores, B. (1991). *Whole language: What's the difference?* Portsmouth, NH: Heinemann.

Elliott, L. L., & Hammer, M. A. (1988). Longitudinal changes in auditory discrimination in normal children and children with language-learning problems. *Journal of Speech and Hearing Disorders, 4,* 467–474.

Ferreiro, E. (1986). The interplay between information and assimilation in beginning literacy. In W. H. Teale & E. Sulzby (Eds.), *Emergent literacy: Writing and reading* (pp. 15–49). Norwood, NJ: Ablex.

Ferreiro, E., & Teberosky, A. (1982). *Literacy before schooling.* Portsmouth, NH: Heinemann.

Fey, M. E. (1986). *Language intervention with young children.* San Diego, CA: College-Hill Press.

Fey, M. E. (1988). Generalization issues facing language interventionists: An introduction. *Language, Speech and Hearing Services in Schools, 19,* 272–281.

Flood, J. (1986). The text, the student, and the teacher: Learning from exposition in middle schools. *The Reading Teacher, 39,* 784–791.

Flood, J., Lapp, D., & Farnan, N. (1986). A reading writing procedure that teaches expository text structure. *The Reading Teacher, 39,* 556–561.

Forester, A. D., & Mickelson, N. I. (1979). Language acquisition and learning to read. In R. Shafer (Ed.), *Applied linguistics and reading* (pp. 74–88). Newark, DE: International Reading Association.

French, L., & Nelson, K. (1985). *Young children's knowledge of relational terms: Some ifs, ors, and buts.* New York: Springer-Verlag.

Gallagher, T. M. (1991). Language and social skills: Implications for clinical assessment and intervention with school-age children. In T. M. Gallagher (Ed.), *Pragmatics of language: Clinical practice issues* (pp 11–43). San Diego, CA: Singular Publishing Group.

Gallagher, T. M., & Prutting, C. A. (1983). *Pragmatic assessment and intervention issues in language.* San Diego, CA: College-Hill Press.

Gentry, J. R. (1982). An analysis of developmental spelling in GYNS AT WRK. *The Reading Teacher, 36,* 192–200.

Gentry, J. R. (1989). *SPEL . . . is a four letter word.* Portsmouth, NH: Heinemann.

Gibbs, D. B., & Cooper, E. B. (1989). Prevalence of communication disorders in students with learning disabilities. *Journal of Learning Disabilities, 22,* 60–63.

Golden, J. M. (1990). *The narrative symbol in childhood literature: Explorations in the construction of text.* New York: Mouton de Gruyter.

Good, T., & Stipek, D. (1983). Individual differences in the classroom: A psychological perspective. In M. Fernstermacher & J. Goodlad (Eds.), *National Society for the Study of Education 18th Yearbook* (pp. 9–43). Chicago: University of Chicago Press.

Goodman, K. (1985). Transactional psycholinguistic model: Unity in reading. In H. Singer & R. B. Ruddell (Eds.), *Theoretical models and processes of reading* (pp. 813–840). Newark, DE: International Reading Association.

Goodman, K. S. (1986). *What's whole in whole language?* Portsmouth, NH: Heinemann.

Goodman, K. S., & Goodman, Y. M. (1977). Learning about psycholinguistic processes by analyzing oral reading. *Harvard Educational Review, 47,* 317–333.

Goodman, K. S., Goodman, Y. M., & Burke, C. L. (1987). *Reading miscue inventory: Alternative procedures.* New York: Richard C. Owen.

Goodman, Y. M. (1980). The roots of literacy. In M. T. Douglass (Ed.), *The Claremont Reading Conference: 44th Yearbook* (pp. 1–32). Claremont, CA: Claremont Reading Conference, Center for Developmental Studies.

Graesser, A. C., Magliano, J. P., & Tidwell, P. M. (1992). World knowledge, inferences, and questions. In R. Beach, J. L. Green, M. L. Kamil, & T. Shanahan (Eds.), *Multidisciplinary perspectives on literacy research* (pp. 245–274). Urbana, IL: National Council of Teachers of English.

Graesser, A. C., Millis, K. K., & Long, D. L. (1986). The construction of knowledge structures and inferences during text comprehension. In N. E. Sharkey (Ed.), *Advances in cognitive science* (pp. 125–157). New York, NJ: Ellis Horwood.

Graves, M. F. (1986). Vocabulary learning and instruction. In E. Z. Rothkopf (Ed.), *Review of research in education, 13* (pp. 49–89). Washington: American Educational Research Association.

Hall, P. K., & Tomblin, J. B. (1978). A follow-up study of children with articulation and language disorders. *Journal of Speech and Hearing Disorders, 43,* 227–241.

Hall, R. J. (1984). Orthographic problem-solving. *Academic Therapy, 20,* 67–75.

Halliday, M. A. K. (1985). *Learning to mean: Explorations in the development of language.* London: Arnold.

Halliday, M. A. K., & Hasan, R. (1976). *Cohesion in English.* London: Longman Group.

Harste, J. C., Woodward, V. A., & Burke, C. L. (1984). *Language stories and literacy lessons.* Portsmouth, NH: Heinemann.

Heath, S. B. (1982). What no bedtime story means: Narrative skills at home and school. *Language in Society, 11,* 49–76.

Hillocks, G. (1986). *Research on written composition: New directions for teaching.* Urbana, IL: ERIC Clearinghouse on Reading and Communication Skills and the National Conference on Research in English.

Hoffman, P. R., Schuckers, G., & Daniloff, R. G. (1989). *Children's phonetic disorders: Theory and practice.* Austin, TX: PRO-ED.

Hoffman, P. R. (1990). Spelling, phonology, and the speech-language pathologist: A whole language perspective. *Language, Speech, and Hearing Services in Schools, 21,* 238–243.

Hoffman, P. R., & Norris, J. A. (1989). On the nature of phonological processes: Evidence from normal children's spelling errors. *Journal of Speech and Hearing Research, 32,* 787–794.

Hudson, J. A., & Shapiro, L. R. (1991). From knowing to telling: The development of children's scripts, stories, and personal narratives. In A. McCabe & C. Peterson (Eds.), *Developing narrative structure* (pp. 89–136). Hillsdale, NJ: Lawrence Erlbaum.

Huey, E. B. (1908, reprinted 1968). *The psychology and pedagogy of reading.* Cambridge, MA: MIT Press.

Indrisano, R., & Paratore, J. R. (1991). Classroom contexts for literacy learning. In J. Flood, J. M. Jensen, D. Lapp, & J. R. Squire (Eds.), *Handbook of research on teaching the English language arts* (pp. 477–488), New York: Macmillan.

Jackson, T. (1990). *The wonderhair hair restorer.* Bothell, WA: The Wright Group.

Jalongo, M. R. (1988). *Young children and picture books: Literature from infancy to six.* Washington, DC: National Association for the Education of Young Children.

Jastak, S., & Wilkinson, G. S. (1984). *Manual: Wide Range Achievement Test Level I (Revised).* Wilmington, DE: Jastak Associates.

Jones, E. (1986). Old Nelson Godon. In *Tales of the Caribbean: The beginnings of things* (pp. 16–26). Bothell, WA: The Wright Group.

King, M., & Rentel, V. (1981). *Transition to writing.* Columbus, OH: Ohio State University.

Labov, W. (1972). *Language in the inner city.* Philadelphia: University of Pennsylvania Press.

Lahey, M. (1988). *Language disorders and language development.* New York: Macmillan.

Langer, J. (1986). *Children's reading and writing: Structures and strategies.* Norwood, NJ: Ablex.

Lee, D. & Allen, R. V. (1963). *Learning to read through experience* (2nd ed.). New York: Appleton Century Crofts.

Lehr, F. (1985). Instructional scaffolding. *Language Arts, 62,* 667–672.

Liles, B. Z. (1987). Episode organization and cohesive conjunctives in narratives of children with and without language disorder. *Journal of Speech and Hearing Research, 30,* 185–196.

Loban, W. (1976). *Language development: Kindergarten through grade twelve.* Urbana, IL: National Council of Teachers of English.

Lovett, S. (1992). *Extremely weird frogs.* Bothell, WA: The Wright Group.

MacLachlan, B., & Chapman, R. (1988). Communication breakdowns in normal and language learning-disabled children's conversation and narration. *Journal of Speech and Hearing Disorders, 53,* 2–7.

Mahler, M. S., Pine, F., & Bergman, A. (1975). *The psychological birth of the human infant.* New York: Basic Books.

Mahy, M. (1986). *The man who enjoyed grumbling.* Bothell, WA: The Wright Group.

Mahy, M. (1987a). *The king's jokes.* Bothell, WA: The Wright Group.

Mahy, M. (1987b). *Tai Taylor and the sweet Annie.* Bothell, WA: The Wright Group.

Mahy, M. (1990). *Crocodile! Crocodile!* Bothell, WA: The Wright Group.

Mandler, J. M., & Johnson, N. S. (1977). Remembrance of things parsed: Story structure and recall. *Cognitive Psychology, 9,* 111–151.

Martinez, M. (1983). Exploring young children's comprehension through story-time talk. *Language Arts, 60,* 202–209.

Martinez, M., & Rozer, N. (1985). Read it again: The value of repeated readings during storytime. *The Reading Teacher, 38,* 782–786.

Marzano, R. J. (1991). Language, the language arts, and thinking. In J. Flood, J. M. Jensen, D. Lapp, & J. R. Squire (Eds.), *Handbook of research on teaching the English language arts* (pp. 559–590). New York: Macmillan.

Mason, J. M., & Allen, J. (1986). A review of emergent literacy with implications for research and practice in reading. In E. Z. Rothkopf (Ed.), *Review of research in education* (Vol. 13, pp. 3–47). Washington, DC: American Educational Research Association.

Maxwell, S. E., & Wallach, G. P. (1984). The language-learning disabilities connection: Symptoms of early language disability change over time. In G. Wallach & K. Butler (Eds.), *Language learning disabilities in school-age children* (pp. 15–34). Baltimore: Williams and Wilkins.

McCabe, A., & Peterson, C. (1991). *Developing narrative structure.* Hillsdale, NJ: Lawrence Erlbaum.

McGee, L. M., & Richgels, D. J. (1990). *Literacy's beginnings: Supporting young readers and writers.* Boston: Allyn and Bacon.

McKeown, M. G., & Beck, I. L. (1988). Learning vocabulary: Different ways for different goals. *Remedial and Special Education, 9,* 42–46.

McLeish, K. (1986a). Merpeople. In *Tales of the British Isles* (pp. 50–58). Bothell, WA: The Wright Group.

McLeish, K. (1986b). Guher and Suher. In *Tales of the Mediterranean: Turkey* (pp. 11–17). Bothell, WA: The Wright Group.

Melser, J. (1981). *Little pig.* Bothell, WA: The Wright Group.

Melser, J. (1985). *One, one, is the sun.* Bothell, WA: The Wright Group.

Melser, J., & Cowley, J. (1980). *The big toe.* Bothell, WA: The Wright Group.

Melser, J., & Cowley, J. (1990a). *Boo hoo.* Bothell, WA: The Wright Group.

Melser, J., & Cowley, J. (1990b). *Obadiah.* Bothell, WA: The Wright Group.

Merritt, D., & Liles, B. (1987). Story grammar ability in children with and without language disorder: Story generation, story retelling, and story comprehension. *Journal of Speech and Hearing Research, 30,* 539–552.

Merritt, D., & Liles, B. (1989). Narrative analysis: Clinical application of story generation and story telling. *Journal of Speech and Hearing Disorders, 54,* 438–447.

Miller, J. (1991). *Research on child language disorders: A decade of progress.* Austin, TX: Pro-Ed.

Monroe, M. (1951). *Growing into reading: How readiness for reading develops at home and at school.* New York: Scott Foresman.

Moon, C. (1988a). *Goldilocks and the three bears.* Bothell, WA: The Wright Group.

Moon, C. (1988b). *Jack and the beanstalk.* Bothell, WA: The Wright Group.

Moon, C. (1988c). *Little red riding hood.* Bothell, WA: The Wright Group.

Moon, C. (1988d). *The three pigs.* Bothell, WA: The Wright Group.

Moon, C., & Moon, B. (1986). *Look at an ice lolly.* Bothell, WA: The Wright Group.

Morrow, L. M. (1988). Young children's responses to one-to-one story readings in school settings. *Reading Research Quarterly, 23,* 89–107.

Morrow, L. M., & Smith, J. K. (1990). The effects of group setting on interactive storybook reading. *Reading Research Quarterly, 25,* 213–231.

Nagy, W. E. (1988). *Teaching vocabulary to improve reading comprehension.* Newark, DE: International Reading Association.

Nagy, W. E., & Herman, P. A. (1987). Breadth and depth of vocabulary knowledge: Implications for acquisition and instruction. In M. G. McKeown & M. E. Curtis (Eds.), *The nature of vocabulary acquisition* (pp. 19–35). Hillsdale, NJ: Lawrence Erlbaum.

Neidecker, E. A. (1980). *School programs in speech-language: Organization and management.* Englewood Cliffs, NJ: Prentice-Hall.

Nelson, K. (1985). *Making sense: The acquisition of shared meaning.* New York: Academic Press.

Nelson, K. (1986). *Event knowledge: Structure and function in development.* Hillsdale, NJ: Lawrence Erlbaum.

Nelson, K. (1991). Event knowledge and the development of language functions. In J. Miller (Ed.), *Research on child language disorders: A decade of progress* (pp. 125–142). Austin, TX: Pro-Ed.

Nelson, N. W. (1989). Curriculum-based language assessment and intervention. *Language, Speech, and Hearing Services in Schools, 20,* 170–184.

Nelson, N. W. (1992). Targets of curriculum-based language assessment. In W. A. Secord & J. S. Damico (Eds.), *Best practices in school speech-language pathology: Descriptive/nonstandardized language assessment* (pp. 73–86). San Antonio, TX: The Psychological Corporation.

Newcomer, P. L., & Hammill, D. D. (1988). *Test of Language Development-Primary 2.* Austin, TX: Pro-Ed.

Ninio, A., & Bruner, J. (1978). The achievement and antecedents of labeling. *Journal of Child Language, 55,* 5–15.

Norris, J. A. (1988). Using communication strategies to enhance reading acquisition. *The Reading Teacher, 41,* 368–373.

Norris, J. A. (1989). Providing language remediation in the classroom: An integrated language-to-reading intervention method. *Language, Speech & Hearing Services in Schools, 20,* 205–219.

Norris, J. A. (1991). From frog to prince: Using written language as a context for language learning. *Topics in Language Disorders, 12,* 66–81.

Norris, J. A. (1992). Learning to talk through literacy: Whole language for handicapped preschoolers. In *Perspectives on whole language: Past, present, potential* (pp. 148–156). Columbia, MO: Instructional Materials Laboratory, University of Missouri.

Norris, J. A. (1992). Assessment of infants and toddlers in naturalistic contexts. In W. A. Secord & J. S. Damico (Eds.), *Best practices in school speech-language pathology: Descriptive/nonstandardized language assessment* (pp. 21–32). San Antonio, TX: The Psychological Corporation.

Norris, J. A., & Bruning, R. H. (1988). Cohesion in the narratives of good and poor readers. *Journal of Speech and Hearing Disorders, 53,* 416–424.

Norris, J. A., & Damico, J. S. (1990). Whole language in theory and practice: Implications for language intervention. *Language, Speech, and Hearing Services in Schools, 21,* 212–220.

Norris, J. A., & Hoffman, P. R. (1990). Language intervention within naturalistic environments. *Language, Speech & Hearing Services in Schools, 21,* 102–109.

Norris, J. A., & Hoffman, P. R. (1991). Alphabet knowledge: Collections versus hierarchies. Louisiana Educational Quality Support Fund Grant.

Norris, J. A., & Hoffman, P. R. (1992a). *A narrative centered curriculum guide for a whole language kindergarten.* Baton Rouge: Louisiana State University.

Norris, J. A., & Hoffman, P. R. (1992b). Whole language strategies for language and literacy. Videotape and viewers guide. Baton Rouge: Louisiana State University.

O'Donnell, R. C., Griffin, W. J., & Norris, R. C. (1967). *Syntax of kindergarten and elementary school children: A transformational analysis.* Urbana, IL: National Council of Teachers of English.

Pearson, P. D., & Fielding, L. (1982). Research update: Listening comprehension. *Language Arts, 59,* 617–629.

Pellegrini, A. D. (1984). The effect of dramatic play on children's generation of cohesive text. *Discourse Processes, 7*(1), 57–67.

Pellegrini, A. D. (1985). The relations between symbolic play and literate behavior: A review and critique of the empirical literature. *Review of Educational Research, 55*(1), 107–121.

Peterson, C., & McCabe, A. (1983). *Developmental psycholinguistics: Three ways of looking at a child's narrative.* New York: Plenum Press.

Piaget, J. (1952). *The language and thought of the child.* London: Routledge and Kegan Paul.

Piaget, J. (1954). *The construction of reality in the child.* New York: Basic Books.

Piaget, J. (1960). *The child's conception of physical causality.* Totowa, NJ: Little-field, Adams.

Piaget, J. (1970). *Structuralism.* New York: Basic Books.

Pikulski, J. J. (1990). Assessment: Informal reading inventories. *The Reading Teacher, 43,* 514–516.

Purves, A. C. (1991). *The idea of difficulty in literature.* New York: State University of New York Press.

Raphael, T. (1982). Question-answering strategies for children. *The Reading Teacher, 36,* 186–190.

Raphael, T. E. (1986). Teaching question-answer relationships, revisited. *The Reading Teacher, 39,* 516–523.

Read, C. (1971). Preschool children's knowledge of English phonology. *Harvard Educational Review, 41,* 1–34.

Read, C. (1986). *Children's creative spelling.* Boston: Routledge and Kegan.

Ripich, D. N., & Griffith, P. L., (1988). Narrative abilities of children with learning disabilities and nondisabled children: Story structure, cohesion, and propositions. *Journal of Learning Disabilities, 21,* 165–173.

Rosenblatt, L. M. (1985). The transactional theory of the literary work: Implications for research. In C. R. Cooper (Ed.), *Researching response to literature and the teaching of literature: Points of departure* (pp. 33–53). Norwood, NJ: Ablex.

Roser, N., & Martinez, M. (1985). Roles adults play in preschoolers' response to literature. *Language Arts, 62,* 485–490.

Roth, F. P., & Spekman, N. J. (1986). Narrative discourse: Spontaneously generated stories of learning disabled and normally achieving students. *Journal of Speech and Hearing Disorders, 51,* 8–23.

Roth, F. P., & Spekman, N. J. (1989). The oral syntactic proficiency of learning disabled students: A spontaneous story sampling analysis. *Journal of Speech and Hearing Research, 32,* 67–77.

Rumelhart, D. E. (1977). Toward an interactive model of reading. In S. Dormic (Ed.), *Attention and performance, VI* (pp. 573–603). Hillsdale, NJ: Lawrence Erlbaum.

Rumelhart, D. E., & McClelland, J. L., (and the PDP Research Group). (1986). *Parallel distributed processing: Explorations in the microstructures of cognition.* Cambridge, MA: The MIT Press.

Scott, C. M., & Erwin, D. L. (1992). Descriptive assessment of writing: Process and products. In W. A. Secord & J. S. Damico (Eds.), *Best practices in school speech-language pathology: Descriptive/nonstandardized language assessment* (pp. 87–98). San Antonio, TX: The Psychological Corporation.

Schank, R., & Abelson, R. (1977). *Scripts, plans, goals and understanding.* Hillsdale, NJ: Lawrence Erlbaum.

Secord, W. A. (Ed.). (1990). *Best practices in school speech-language pathology: Collaborative programs in the schools: Concepts, models, and procedures* (pp. 11–41). San Antonio, TX: The Psychological Corporation.

Secord, W. A., & Wiig, E. H. (1991). *Developing a collaborative language intervention program.* Buffalo, NY: Educom Assoc.

Shavelson, R. J., & Stern, P. (1981). Research on teachers' pedagogical thoughts, judgments, decisions, and behavior. *Review of Educational Research, 51,* 455–498.

Shriberg, L. D., & Kwiatkowski, J. (1988). A follow-up study of children with phonologic disorders of unknown origin. *Journal of Speech and Hearing Disorders, 53,* 144–155.

Simon, C. S. (1987). Out of the broom closet and into the classroom: The emerging SLP. *Journal of Childhood Communication Disorders, 11,* 41–66.

Sinatra, G. M. (1990). Convergence of listening and reading processing. *Reading Research Quarterly, 15,* 115–130.

Slavin, R. E. (1986). *Ability grouping and student achievement in elementary school: A best evidence synthesis.* Baltimore: Johns Hopkins University, Center for Research on Elementary and Middle Schools.

Smith, F. (1983). Reading like a writer. *Language Arts, 60,* 558–567.

Smith, F. (1985). *Reading without nonsense.* New York: Teachers College Press.

Smith, F. (1990). *To think.* New York: Teacher's College Press.

Snow, C. E. (1972). Mothers' speech to children learning language. *Child Language, 43,* 549–565.

Snow, C. E., & Goldfield, B. A. (1983). Turn the page, please: Situation-specific language acquisition. *Journal of Child Language, 10,* 535–549.

Snow, C. E., Nathan, D., & Perlman, R. (1985). Assessing children's knowledge about book reading. In L. Galda & A. Pellegrini (Eds.), *Play, language and stories* (pp. 167–181). Norwood, NJ: Ablex.

Sorensen, A. B., & Hallinan, M. T. (1986). Effects of ability grouping on growth in academic achievement. *American Educational Research Journal, 23,* 519–542.

Spekman, N. J. (1983). Discourse and pragmatics. In C. Wren (Ed.), *Language learning disabilities: Diagnosis and remediation* (pp. 157–216). Rockville, MD: Aspen.

Stanovich, K. E. (1988). *Children's reading and the development of phonological awareness.* Detroit: Wayne State University Press.

Staton, J., Shuy, R., Peyton, J., & Reed, L. (1988). *Dialogue journal communication.* Norwood, NJ: Ablex.

Stein, N. L., & Glenn, C. G. (1979). An analysis of story comprehension in elementary school children. In R. O. Freedle (Ed.), *Advances in discourse processing (Vol. 2): New directions* (pp. 53–120). Norwood, NJ: Ablex.

Straw, S. B. (1990). Reading and response to literature: Transactionalizing instruction. In S. Hynds & D. L. Rubin (Eds.), *Perspectives on talk and learning* (pp. 129–148). Urbana, IL: National Council of Teachers of English.

Strickland, D., Dillon, R., Funkhouser, L., Glick, M., & Rogers, C. (1989). Research currents: Classroom dialogue during literature response groups. *Language Arts, 66,* 192–200.

Sulzby, E. (1985). Children's emergent reading of favorite storybooks: A developmental study. *Reading Research Quarterly, 20,* 458–481.

Sulzby, E. (1986). Writing and reading: Signs of oral and written language organization in the young child. In W. H. Teale & E. Sulzby (Eds.), *Emergent literacy: Writing and reading* (pp. 50–89). Norwood, NJ: Ablex.

Sulzby, E., & Zecker, L. B. (1991). The oral monologue as a form of emergent reading. In A. McCabe & C. Peterson (Eds.), *Developing narrative structure* (pp. 175–214). Hillsdale, NJ: Lawrence Erlbaum.

Teale, W. H. (1984). Reading to young children: Its significance for literacy development. In H. Goelman, A. A. Oberg, & F. Smith (Eds.), *Awakenings to literacy* (pp. 110–130). London: Heinemann.

Teale, W. H., & Sulzby, E. (1986). *Emergent literacy: Writing and reading.* Norwood, NJ: Ablex.

Temple, C., Nathan, R., Burris, N., & Temple, F. (1988). *The beginnings of writing* (2nd ed.). Boston: Allyn and Bacon.

van Dijk, T. A., & Kintsch, W. (1983). *Strategies of discourse comprehension.* New York: Academic Press.

van Kleeck, A. (1982). The emergence of linguistic awareness: A cognitive framework. *Merrill-Palmer Quarterly, 28,* 237–265.

van Kleeck, A. (1984). Metalinguistic skills: Cutting across spoken and written language and problem-solving abilities. In G. P. Wallach & K. G. Butler (Eds.), *Language learning disabilities in school-age children* (pp. 128–153). Baltimore: Williams & Wilkins.

Vellutino, F. R., & Scanlon, D. M. (1987). Phonological coding, phonological awareness and reading ability: Evidence from a longitudinal and experimental study. *Merrill-Palmer Quarterly, 33,* 321–363.

Vickers, K. (1987). *A wizard came to visit.* Bothell, WA: The Wright Group.

Vygotsky, L. S. (1962). *Thought and language.* (E. Hanfmann & G. Vakar, Ed. and Trans.). Cambridge, MA: MIT Press.

Vygotsky, L. S. (1967). Play and its role in the mental development of the child. *Soviet Psychology, 12,* 62–76.

Vygotsky, L. S. (1978). *Mind in society: The development of higher psychological processes.* Cambridge; MA: Harvard University Press.

Vygotsky, L. (1986). *Thought and language.* Cambridge, MA: MIT Press.

Wagner, B. J. (1991). Imaginative expression. In J. Flood, J. M. Jensen, D. Lapp, & J. R. Squire (Eds.), *Handbook of research on teaching the English language arts* (pp. 787–804). New York: Macmillan.

Walker, C. (1992a). *Ecology — Plants and animals.* Bothell, WA: The Wright Group.

Walker, C. (1992b). *Forests forever.* Bothell, WA: The Wright Group.

Walker, C. (1992c). *Oceans of fish.* Bothell, WA: The Wright Group.

Walker, C. (1992d). *Our changing atmosphere.* Bothell, WA: The Wright Group.

Watson, K. (1987). *English teaching in perspective* (2nd ed.). Milton Keynes: Open University Press.

Wells, G. (1985). *Language, learning and education.* England: NFER-NELSON.

Wells, G. (1986). *The meaning makers: Children learning language and using language to learn.* Portsmouth, NH: Heinemann.

Westby, C. E. (1984). Development of narrative language abilities. In G. P. Wallach & K. G. Butler (Eds.), *Language learning disabilities in school-age children* (pp. 103–127). Baltimore: Williams & Wilkins.

Westby, C. E. (1985). Learning to talk — talking to learn: Oral-literate language differences. In C. Simon (Ed.), *Communication skills for classroom success: Therapy methodologies* (pp. 183–213). San Diego, CA: College-Hill Press.

Westby, C. E. (1991). A scale for assessing children's pretend play. In I. B. Weiner (Ed.), *Play diagnosis and assessment* (pp. 131–161). New York: John Wiley and Sons.

Westby, C. E. (1992). Narrative analysis. In W. A. Secord & J. S. Damico (Eds.), *Best practices in school speech-language pathology: Descriptive/nonstandardized language assessment* (pp. 53–64). San Antonio, TX: The Psychological Corporation.

White, T. G., Graves, M. F., & Slater, W. H. (1989). Growth of reading vocabulary in diverse elementary schools. *Journal of Educational Psychology, 82,* 281–290.

Wiig, E. H., & Semel, E. M. (1984). *Language assessment and intervention for the learning disabled.* Columbus, OH: Charles E. Merrill.

Williams, R. (1990a). *Underground.* Bothell, WA: The Wright Group.

Williams, R. (1990b). *Who lives in this hole?* Bothell, WA: The Wright Group.

Wren, C. T. (1983). *Language learning disabilities: Diagnosis and remediation.* Rockville, MD: Aspen.

Wong, B. (1986). A cognitive approach to spelling. *Exceptional Children, 53,* 169–173.

Yaden, D. B. (1988). Understanding stories through repeated read-abouts: How many does it take? *Reading Teacher, 41,* 556–560.

Yaden, D. B., & Templeton, S. (1986). *Metalinguistic awareness and beginning literacy: Conceptualizing what it means to read and write.* Portsmouth, NH: Heinemann.

Yaden, D. B., Smoklin, L. B., & Conlon, A. (1989). Preschoolers' questions about pictures, print convention, and story text during reading aloud at home. *Reading Research Quarterly, 24,* 188–214.

Young, C. (1988a). *The gingerbread man.* Bothell, WA: The Wright Group.

Young, C. (1988b). *The little red hen.* Bothell, WA: The Wright Group.

Young, C. (1988c). *Shopping.* Bothell, WA: The Wright Group.

Zakaluk, B. L., & Samuels, S. J. (Eds.) (1988). *Readability: Its past, present, and future.* Newark, DE: International Reading Association.

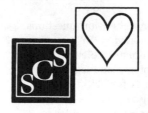

Index